SI2 60   WL520

D1634280

(3)

...ed on or before
...ed below.

SWNHS

C20091496

Neuropsychological Management of Mild Traumatic Brain Injury

Neuropsychological Management of Mild Traumatic Brain Injury

Edited by

SARAH A. RASKIN, PH.D.

Department of Psychology and Neuroscience Program
Trinity College
Hartford, Connecticut

CATHERINE A. MATEER, PH.D.

Department of Psychology
University of Victoria
Victoria, British Columbia
Canada

Medical Library
Cornwall Postgraduate Centre
Royal Cornwall Hospital
Truro TR1 3LJ

New York   Oxford
OXFORD UNIVERSITY PRESS
2000

Oxford University Press

Oxford   New York
Athens   Auckland   Bangkok   Bogotá   Buenos Aires   Calcutta
Cape Town   Chennai   Dar es Salaam   Delhi   Florence   Hong Kong   Istanbul
Karachi   Kuala Lumpur   Madrid   Melbourne   Mexico City   Mumbai
Nairobi   Paris   São Paulo   Singapore   Taipei   Tokyo   Toronto   Warsaw

and associated companies in
Berlin   Ibadan

Copyright © 2000 by Oxford University Press, Inc.

Published by Oxford University Press, Inc.,
198 Madison Avenue, New York, New York, 10016
http://www.oup-usa.org

All rights reserved. No part of this publication may be reproduced,
stored in a retrieval system, or transmitted, in any form or by any means,
electronic, mechanical, photocopying, recording, or otherwise,
without the prior permission of Oxford University Press.

Library of Congress Cataloging-in-Publication Data
Raskin, Sarah A.
Neuropsychological management of mild traumatic brain injury /
Sarah A. Raskin, Catherine A. Mateer.
p. cm.)
Includes bibliographical references and index.
ISBN 0-19-508527-2
1. Brain damage—Patients—Rehabilitation.
2. Clinical neuropsychology.
I. Mateer, Catherine A.   II. Title.
[DNLM: 1. Brain Injuries—rehabilitation.   2. Brain Injuries— complications.
3. Brain Injuries—psychology.
WL 354 R225n 2000]   RC387.5.R37   2000   617.4'81044—dc21
DNLM/DLC for Library of Congress   99-13808

1 2 3 4 5 6 7 8 9

Printed in the United States of America
on acid-free paper

To Brian and Julian
SR

To Kim
CM

Preface

This book is intended for use by rehabilitation professionals, including neurologists, psychologists, neuropsychologists, counselors, speech pathologists, occupational therapists and physical therapists, and vocational counselors who are already familiar with the sequelae and treatment of various forms of brain injury. Its aim is to present guidelines for the application of rehabilitation techniques to the cognitive and emotional effects of mild traumatic brain injury (MTBI). It is not intended to be an academic review of either MTBI or cognitive rehabilitation; many such works are already in print. Instead, we believe there is a need for a clear, pragmatic guide to the actual practice of rehabilitation with this population.

The techniques and approaches we describe are derived from the literature and from our own experience in working with individuals who have sustained MTBI. We have focused on theories and strategies of treatment that are well-founded in research. This has been a challenge as the great majority of research in the area of MTBI is on issues related to assessment rather than treatment.

Preparation of a book about treatment strategies has also been challenging in light of the pervasive questions about the nature and origins of persistent symptoms after what appear to be relatively mild injuries. We take no exception to the well-documented finding that the great majority of individuals who sustain MTBI go on to make essentially full recovery and return to their former levels of work, daily living, and leisure activity. It is equally well-documented, however, that a small minority of individuals who sustain MTBI, estimated from between 5 and 20 percent, do not make full recovery and report disruptive symptoms for many months, or even years, after injury. While the reasons for this are undoubtedly multifaceted, there are no simple explanations that can account for the findings across all affected individuals. Possible explanations include more severe injury than was initially diagnosed, MTBI complicated by other injuries, or greater individual vulnerability. Many of these individuals have been shown to benefit from structured rehabilitation programs that address changes in cognitive ability, alterations in mood, and problems with adjustment and reintegration to home, work, and social activity. It is for these individuals that this book is intended.

We acknowledge that, in some cases, symptoms seen after accident or injury are exaggerated in response to various forms of conscious and unconscious secondary gain. We support careful evaluation and diagnosis to identify such situations. While overt malingering is not a target for treatment, psychologists and other rehabilitation professionals can play an important role in working with individuals who are demonstrating conversion or psychosomatic disorders. Careful investigation of the nature of persistent symptoms following MTBI is necessary and applauded, failure to find convincing "organic" underpinnings has too often resulted in a minimization of the need to develop effective interventions to assist affected individuals. Indeed, acknowledgment of psychological correlates of the disorder should not cause rehabilitation specialists, and especially psychologists to abandon efforts to provide effective interventions.

This book is intended to be an integrated guide to dealing with both cognitive and emotional sequelae, and with the beliefs about and reactions to these sequelae that often serve to exacerbate and maintain these sequelae. Presenting symptoms are commonly cognitive and physical in nature but often are shaped by depression, anxiety, frustration, and feelings of anger. In assessment, there is usually an attempt to dissociate these various factors and to identify specific impairments in different cognitive and emotional domains. This is appropriate and useful in the diagnostic process but may be only partially valid in treatment. Cognitive and emotional factors interact with each other and with the injured person's own history, background, personality, and social context. While we have written separate chapters on specific cognitive and emotional domains, we recognize their complex interactions and the need to address these interactions in treatment. The rehabilitation specialist and/or team working with individuals who have sustained MTBI should be versed in or have available an eclectic mix of treatment strategies.

Throughout the book we have tried to provide enough theory, information, and case examples so that trained professionals can begin to understand and use the intervention techniques in their practices. As will be emphasized throughout, these techniques work best when individualized for each client. This can be done with regard not only to the individual's unique constellation of cognitive and emotional strengths and deficits, but also to their life experiences, goals, and interests. The form, time frames, and settings for rehabilitation of individuals with MTBI need to be variable and flexible.

Each chapter follows approximately the same general format. First, there is a review of the relevant theories and research findings for the various cognitive and emotional processes with respect to MTBI. This is followed by suggestions for assessment, including questionnaires and standard neuropsychological and psychological measures. The primary focus of each chapter will be on treatment strategies, augmented by case examples and treatment materials. Materials can be copied or adapted as appropriate to the reader's setting.

The first section of the book deals with concepts of MTBI and its effects, neurological and medical aspects, and assessment. Chapter 1 gives an overview of various factors that may contribute to persistent disability following MTBI and their interactions. Problems of definition and diagnosis are discussed. Chapter 2, written by a neurologist, covers medical aspects of the syndrome, including visual and vestibular disturbances, headache, and chronic pain. It provides information on the diagnosis of physical signs and symptoms and on current treatment approaches. Chapter 3 focuses on issues of assessment, and includes a discussion of various challenges in the selection and interpretation of assessment tools in this population. The chapter stresses issues in the assessment of cognitive and emotional functioning and includes a discussion of problems related to assessment of motivation and symptom validity.

The next section deals with cognitive symptoms common to individuals with MTBI. The chapters are divided by type of cognitive process—attention, memory, and executive functions. Research has shown that each of these areas is commonly affected by MTBI. Each chapter begins by reviewing the relevant research literature and then discusses specific treatment strategies. These include techniques for demonstrating generalization of training to everyday activities. The strategies we describe represent a mix of process-specific interventions, compensation strategies, and psychological interventions to assist clients in gaining a sense of mastery and control over their cognitive performance.

The next section of the book addresses the emotional sequelae of MTBI. It begins with a discussion of principles of psychotherapy that emphasizes how they can be used with this population. The following four chapters cover management strategies for dealing with depression, anxiety, and irritability and anger. They review relevant research on MTBI in each of these emotional domains. The treatment strategies presented are eclectic but for the most part build on empirically validated cognitive behavioral principles and strategies.

Posttraumatic stress disorder is far more prevalent in individuals with MTBI than in those with more severe brain injuries, and its evaluation and treatment are discussed in the chapter on anxiety disorders. The chapter on irritability and anger points out the subtle interactions between brain injury, which often results in diminished self-control, and the emotional response, manifested in frustration, blame, and diminished coping ability.

Chapter 11 deals with the effects of MTBI on work performance and discusses the critical elements of vocational rehabilitation in this population. Vocational outcomes are reviewed with emphasis on integrating vocational skills and skill training with other areas of rehabilitation.

The final section deals with particular populations. There are chapters on the special needs of children and of the elderly who have sustained MTBI. Relevant literature and intervention strategies for these populations are presented, along with case examples and discussions of outcome. The final chapter deals with issues related to gender, socioeconomic status, and culture that are often missing from rehabilitation texts but that we have found to be important in working with brain-injured individuals, their families, and their communities.

Interest in and knowledge of neuropsychological disorders and syndromes, like MTBI, have continued to expand. It is important that the development of effective management and rehabilitation strategies keep abreast of our emerging knowledge. Our role as health care specialists requires that we continue trying to bridge the gaps between theory, assessment, and intervention. Rehabilitation, perhaps more than any other area of medical practice, is most effective when there is a partnership between client and rehabilitation specialist. The great majority of clients with MTBI with whom we have worked are eager and motivated to improve their cognitive and emotional functioning, and have been dynamic partners in the rehabilitation process. We hope that this book will provide information, tools, and support for the rehabilitation specialist who is working in this area.

March 1999   S.A.R.
                                                               C.A.M.

Acknowledgments

First, we thank those individuals with mild traumatic brain injury who shared their time and their lives with us. In particular, we thank the members of the Seattle women's mild traumatic brain injury group: Leela, Louisa, and Erin.

We also thank the staff at Good Samaritan Neuropsychological Services. Shirlee Crain typed most of the manuscript and created most of the figures and tables. Cindy Hacker, Betty Branton, and Elizabeth Rearick contributed to the completion of this text.

The team at Good Samaritan's Center for Continuing Rehabilitation-II also made this book possible. Many of them contributed chapters to the volume. Others, including Lori Johnson, Laurie Paule, and Jamie Hatleberg contributed information used in chapters.

We are grateful to Carol Buckheit who read and edited the entire manuscript. Some of the data presented in this text was collected with help from a grant to SR from the Trinity College Faculty Research Committee. This included providing funding for student research assistants, some of whom are: Laura O'Sullivan, Marsha Byrne, Andria Reyes, Andrew Burke, Sara Levy, Suzanne Fallon, Brian Harel, Celia Heck, Kim Mendell, Chloe Zaug, and Kaja LeWinn. Dawn Zorgdrager, Tracy Knight, and Elizabeth Adorno at Trinity College provided word processing, printing, photocopying and support in many ways.

Many people who read individual chapters and provided valuable insights include Allen Raskin, Patricia Paddison, Tammy Nicol, Karl Haberlandt, Priscilla Kehoe, Theol Raskin, Carolyn Prouty, and Christina Ciocca. The comments of an anonymous reviewer were helpful in redirecting the focus of the text.

Jeffrey House at Oxford University Press first presented the idea for this volume, provided considerable guidance throughout the project, and then demonstrated patience in waiting for its completion.

Brian Waddell read and edited virtually the entire manuscript and provided hours of discussion, critique, and support. SR thanks him for his unfailing confidence and contagious energy, which were essential to this volume. She thanks Julian for his constant affection and joyfulness.

CM thanks Kim Kerns for her humor, patience, advice, and support.

Contents

Part IV Vocational and Community Integration

Part V Special Populations

Contributors

RYAN C.N. D'ARCY, M.SC.
Graduate Student
Cognitive/Clinical Neuroscience Unit
Department of Psychology and
  Neuroscience
Dalhousie University
Halifx, Nova Scotia

DAVID HOVLAND, M.S.W.
Psychosocial Therapist
Good Samaritan's Center for
  Continuing Rehabilitation
Puyallup, Washington

GINGER D. HURT, M.A., C.R.C
Vocational Rehabilitation Counselor
Good Samaritan Rehabilitation Center
Puyallup, Washington

KIMBERLY A. KERNS, PH.D.
Associate Professor
Department of Psychology
University of Victoria
Victoria, British Columbia

CATHERINE A. MATEER, PH.D.,
  ABPP/ABCN
Professor
Deparment of Psychology
University of Victoria
Victoria, British Columbia

SARAH A. RASKIN, PH.D.,
  ABPP/ABCN
Associate Professor
Department of Psychology and
  Neuroscience Program
Trinity College
Hartford, Connecticut

MCKAY MOORE SOHLBERG, PH.D.
Assistant Professer
Communication Disorders and Sciences
University of Oregon
Eugene, Oregon

PAULA N. STEIN, PH.D.
Fishkill Consultation Group
Fishkill, New York

JENNIFER BLAIR THOMSON, PH.D.
Educational Psychology
University of Washington
Seattle, Washington

NATHAN D. ZASLER, M.D.
Concussion Care Centre of Virginia
Medical Director
Tree of Life, LLC
Richmond, Virginia

I

INTRODUCTION

1

Current Concepts and Approaches to Management

CATHERINE A. MATEER AND
RYAN C.N. D'ARCY

There is much controversy about the origins of persistent disability following what initially seem to be mild brain injuries. Nevertheless, persistent symptoms do occur in some individuals and rehabilitation efforts can often mitigate these symptoms and improve adaptive functioning. The purpose of this chapter is to give readers a brief, up-to-date framework for defining and conceptualizing mild traumatic brain injury (MTBI). We also discuss the various perspectives on both the causes of persisting symptoms and disability after MTBI and the most effective approaches to their management.

Mild traumatic brain injury is typically defined as an injury to the head resulting in a brief loss of consciousness or a period of being dazed with no loss of consciousness, posttraumatic amnesia of less than 1 hour, Glasgow Coma Scale (GCS) greater than 13, and a negative neuroimaging scan (Alexander, 1995; Williams et al., 1990). The most common complaints following MTBI are headaches, dizziness, nausea, memory problems, fatigue, irritability, anxiety, insomnia, difficulty with concentration, and increased sensitivity to light and sound (Alves, 1992; Alves et al., 1993; Binder, 1986; Bohnen and Jolles, 1992; Dikmen et al., 1986). Mild traumatic brain injury has also been called mild head injury, minor head injury, minor traumatic brain injury, and concussion. The persisting symptom complex seen in some individuals who have sustained MTBI has also been referred to as persisting postconcussive syndrome (PPCS).

Few neurological disorders are as prevalent as MTBI, which has an estimated incidence of 290,000–325,000 new cases each year and approximately 131 per 100,000 population requiring hospitalization (Katz and DeLuca, 1992). According to the National Center of Health Statistics, approximately 85% of all traumatic brain injuries are classified as mild.

Most individuals with MTBI have relatively uneventful recoveries and return to their former level of functioning. However, it has been estimated that 25%–35% individuals who sustain MTBI continue to report symptoms when reevaluated 3 to 6 months later, and about 10%–15% report persisting symptoms for periods longer than 6 months post injury (Alves et al., 1993; Bohnen et al., 1992; Brown et al., 1994; Evans, 1992; Kraus and Nourjah, 1988; Leninger et al., 1990; McAllister, 1992; Ruff et al., 1989; Rimel et al., 1981). Many individuals with persisting complaints report difficulties with efficiency of task completion at work and at home, and describe changes in emotional and social functioning (Dikmen et al., 1986; Fenton et al., 1993).

In individuals who have not substantially resumed premorbid levels of functioning more than 6 months post injury there are typically few, if any, neurological findings or neuropsychological indicators consistent with the degree of reported symptomatology. Accordingly, a psychogenic as opposed to physiogenic basis for persisting symptomatology is often proposed.

Mild traumatic brain injury like more severe traumatic brain injury, commonly results from motor vehicle accidents, falls, assaults, and sport-related injuries. The mechanical aspects of MTBI are believed to be similar to those of more severe forms of traumatic brain injury (TBI), the distinguishing factor being lower inertial forces on the head and neck (Alexander, 1995). The severity of brain insult is related to the direction of motion, the surface of the skull surrounding the brain, and the violence of the impact (Dixon et al., 1993).

Pathophysiology of Mild Traumatic Brain Injury

Magnetic resonance imaging reveals the majority of MTBI lesions to be localized to the frontal and temporal regions (Levin et al., 1987). In particular, due to bony protrusions on the skull, the orbitofrontal region of the frontal lobes is particularly likely to be injured (Jennett and Teasdale, 1981). These lesions are not usually overt contusions in cases of MTBI, but are rather hypothesized to represent precontusional changes associated with abnormalities of the blood–brain barrier (Hayes et al., 1992). With such an opening of the blood–brain barrier, serum proteins and circulating neurotransmitters can enter the brain parenchyma (Hayes et al., 1992).

Besides these focal changes, there is considerable evidence to suggest diffuse axonal injury (DAI) throughout the brain following MTBI (Oppenheimer, 1968; Pilz, 1983). Diffuse axonal injury is due to gradients of stress within the brain following acceleration–deceleration forces (Adams et al., 1982) and has been demonstrated in individuals with a loss of consciousness of less than 5 minutes (Pilz, 1983). While fiber tracts throughout the brain are involved, the frontal lobes, and in particular orbitofrontal regions, are usually severely affected (Gentry et al., 1988; Nevin, 1967). There is also evidence of diffuse cortical/subcortical disconnection phenomena involving the prefrontal cortex (Ommaya and Gennarelli, 1974).

Axonal degeneration has been noted in animals subjected to acceleration–deceleration injury with brief loss of consciousness (Jane et al., 1985). In a study of human MTBI cases who died shortly after the injury (2–99 days), Blumbergs et al. (1994) demonstrated axonal injury in all cases in the fornices. In contrast, controls showed almost no axonal immunostaining with amyloid precursor protein, suggesting no axonal injury. In a follow-up study (Blumbergs et al., 1995), the findings in MTBI were replicated, and it was demonstrated that increased axonal injury occurred with increased injury severity.

Widespread neuronal depolarization can produce a large release of acetylcholine (ACh) (Hayes et al., 1992). Hippocampal ACh levels have been reported to increase 74% above normal after TBI (Gorman et al., 1989). Hippocampal tissue may be especially vulnerable to MTBI (Phillips and Belardo, 1992), possibly due to enhanced coupling between muscarinic receptors and phosphoinositide hydrolysis (Delahunty, 1992).

Concussive brain trauma also leads to transient increases in extracellular excitatory amino acid concentrations, suggesting that glutamate receptor-associated ion channels may be open for prolonged periods, allowing the influx of Ca^{2+} (McIntosh et al., 1997). This influx induces the release of free radicals from mitochondria which then can attack both the neuronal membranes and the cerebrovasculature.

Diagnostic Criteria

The diagnosis of MTBI rests on the presence of various objective indicators of acute injury status. Current measures used to quantify the severity of injury are the duration of loss of consciousness (LOC), the Glasgow Coma Scale (GCS), and the duration of posttraumatic amnesia (PTA).

In most definitions, the duration of LOC must be 20 minutes or less for classification as an MTBI. Any injury associated with a duration of LOC longer than this would be classified as at least moderate in severity. While some view LOC as an absolute requirement for indicating possible brain injury, others point out that there are many reported instances of clear injury to the brain without LOC. In addition, it is often difficult, if not impossible, to ascertain if there has been a brief LOC or not. Some definitions consider an altered state of consciousness to be as indicative of possible injury as an apparently total LOC. Descriptions of the injured individual being dazed, confused, or disoriented immediately after injury would be suggestive of an altered state of consciousness. The duration of LOC has been shown to be an effective prognosticator of functional recovery in only moderate to severe injuries (Stevens, 1984).

The GCS is a 15-point scale used to determine levels of consciousness. A patient with head trauma with a GCS score between 13 and 15 within a short time following the injury normally would be diagnosed with MTBI. Usually this means that the person has spontaneous eye opening and is likely to be able to obey commands, but may be disoriented and/or demonstrate confusion. The scale and the equation used to determine the score are shown in Table 1.1. It is important, however, to recognize the limitations of the GCS. For example, in a sample of 690 cases of apparent MTBI with GCS > 13, over 23% of patients had an intracerebral lesion

Table 1-1 The glasgow coma scale and posttraumatic amnesia index

GCS	
Eye Opening	
Spontaneous	E4
To speech	3
To pain	2
Nil	1
Best Motor Response	
Obeys	M6
Localizes	5
Withdraws	4
Abnormal flexion	3
Exterior response	2
Nil	1
Verbal Response	
Oriented	V5
Confused conversation	4
Inappropriate words	3
Incomprehensible sounds	2
Nil	1
PTA	
Less than 5 minutes — very mild	
5 – 60 minutes — mild	
1 – 24 hours — moderate	
1 – 7 days — severe	
1 – 4 weeks — very severe	
More than 4 weeks — extremely severe	

(Coma score = $(E + M + V)$ = 3 to 15)
GCS, Glasgow Coma Scale; PTA, Posttraumatic amnesia.

identified on their CT scan (Stein et al., 1993). Thus, a subset of patients with apparent MTBI may have sustained significant brain injury.

Following recovery of consciousness, or in some cases without an apparent loss of consciousness, there is often a period during which the injured individual does not seem to be storing memories from moment to moment. This state is called posttraumatic amnesia (PTA). The duration of PTA is defined as the period of time between the injury and the appearance of intact memory for new information (not including any period during which the individual was not conscious or was unresponsive). Posttraumatic amnesia is thought to reflect cognitive disturbances secondary to brain damage and must last less than 1 hour to qualify as indicative of MTBI (see Table 1.1).

Given the guidelines discussed above, it is important to recognize the difficulties faced by researchers and clinicians in classifying the severity of brain injury. First, judgments made about the duration of impaired consciousness and amnesia may be inaccurate. The reliability of the three acute measures of severity (LOC, GCS, and PTA), center on the subjective judgments of both the patient and the examiner as well as potential confounds (e.g., alcohol intoxication) that can affect physical and mental functioning. The lack of sensitivity of the GCS and LOC in predicting outcome in cases of MTBI is well documented (Hugenholtz et al., 1988; Kraus and Nourjah, 1988; Vilkki et al., 1994), and the need for more comprehensive definitional schemas is recognized.

Definitions of Mild Traumatic Brain Injury

The *DSM-IV* (American Psychiatric Association, 1994) does not have an established category for traumatic brain injury per se. However, a set of proposed criteria and axes for postconcussional disorder is given in its Appendix B. The features of postconcussional disorder are, "an acquired impairment in cognitive functioning, accompanied by specific neurobehavioral symptoms, that occurs as the consequence of closed head injury of sufficient severity to produce significant cerebral concussion. The manifestations of concussion include loss of consciousness, posttraumatic amnesia, and less commonly, posttraumatic onset of seizures." The research criteria set out in the *DSM-IV* for postconcussional disorder are given in Table 1.2.

In an effort to foster consideration of MTBI as a distinctive clinical entity, a working definition was put forth by the Mild Traumatic Brain Injury Committee of the Head Injury Interdisciplinary Special Interest Group (HIISIG) of the American Congress of Rehabilitation Medicine (ACRM) in 1993 (Table 1.3). The purpose of this definition was to provide health care professionals with a more specific set of clinical and research criteria for MTBI. One major advantage of the system was that whereas the prior definitions were exclusive in nature (i.e., what level of

Table 1-2 The *DSM-IV* Appendix B — criteria sets and axes provided for further study

---

Research criteria for postconcussional disorder

    A. A history of head trauma that caused significant cerebral concussion.

      Note: The manifestations of concussion include loss of consciousness, post-traumatic amnesia, and less commonly, posttraumatic onset of seizures. The specific method of defining this criterion needs to be established by further research.

    B. Evidence from neuropsychological testing or quantified cognitive assessment of difficulty in attention (concentrating, shifting focus of attention, performing simultaneous cognitive tasks) or memory (learning or recalling information).

    C. Three (or more) occur shortly after the trauma and last at least 3 months:

        1. becoming fatigued easily

        2. disordered sleep

        3. headache

        4. vertigo or dizziness

        5. irritability or aggression on little or no provocation

        6. anxiety, depression, or affective lability

        7. changes in personality (e.g., social or sexual inappropriateness)

        8. apathy or lack of spontaneity

    D. The symptoms in the Criterion B and C have their own onset following head trauma or else represent a substantial worsening of preexisting symptoms.

    E. The disturbance causes significant impairment in the social or occupational functioning and represents a significant decline from a previous level of functioning. In school-age children, the impairment may be manifested by a significant worsening in school or academic performance dating from the trauma.

    F. The symptoms do not meet the criteria for Dementia Due to Head Trauma and are not better accounted for by another mental disorder (e.g., Amnestic Disorder Due to Head Trauma, or Personality Change Due to Head Trauma).

Published in the Diagnostic and Statistical Manual of Mental Disorders-IV in 1994.

injury would be too much to be categorized as more than MTBI), the ACRM criteria specified some of the features that would be expected to be present at the time of injury. This is important if the diagnosis is not to rest solely on symptoms that are reported many weeks, months, or even years later. The committee also recommended the adoption of a grading system that classifies TBI in terms not only of injury severity, but also of impairment severity, and relative disability.

Table 1-3 Mild traumatic brain injury—definition, comments, and symptomatology

---

Definition

A patient with mild traumatic brain injury is a person who has had a traumatically induced physiological disruption of the brain functions, as manifested by at least one of the following:

1. any period of loss of consciousness;
2. any loss of memory for the events immediately before or after the accident;
3. any alteration in mental state at the time of the accident (e.g., feeling dazed, disoriented, or confused); and
4. focal neurologic deficit(s) that may or may not be transient;

but where the severity of the injury does not exceed the following:

- loss of consciousness for approximately 30 minutes or less;
- after 30 minutes, an initial Glasgow Coma Scale (GCS) of 13–15; and
- posttraumatic amnesia (PTA) not greater than 24 hours.

Comments

This definition includes: (1) the head being struck, (2) the head striking an object, and (3) the brain undergoing an acceleration/deceleration movement (i.e., whiplash) without direct external trauma to the head. It excludes stroke, anoxia, tumor, encephalitis, etc. Computed tomography, magnetic resonance imaging, electroencephalogram, or routine neurologic evaluation may be normal. Due to the lack of medical emergency, or the realities of certain medical systems, some patients may not have the above factors medically documented in the acute stage. In such cases it is appropriate to consider symptomatology that, when linked to the traumatic head injury, can suggest the existence of mild traumatic brain injury.

Symptomatology

The above criteria define the event of a mild traumatic brain injury. Symptoms of brain injury may or may not persist, for varying lengths of time, after such a neurological event. It should be recognized that patients with mild traumatic brain injury can exhibit persistent emotional, cognitive, behavioral, and physical symptoms, alone or in combination, which may produce a functional disability. These symptoms generally fall into one of the following categories, and are additional evidence that mild traumatic brain injury has occurred:

1. Physical symptoms of brain injury (e.g., nausea, vomiting, dizziness, headache, blurred vision, sleep disturbance, quickness to fatigue, lethargy, or other sensory loss) that cannot be accounted for by peripheral injury or other causes;
2. Cognitive deficits (e.g., involving attention, concentration, perception, memory, speech/language, or executive functions) that cannot be completely accounted for by emotional state or other causes; and

(continued)

Table 1-3 Mild traumatic brain injury—definition, comments, and symptomatology (*continued*)

---

3. Behavioral change(s) and/or alteration in degree of emotional responsivity (e.g., irritability, quickness to anger, disinhibition, or emotional lability) that cannot be accounted for by psychological reaction to physical or emotional stress or any other causes.

Defition developed by the Mild Traumatic Brain Injury Committee of the Head Injury Interdisciplinary Special Interests Group of the american Congress of Rehabilitation Medicine, published in *The Journal of Head Trauma and Rehabilitation* in 1993.

Natural History of Mild Traumatic Brain Injury and the Postconcussive Syndrome

In the acute period after MTBI, physical complaints tend to be most prominent. Headaches are a very common complaint; these may be attributable to scalp injury, neck injury, neural injury, or a mixture of causes. Patients often report noticeable increases in fatigue and sleep disturbances during this period. Other commonly reported physical symptoms include increased sensitivity to light and sound, ringing in the ears (tinnitus), dizziness, difficulties with balance, and nausea. Moreover, headaches, dizziness, nausea, and memory problems appear to be symptoms that are unique to head injury patients compared to nonhead injured hospitalized controls (Barth et al., 1989; Bohnen et al., 1992). By 1 month post injury, there is a noticeable reduction in the number of physical complaints, although some, particularly headaches and vertigo, can persist for many months (Alves 1992). These physical symptoms and their management are described in detail in Chapter 2.

Cognitive difficulties, particulary in the areas of concentration and memory, are also frequently reported after mild traumatic brain injury. In support of such complaints, neuropsychological investigations have documented impairments in speed of information processing, complex attention, and concentration in the acute period following injury (Gronwall, 1991). Many patients with MTBI also report difficulties with memory, as well as changes in the ability to initiate and organize complex activities. The simple clinical tests used in neurological screening are unlikely to reveal these impairments and when symptoms persist more than 6 months post injury, a neuropsychological evaluation is advisable. Reviews of the nature of difficulties with attention, memory, and executive function that are commonly associated with MTBI are presented in Chapters 4, 5, and 6.

In addition, a number of behavioral, affective, and emotional effects of MTBI are well documented. They are often characterized by an insidious onset and are potentially quite incapacitating. Common emotional symptoms are irritability, anger, depression, anxiety, frustration, and affective lability. Socially, individuals with MTBI often isolate themselves and withdraw from friends, family, and social activities.

Conceptualization regarding the temporal aspects of symptoms associated with MTBI was assisted by a distinction between early and late postconcussive symptoms (PCS)(Rutherford, 1989). It is fairly widely accepted that early postconcussive symptoms, including headache, dizziness, and concentration problems are a result of neurophysiological/ neurological influences. There is more controversy about the etiology of persisting or late-onset symptoms. Both preinjury and postinjury psychological factors are often seen as contributing to the maintenance and possible exaggeration of symptoms. Stressful life events, poor coping mechanisms, stress, depression, and individual vulnerability have been proposed to contribute to the psychogenesis of persistent postconcussion syndrome (PPCS), although concrete, objective evidence for such claims is limited (Bohnen et al., 1992; Cicerone, 1991; Fenton et al., 1993; Lishman, 1988; Middleboe et al., 1991; Rutherford, 1989). While many clinicians and researchers recognize the importance of psychological factors in recovery from MTBI, a detailed understanding of these factors and the role they play in recovery is still lacking.

Premorbid Risk Factors

Several studies have looked at the potential role of a variety of demographic variables, preexisting conditions, and premorbid factors in recovery from MTBI. While early studies reported that women were more likely than men to develop PPCS after MTBI (Lishman, 1988), more recent studies have not confirmed this finding (Fenton et al., 1993; Mittenberg et al., 1992). (See Chapter 14 for a review of considerations regarding gender in rehabilitation.)

Some studies have found older individuals (i.e., > 50 years) to be more susceptible to more severe and persistent symptomatology following MTBI than younger individuals (Fenton, et al., 1993; Radanov et al., 1991; Williams, et al., 1990), though others have not (Alves et al., 1993; Hugenholtz et al., 1988; Mittenerg et al., 1992) (See Chapter 13 for a review of MTBI in older individuals.)

Studies exploring such factors as a dysfunctional family history, a history of abuse, a preexisting pattern of difficult social interactions, and such personality variables as "neuroticism," or state and trait anxiety have generally failed to reveal any significant relationships that differentiate individuals with MTBI from controls (Fenton et al., 1993; Radanov et al., 1991; Robertson et al., 1994; Schoenhuber and Gentilini, 1988). Indeed, in a study of late PPCS, Karzmark et al., (1995) found that neither premorbid variables nor severity of injury were associated with level of PPCS, while level of current psychological distress was strongly associated with PPCS. Results such as these have been used to support the importance of addressing postinjury psychological factors in managing persistent complaints following MTBI. These issues are discussed in greater depth in later chapters on assessment and on the management of depression and anxiety in individuals with persisting disability following MTBI.

A number of other postinjury factors may play a significant role in recovery. For example, individuals whose work requires a high level of cognitive ability often find it difficult to return to their previous level of productivity. Work environments which require managing multiple sources of information, prioritizing work-related activities, divided attention skills, and a high degree of mental flexibility may pose particular problems for an individual with MTBI.

Other postinjury factors such as a family member who overfocuses on injury, financial pressures, chronic pain, and/or feelings of resentment and/or entitlement regarding the accident itself can also impede recovery. Many professionals working in this field are also concerned that recovery may be hampered by the entanglement of clinical issues with litigation. While some studies have suggested that the presence of persistent symptoms is as common in those individuals with MTBI who have never pursued litigation as in those pursuing or receiving compensation, others have argued that involvement in litigation tends to be associated with prolonged or magnified symptom reporting (Fenton, et al, 1993; Gfleller et al., 1994; Hugenholtz et al., 1988; Leninger et al., 1989; Mendelson, 1982; Tarsh and Royston, 1985).

Clinical Perspectives and Management Issues

Not surprisingly, the various perspectives regarding the origin of persistent symptoms following MTBI have engendered significant controversy about when and how to manage symptoms associated with MTBI. The key issue often hinges on whether impairments are viewed as physiogenic or psychogenic in nature. The two are not, however, mutually exclusive and interventions need to consider various etiologies in different individuals and at different times post injury.

Sources of Variation in Functional Outcome

As mentioned above, much of the debate surrounding MTBI has risen out of disagreements about the relative effect of the injury itself vs. the role of extraneous factors. These latter factors include both premorbid characteristics of the injured person (e.g., personality characteristics, psychosomatic tendencies, cognitive and emotional functioning) and postinjury variables (e.g., pain, fatigue, depression, motivational issues).

If one takes a strong biological perspective, physical, cognitive, and behavioral changes are viewed as a direct consequence of structural changes in the brain and a course of natural recovery is anticipated. Residual difficulties are anticipated to be minimal, though in some cases more severe and persistent. Psychological manifestations are acknowledged but seen to be a direct consequence of the organic disruption and the impact of dealing with physical and cognitive limitations. Lesser emphasis is placed on premorbid conditions and personality characteristics.

Alternatively, if one takes a strong psychological perspective, any physiologically based symptoms of MTBI are believed to resolve quickly and thus have relatively little impact on functional outcomes. Instead, symptoms lasting beyond the initial recovery stage are believed to reflect premorbid psychological factors, normal variations in ability, personality variables, psychological responses to the injury, and/or motivation. An extreme view is that much of the prolonged symptomatology is primarily iatrogenic, based on perceptions deriving from exposure to health care professionals or other sources of information about brain injury.

An interactional perspective is more holistic and incorporates features of both perspectives. It supports the premise that early symptoms are primarily organic in nature and resolve to a great extent over a relatively short period of time. However, it is acknowledged that a complete resolution of symptoms does not always occur and those residual difficulties with cognitive efficiency and emotional stability may persist. Functional recovery varies from case to case, and adjustment depends on both the degree to which physical and cognitive symptoms improve and the degree to which emotional reactions and beliefs about the impact of the injury interfere with return to premorbid activities. Other external factors, such as premorbid personality and emotional functioning, and the demands placed on the individuals at home and at work, are seen to impact on the interaction and can function to prolong disability.

According to a model proposed by Kay (1993), individuals respond to injury in a variety of manners depending on personality and social and environmental factors. The neurocognitive and neurobehavioral deficits can produce "a shaken sense of self" and this psychological overlay can become functionally disabling. The degree of functional disability results from the interaction of personality and environmental factors with the primary deficits.

Increasingly, researchers are adopting a multideterministic view of prolonged sequelae of MTBI. Cicerone and Kalmar (1995) examined the structure of PPCS in a sample of 50 patients who had sustained MTBI. Four factors, each consisting of multiple symptoms, were identified. These included cognitive, affective, somatic, and sensory factors. Patient clusters consisted of those with minimal symptoms, those with primarily cognitive–affective symptoms, those with prominent somatic symptoms, and those with severe global symptoms. Outcomes differed significantly across the groups; the great majority of those with minimal or primarily cognitive–affective symptoms resumed productive functioning, while those with prominent somatic or global symptoms did not.

Approaches to Management and Treatment

There are many different approaches to the management of MTBI, in part, dependent on the perspectives on etiology described above. Some health care professionals would argue for the most minimal of intervention in individuals with MTBI aside from needed emergency care. This philosophy has risen out of a primarily psychological perspective on MTBI and a premise that complete recovery should always be anticipated and prolonged symptomatology is often iatrogenic. In this model, it is argued that only the physical symptoms should be treated and that any suggestion of a possible brain insult should be deemphasized. The rationale is that by informing patients of potential problems, the professional increases the likelihood that they will experience and/or report these specific symptoms in the future as a consequence of suggestibility and/or expectancy.

Emergency room personnel often avoid informing patients about the possible effects of concussion or MTBI as a precaution against later psychosomatic endorsement of these symptoms. This form of intervention, by definition, begins and ends in the acute-care stage, resolving the need for future long-term care. It is a relatively hassle free and economically advantageous approach. Many professionals would argue, however, that patients should at least be informed about what they might expect and what resources are available should problems arise. There is certainly no data to support that not mentioning potential symptoms will prevent their development.

Other professionals propose that an individual with MTBI should be identified, provided with information about symptoms he/she might experience, monitored in the acute stages for physical and possible cognitive or emotional symptoms, and then followed to ensure that recovery proceeds in an orderly fashion. The benefit of this approach is that it attempts to maintain contact while keeping the suggestibility factor to a minimum. The procedure entails telephone or face to face contacts to monitor the patient's progression through the recovery stages. In the event that symptoms worsen during these stages, they can potentially be addressed quickly so as not to disrupt the patient's recovery. Unfortunately, most of the monitoring during the early phases of recovery is done by general or family practice physicians who may not have adequate information about MTBI to recognize or appropriately manage symptoms.

In support of this approach, several studies have documented that the number and frequency of postconcussional sequelae were markedly reduced by treatment that included information, explanation, and encouragement (Minderhoud et al., 1980; Mittenberg et al., 1992). Examples of materials that can be used in this way have been provided by several clinical and research groups (Lawler and Terregino, 1996). Mateer (1992) described the use of an information sheet that was given to a series of consecutive cases of patients with MTBI seen in an emergency room. This sheet addressed a variety of concerns and issues relevant to recovery following MTBI, including the need for rest, the potential for difficulties with concentration and memory, irritability, the danger of alcohol use during recovery, and the potential need for a graduated return to work. The sheet provided both information and recommendations for management of potential difficulties. At the same time, strong messages about the expectancy of full recovery were stressed.

Results from a large-scale study of 579 patients, most of whom had suffered MTBI, indicated that the majority of patients seen at 6 months post injury needed reassurance, advice, or other services. The authors concluded that monitoring of patients for some time after even mild injury appeared warranted (King et al., 1997).

The utility of more intensive cognitive screening, an extension of this approach, was investigated by Veltman and her colleagues in 1993. These researchers assessed 166 MTBI patients with a cognitive screening tool during the acute-care stage and then followed them through recovery. Statistically significant results supporting the efficacy of cognitive screening tests as predictors of later impairments were reported. The authors concluded that cognitive screening in the acute stages was beneficial in that it was likely to identify those individuals who may experience difficulties later.

In the first 6 months after injury, individuals with MTBI commonly receive physiotherapy for management of pain and other physical injuries. They are also often prescribed medications for pain relief, sleep difficulty and/or depression. For many, this regime is sufficient. If, however, cognitive, emotional, and behavioral changes persist, and the individual has not resumed his/her daily routine and activities, further evaluation and possible intervention probably are warranted. Intervention might include pharmacological therapies, cognitive rehabilitation strategies (work on attention, compensatory memory techniques, and organizational skills), various psychological therapies (i.e., supportive psychotherapy, cognitive–behavioral intervention), and/or vocational intervention (Conboy et al., 1986).

Gronwall (1986) pioneered research in this area describing a program that offered counseling, cognitive remediation, stress management, and vocational support. Although involvement in an active treatment program of this nature is unlikely to begin until at least 6 months post injury, in many cases, earlier intervention might decrease the development of maladaptive behaviors and psychological states.

A number of clinical research teams have described the efficacy of programs designed specifically for management of protracted symptoms following MTBI. Mateer (1992) and Mateer et al. (1990) describe cognitive and vocational outcomes for a small group of consecutive patients involved in a program consisting of cognitive rehabilitation, counseling for anxiety, depression, and pain management, and vocational reintegration services. All patients made significant improvement in cognitive function and 86% were employed at their preinjury level when contacted 3 months after discharge. Ho and Bennett (1997) also found improvements in cognitive functions after clients were involved in a program designed for MTBI. However, they stressed that reliance on such measures as indicators of outcomes is problematic, since a major feature of rehabilitation is a focus on compensatory and adjustment strategies.

Cicerone and his colleagues (1996) described a program based on education, stress management, cognitive remediation, psychotherapy, and structured resumption of activities. In a recent report of outcomes following such a program for 20 patients with MTBI, Cicerone described mixed results. Ten patients with good outcomes made significant improvement on measures of cognitive functioning and self-reported PCS symptomatology, while 10 others had poor outcomes and showed little improvement, and in some cases decline, in these areas. The authors stressed the importance of individual variability in both recovery and response to treatment. Poor outcomes may reflect either person-specific variables or differences in the level of injury severity that may not have been detected in the early stages after injury (Ruff et al., 1994).

Categories of Intervention

Specific approaches to intervention discussed in the remainder of this book address the cognitive, behavioral, and emotional symptomatology commonly associated with MTBI. In terms of cognitive disorders, the rehabilitation professional typically takes one or more of four broad approaches. In the first, the focus is on changing the environment in some way to provide more support to the individual or on changing the expectations placed upon the individual for a period of time. In the second, there is an attempt to compensate for the impaired ability by helping the individual to accomplish tasks in some other way or by using some sort of compensatory strategy. The third approach involves working directly to improve the impaired abilities and bring them closer to the premorbid condition. In the fourth, the focus is on altering the client's emotional response to and beliefs about their cognitive difficulties. The approach taken depends, in part, on the rehabilitation specialist's perspective on the individual and the symptom presentation (Harrington et al., 1993).

Intervention programs should also address the alterations in mood, affective response, self-regulation and self-image that frequently accompany MTBI. Behavioral, cognitive, and psychotherapeutic strategies for the management of these changes are discussed in detail. Response to injury and to change will, in part, be shaped by premorbid variables. Pre-existing risk factors, including personality profiles and individual coping styles, should not provide reasons for denying treatment, but should be taken into account in conceptualizing and carrying out treatment approaches (Ruff et al., 1996).

Before discussing specific rehabilitation strategies in the remainder of the book, some general principles of therapeutic interaction should be considered:

1. Every individual has rights, including their right to choose and consent to treatment;
2. Effective rehabilitation is modeled as a partnership in which the therapist and client work to achieve specific goals;
3. Interactions between client and therapist are based on honesty and mutual respect;
4. Clients are afforded confidentiality;
5. Treatment efficacy is evaluated and treatment is modified or terminated as indicated.

The therapeutic intervention itself begins with a comprehensive assessment, including review of records, interview, and testing. From this, a set of diagnostic impressions and clinical recommendations are developed. Interventions are based on objective findings and reported areas of concern. Specific treatment goals are developed and mutually agreed upon. Ongoing assessment and data-based treatment planning are used to assure that goals are being met. The goals of therapy are to help patients function more effectively in their home and work environments and to support their emotional and social adjustment.

Summary

The diagnosis of mild traumatic brain injury relies on specific criteria as measured by acute indicators (i.e., GCS, LOC, PTA). These measures ensure that the severity of insult is on the mild end of the continuum of TBI. While it may be true that the resulting deficits are also less severe, one must not equate the degree of pathology with the real and perceived impact on physical, cognitive, and emotional functioning.

Many issues affect functional outcomes, and the interactions among these different factors may give rise to countless variations in patterns of recovery. Following the injury, a patient may experience various physical symptoms, cognitive impairment, and psychological difficulties, which together have commonly been referred to as postconcussion symptoms or PCS. In the majority of MTBI cases, PCS symptoms subside over time. However, there is evidence that a small proportion of individuals who sustain MTBI may suffer from PCS for extended periods of time. The clinician's task is to understand the panoply of influences on adaptive functioning following MTBI and to make recommendations and treatment plans accordingly. It is the small but consistently reported subset of patients with MTBI who demonstrate persisting disability, and for whom the interventions described in this book are intended.

There is a growing body of literature that addresses the efficacy of various rehabilitation and management strategies for working with individuals who have persisting problems after MTBI. Coupled with this is increasing support for early provision of information, access to appropriate and timely services, and a holistic, multidisciplinary approach to evaluation and management of individuals who report persistent and disabling symptoms following MTBI.

References

Adams, J., Graham, D., and Murray, L. (1982). Diffuse axonal injury due to nonmissile head injury in humans: An analysis of 45 cases. *Annals of Neurology, 12,* 557–563.

American Psychiatric Association. (1994). *Diagnostic and Statistical Manual of Mental Disorders,* 4th Ed. Washington, DC. American Psychiatric Association.

Alexander, M.P. (1995). Mild traumatic brain injury: Pathophysiology, natural history, and clinical management. *Neurology, 45,* 1253–1260.

Alves, W.M. (1992). Natural history of postconcussive signs and symptoms. *Physical Medicine and Rehabilitation: State of the Art Reviews, 6*(1), 21–32.

Alves, W., Macciocchi, S.N., and Barth, J.T. (1993). Postconcussive symptoms after uncomplicated mild head injury. *The Journal of Head Trauma and Rehabilitation, 8*(3), 48–59.

Barth, J.T., Alves, W., Ryan, T.V., Macciocchi, S.N., Rimel, R.W., Jane, J.A., and Nelson, W.E. (1989). Mild head injury in sports: Neurolopsychological sequelae and recovery of function. In H.S. Levin, H.M. Eisenberg, and A.L. Benton (Eds.), *Mild Head Injury,* New York, NY: Oxford University Press, pp. 257–275.

Binder, L.M. (1986). A review of mild head trauma. Part II: Clinical implications. *Journal of Clinical and Experimental Neuropsychology, 19*(3), 432–457.

Blumbergs P.C., Scott G., Manavis J., Wainwright H., Simpson D.A., and McLean A.J. (1994). Staining of amyloid precursor protein to study axonal damage in mild head injury. *Lancet, 344*(8929), 1055–1056.

Blumbergs, P.C., Scott, G., Manavis, J., Wainwright, H., Simpson, D.A., and McLean, A.J. (1995). Topography of axonal injury as defined by amyloid precursor protein and the sector scoring method in mild and severe closed head injury. *Journal of Neurotrauma, 12*(4), 565–572.

Bohnen, N., and Jolles, J. (1992). Neurobehavioral aspects of postconcussive symptoms after mild head injury. *The Journal of Nervous and Mental Disease, 180*(11), 683–692.

Bohnen, N., Jolles, J., and Twijnstra, A. (1992). Neuropsychological deficits in a patient with persistent symptoms six months after mild head injury. *Neurosurgery, 30,* 692–696.

Brown, S.J., Fann, J.R. and Grant, I. (1994). Postconcussive disorder: Time to acknowledge a common source of neurobehavioral morbidity. *Journal of Neuropsychiatry and Clinical Neurosciences, 6,* 15–22.

Cicerone, K.D. (1991). Psychotherapy after mild traumatic brain injury: Relation to the nature and severity of subjective complaints. *Journal of Head Trauma Rehabilitation, 4,* 30–43.

Cicerone, K.D., Smith, L.C., Ellmo, W., and Mangle, H.R. (1996). The neuropsychological rehabilitation of mild traumatic brain injury. *Brain Injury,10*(4), 277–286.

Conboy, T.J., Barth, J., and Boll, T.J. (1986). Treatment and rehabilitation of mild and moderate head trauma. *Rehabilitation Psychology, 31*(4), 203–215.

Dikmen, S.S., McLean, A., and Temkin, N. (1986). Neuropsychological and psychosocial consequences of minor head injury. *Journal of Neurology, Neurosurgery and Psychiatry, 49,* 1227–1232.

Delahunty, T.M. (1992). Mild traumatic brain injury enhances muscarinic receptor-linked inositol phosphate production in rat hippocampus. *Brain Research, 594*(2), 307–310.

Dixon, E.C., Taft, W.C., and Hayes, R.L. (1993). Mechanisms of mild traumatic brain injury. *The Journal of Head Trauma and Rehabilitation, 8*(3), 1–12.

Evans, R.W. (1992). The postconcussion sundrome and the sequeale of mild head injury. *Neurologic Clinics, 10,*(4), 815–847.

Fenton, G., McClelland, R., Montgomery, A., MacFlynn, G. and Rutherford, W. (1993). The postconcussional syndrome: Social antecedents and psychological sequelae. *British Journal of Psychiatry, 162,* 493–497.

Gentry, L., Godersky, J., and Thompson, B. (1988). MR imaging of head trauma: Review of the distribution and radiopathologic features of traumatic lesions. *American Journal of Neuroradiology, 9,* 101–110.

Gfeller, J.D., Chibnall, J.T., and Duckro, P.N. (1994). Postconcussion symptoms and cognitive functioning in posttraumatic headache patients. *Headache, 34*(9), 503–507.

Gorman, L.K., Fu, K., Hovda, D.A., et al. (1989). Analysis of acetylcholine release following concussive brain injury in the rat. *Journal of Neurotrauma, 6,* 203.

Gronwall, D. (1986). Rehabilitation programs for patients with mild head injury: Components, problems and evaluation. *Journal of Head Trauma Rehabilitation, 1*(2), 53–62.

Gronwall, D. (1991). Minor head injury. *Neuropsychology, 5*(4), 253–265.

Harrington, D.E., Malec, J., Cicerone, K., and Katz, H.T. (1993). Current perceptions of rehabilitation professionals towards mild traumatic brain injury. *Archives of Medical Rehabilitation, 74,* 579–586.

Hayes, R., Povlishock, J., and Singha, B. (1992). Pathophysiology of mild head injury. In L. Horn and N. Zasler (Eds.), *Rehabilitation of Post-Concussive Disorders. Physical Medicine and Rehabilitation: State of the Art Reviews, 6,* 33–67.

Ho, M.R., and Bennett, T.L. (1997). Efficacy of neuropsychological rehabilitation for mild-moderate traumatic brain injury. *Archives of Clinical Neuropsychology, 12*(1), 1–11.

Hugenholtz, H., Stuss, D.T., Stethem, L.L., and Richard, M.T. (1988). How long does it take to recover from a mild concussion. *Neurosurgery, 22*(5), 853–858.

Jane, J.A., Steward, O., and Gennarelli, T. (1985). Axonal degeneration induced by experimental noninvasive minor head injury. *Journal of Neurosurgery, 62*, 96–100.

Jennett, B. and Teasdale, G. (1981). *Management of Head Injuries.* Philadelphia, PA: F.A. Davis.

Katz, R.T., and Deluca, J. (1992). Sequelae of mild brain injury. *American Family Physician, 46*(5), 1491–1498.

Kay, T. (1993). Neuropsychological treatment of mild traumatic brain injury. *The Journal of Head Trauma and Rehabilitation, 8*(3), 74–85.

Karzmark, P., Hall, K., and Englander, J. (1995). Late-onset post-concussion symptoms after mild brain injury: The role of premorbid, injury-related, environmental, and personality factors. *Brain Injury, 9*(1), 21–26.

King, N.S., Crawford, S., Wenden, F.J., Moss, N.E. and Wade, D.T. (1997). Interventions and service needs following mild and moderate injury: The Oxford Head Injury Service. *Clinical Rehabilitation, 11*(1), 13–27.

Kraus, J., and Nourjah, P. (1988). The epidemiology of mild traumatic brain injury. *Brain Injury, 3*, 177–186.

Lawler, K.A., and Terregino, C.A. (1996). Guidelines for evaluation and education of adult patients with mild traumatic brain injuries in an acute care setting. *Journal of Head Trauma Rehabilitation, 11*(6), 18–28.

Leninger, B., Gramling, S., Farrell, A., Kreutzer, J., and Peck, E. (1990). Neuropsychological deficits in symptomatic minor head injury patients after concussion and mild concussion. *Journal of Neurology, Neurosurgery, and Psychiatry, 53*, 293–296.

Levin, H., Gary, H., High, W., et al. (1987). Minor head injury and the postconcussional syndrome: Methodological issues in outcome studies. In H. Levin, J. Grafman, and H. Eisenberg (Eds.). *Neurobehavioral Recovery From Head Injury.* New York, NY: Oxford University Press, pp. 262–276.

Lishman, W.A. (1988). Physiogenesis and psychogenesis in the 'post-concussional syndrome'. *British Journal of Psychiatry, 153*, 460–469.

Mateer, C.A. (1992). Systems of care for post-concussive syndrome. *Physical Medicine and Rehabilitation, 6*(1), 143–155.

Mateer, C.A., Sohlberg, M.M., and Youngman, P. (1990). The management of acquired attention and memory disorders. In R.I. Wood, and I. Fussey (Eds.), *Cognitive Rehabilitation in Perspective.* London: Taylor and Francis, pp. 68–96.

McAllister, T.W. (1992). Neuropsychiatric sequelae of head injuries. *Psychiatric Clinics of North America, 15*(2), 395–413.

McIntosh, T.K., Garde, E., Saatman, K.E., and Smith, D. (1997). Central nervous system resuscitation. *Emergency Medicine Clinics of North America, 15*(3), 527–550.

Mendelson, G. (1982). Not 'cured by a verdict': Effect of legal settlement on compensation claimants. *Medical Journal of Australia, 2*, 132–134.

Middleboe, T., Andersen, H.S., Birket-Smith, M., and Friis, M.L. (1991). Minor head injury: Impact on general health after one year. A prospective follow-up study. *Acta Neurologica Scandinavica, 85*, 5–9.

Minderhoud, J.M., Boelens, M.E., Huizenga, J., and Saan, R.J. (1980). Treatment of minor head injuries. *Clinical Neurology and Neurosurgery, 82*(2), 127–140.

Mittenberg, W., Digiulio, D.V., Perrin, S., and Babs, A.E. (1992). Symptoms following mild head injury: Expectation as aetiology. *Journal of Neurology, Neurosurgery and Psychiatry, 55*, 200–204.

Nevin, N. (1967). Neuropathological changes in white matter following head injury. *Journal of Neuropathology and Experimental Neurology, 26*, 77–84.

Ommaya, A., and Gennarelli, T. (1974). Cerebral concussion and traumatic unconsciousness: Correlation of experimental and clinical observations on blunt head injuries. *Brain, 97*, 633–654.

Oppenheimer, D. (1968). Microscopic lesions in the brain following head injury. *Journal of Neurology, Neurosurgery, and Psychiatry, 31*, 299–306.

Phillips L.L., and Belardo, E.T. Expression of c-fos in the hippocampus following mild and moderate fluid percussion brain injury. (1992). *Journal of Neurotrauma, 9*(4), 323–333.

Pilz, P. (1983). Axonal injury in head injury. *Acta Neurochirogia, 32*, 119–123.

Radanov, B.P., Stefano, G.D., Schnidrig, A., and Ballinari, P. (1991). Role of psychosocial stress in recovery from common whiplash. *The Lancet, 338*, 712–715.

Rimel, R.W., Giordani, B., Barth, J.T., Boll, T.J., and Jane, J.A. (1981). Disability caused by minor head injury. *Neurosurgery, 9*(3), 221–228.

Robertson, E., Rath, B., Fournet, G., Zelhart, P., and Estes, R. (1994). Asessment of mild brain trauma: A preliminary study of the influences of premorbid factors. *The Clinical Neuropsychologist, 8*, 69–74.

Ruff, R.M., Baser, C.A., Johnson, J.W., Marshall, L.F., Klauber, M.R., and Minteer, M. (1989). Neuropsychological rehabilitation: An experimental study with head injured patients. *Journal of Head Trauma and Rehabilitation, 4*(3), 20–36.

Ruff, R.M., Camenzuli, L., and Mueller, J. (1996). Miserable minority: Emotional risk factors that influence the outcome of mild traumatic brain injury. *Brain Injury, 10*(8) 551–565.

Ruff, R.M., Crouch, J., and Troster, A. (1994). Selected cases of poor outcome following a minor brain trauma: Comparing neuropsychological and positron emission tomography assessment. *Brain Injury, 8*(4), 297–308.

Rutherford, W.H. (1989). Post-concussion symptoms: Relationship to acute neurological indices, individual differences, and circumstances of injury. In H.S. Levin, H.M. Eisenberg, and A.L. Benton (Eds.), *Mild Head Injury.* Oxford University Press, New York, pp. 217–228.

Schoenhuber, R., and Gentilini, M. (1988). Anxiety and depression after mild head injury: A case controlled study. *Journal of Neurology, Neurosurgery and Psychiatry, 52*, 722–724.

Stein, S.C., Spettell, D., Young, G., and Ross, S.E. (1993). Limitations of neurological assessment in mild head injury. *Brain Injury, 7*(5), 425–430.

Stevens, M., M. (1984) Postconcussion syndrome. *Maryland Institute of Emergency Medical Service Systems.* [Brochure]. National Head Injury Foundation Inc.

Tarsh, M.J., and Royston, C. (1985). A follow-up study of accident neurosis. *British Journal of Psychiatry, 145,* 18–25.

Veltman, R.H., VanDongen, S., Jones, S., Buechler, C.M., and Blostein, P. (1993). Cognitive screening in mild brain injury. *Journal of Neuroscience Nursing, 25*(6), 367–371.

Vilkki, J., Ahola, K., Holst, P., Ohman, J., Servo, A., and Heiiskanen, O. (1994). Prediction of psychosocial recovery after head injury with cognitive tests and neurobehavioral ratings. *Journal of Clinical and Experimental Neuropsychology, 16*(3), 325–338.

Williams, D.H., Levin, H.S., and Eisenberg, H.M. (1990). Mild head injury classification. *Neurosurgery, 27*(3), 422–428.

2

Medical Aspects

NATHAN ZASLER

Mild traumatic brain injury (MTBI) has been a poorly understood clinical phenomenon and yet one that appears all too frequently in daily health care practice. This chapter is an overview of medical, diagnostic, and treatment issues germane to MTBI and associated injuries.

If treatment is to be successful, the diagnosis must be accurate and this requires a foundation in the mechanics of brain injuries and posttraumatic pathophysiology. With MTBI we must recognize that many impairments may result from injuries other than those to the brain. Specifically, distinctions need to be made between sequelae associated with MTBI, with cranial trauma, and with cervical acceleration/deceleration (CAD) injury. Typically, posttraumatic pathophysiologic sequelae resulting in pain, visual, and vestibular disturbance is inextricably intertwined, making both diagnosis and treatment much more challenging. In addition, psychological factors such as depression and anxiety can interact with the neurologic injury in the creation and/or maintenance of prolonged posttraumatic symptomatology.

Just as it is necessary to understand specifics of the injury mechanisms relative to the presenting impairments and functional disability, health care practitioners must strive to understand their patient's preinjury status to appreciate how they may or may not cope with particular posttraumatic symptoms. Preexisting medical, substance abuse, psychologic and psychiatric conditions may delay recovery from MTBI (Horn, 1992). It is also necessary to delve into the patient's postinjury psychological status in order to rule out such clinical phenomena as posttraumatic stress disorder (see Chapter 9), and to assess a variety of possible behavioral changes. Clinicians should remain sensitized to the possibility of symptom embellishment, malingering, factitious, and somatoform disorders in this patient population (Ruff et al., 1993).

Two extreme camps unfortunately exist within the health care community regarding diagnostic thresholds for MTBI. One camp generally believes that mild brain injury or postconcussive disorders do not occur or do not cause long-term impairment or disability. Those holding such beliefs tend to have nothing to offer this patient population. The other camp, usually found in the field of neurologic rehabilitation, tends to over diagnose and/or "over treat" MTBI and postconcussive disorders, with inadequate consideration of alternative causes. Finding a happy medium requires a critical analysis of the patient's history, a thorough understanding of the disease process, and clinical experience. For example, clinicians would do well to review the discussion of nomenclature and pathophysiology in Chapter 1.

Results of Neuroimaging Studies

Stein et al. (1993) examined two commonly used methods of assessing neurological status in patients with mild head injury to predict intracranial damage as verified by computerized tomography (CT) scan. Despite relatively normal admission neurological exams, 127 of 689 patients had intracranial lesions, and 38 required surgery. A reaction level scale was superior to a coma scale in predicting intracranial pathology (IP), though even this test was normal in 19 subjects with IP, including nine who required surgery.

Gross et al. (1996) conducted a retrospective study of 20 patients with MTBI (aged 12–59 years at the time of injury) to compare positron emission tomography (PET), neuropsychological assessment, and continuing behavioral dysfunction. They conducted the study 1 to 5 years post injury. Abnormal local cerebral metabolic rates (rLCMs) were most prominent in midtemporal anterior cingulate, precuneus, anterior temporal, frontal white, and corpus callosum brain regions. Abnormal rLCMs were significantly correlated with overall clinical complaints, most specifically with attention/concentration, and with overall neuropsychological test results.

Kant et al. (1997) compared single photon emission computerized tomography (SPECT), magnetic resonance imaging (MRI), and CT scans of 43 adult patients with symptoms of persisting postconcussive syndrome (PPCS). They read SPECT as abnormal in 53% of patients and showed a total of 37 lesions, while they read MRI as abnormal in 9%. CT scans were abnormal in only 4.6% of patients after MTBI. The authors concluded that SPECT was more sensitive in detecting cerebral abnormalities in patients with PPCS symptoms, than either CT or MRI. No statistically significant relationship was found between SPECT scan abnormalities and age, past psychiatric history, history of substance abuse, or history of multiple TBI. SPECT scan results also appeared unrelated to current neuropsychiatric symptoms.

Cranial and Cranial Adnexal Trauma

Damage to the cranium and structures within the cranium may occur because of direct impact and/or effects of acceleration/deceleration insults. Facial and scalp lacerations, skull fractures, and ocular contusions can all result from direct trauma. Peripheral vestibular dysfunction, ossicular chain disruption with resultant conductive hearing loss, perilymphatic fistula formation with symptoms of hearing loss and vertigo, smell loss from shearing of the first cranial nerve at the cribriform plate, retinal detachment with vision compromise, as well as myofacial and temporomandibular joint injury may all be seen as a result of cranial acceleration/deceleration insult (Zasler, 1992; Evans, 1992b).

Cervical Acceleration/Deceleration Injury

Probably one of the better studied pathomechanical events associated with vehicular accidents is that of cervical acceleration/deceleration injury secondary to rear-end impacts. In such injuries, the initial direction of head displacement is into extension as the shoulders are propelled anteriorly. Following extension, the inertia of the head is overcome and accelerated forward, subsequently forcing the neck into flexion. Peak accelerations of 12 G have been noted during extension with relatively low rear-end impacts (20 miles per hour) (Severy et al., 1955). Since most cervical acceleration/deceleration injuries are not exclusively in the sagittal plane, the neck may also be damaged from rotational forces. The forces that must be taken into consideration when analyzing cervical injury include extension, flexion, lateral flexion, and shear forces (Barnsley et al., 1993). Cervical symptoms may be related to injury to multiple structures within the neck including intervertebral discs, muscles, ligaments, cervical vertebra, and neurovascular structures (Tollison and Satterthwaite, 1992).

Clinical Presentations

Mild traumatic brain injury can result in a variety of neurologic deficits, many of which may be subtle in nature and often go undiagnosed or misdiagnosed. Some conditions that may be seen following MTBI include cranial nerve dysfunctions, visual system dysfunctions, alterations in audiological and/or vestibular function, balance disorders, sleep disturbances, high-level coordination deficits and even movement disorders (Zasler, 1992). Cognitive–behavioral dysfunctions are also frequently reported in this patient population (Kay, 1992; Gualtieri, 1991). They are discussed in subsequent chapters.

Loss of Consciousness

Loss of consciousness (LOC) is not essential for a diagnosis of traumatic brain injury (see review by Anderson, 1996). In any case, it is usually very difficult to determine for how long there may have been a loss or alteration of consciousness. Other alterations in mental state, such as confusion, disorientation, agitation, or posttraumatic amnesia, which may have been present following injury and may be indicative of MTBI, are often easier to determine.

Olfactory Disturbances

Cranial nerve dysfunctions can be seen with any size brain injury. Cranial nerve I (olfactory nerve) dysfunction is particularly common compared with other cranial nerve disorders following concussion. Appropriate bedside chemosensory assessment of smell should occur, but is often neglected as part of the comprehensive neurologic assessment of patients with MTBI. When taste dysfunction occurs, it is most likely a consequence of peripheral cranial nerve VII involvement and much less likely due to injury to the IXth or Xth cranial nerve. This is because these latter nerves are extremely well protected and therefore not prone to direct injury (Costanzo and Zasler, 1991).

Hearing Disorders

Other cranial nerves commonly injured following MTBI include VII (facial nerve) and VIII (acoustic nerve: auditory and vestibular). Fractures of the temporal bone are often associated with either conductive hearing loss (due either to ossicular chain disruption or traumatic tympanic membrane tears), sensorineural or mixed hearing loss, hemotympanum and dizziness, often in association with peripheral injury to cranial nerve VII (facial nerve) (Williams and Giordano, 1989). The more common audiological deficits observed following MTBI include phonophobia (sensitivity to sound), high frequency sensorineural hearing loss (typically unilateral), and tinnitus (ringing in the ear/s) (Zasler, 1993). Endolymphatic hydrops, also known as Meniere's disease, can be seen following trauma and is associated with ipsilateral low frequency hearing loss, subjective sensation of fullness in the ear, and tinnitus (Brandt, 1991; Zasler, 1993).

Vestibular Disturbances

Balance and coordination problems are also quite common in MTBI. Subclinical vestibular dysfunction of posttraumatic etiology may be present and should be considered in any patient presenting with symptoms of balance dysfunction, even in those with vague symptoms of unsteadiness, "wooziness," and/or lightheadedness (Shumway-Cook and Horak, 1990).

Multiple etiologies exist for these types of disorders, with benign paroxysmal positional vertigo probably being the most common. This phenomenon is thought to occur secondary to dislodging of calcium carbonate crystals from the utricle and attachment to the cupula of the posterior semicircular canal. Another etiology of posttraumatic dizziness is a perilymphatic fistula, which occurs secondary to rupture of the membranes that separate the inner and middle ear resulting in pathologic stimulation of labyrinthine receptors. Patients with such fistulas often present with symptoms of vertigo, fluctuating hearing loss, tinnitus, low grade nausea, and balance problems.

Visual Disturbances

Cranial nerve dysfunction resulting in impaired extraocular motor function may also be seen. Although such impairments are generally believed to be rare following concussion (Baker and Epstein, 1991), certain types of visual system dysfunctions are quite common following MTBI including oculomotor divergence, convergence, and accommodative insufficiency (Kowal, 1992). Hellerstein et al. (1995) compared the visual status of 16 patients with MTBI and 16 controls. Significant differences were found between groups in the areas of refractive status, near point of convergence, stereo acuity, and visual pursuit functions. Such disorders may produce functional impairments in tasks requiring visual attention and concentration and reading (Zasler and Ochs, 1992).

Another common visual complaint is light sensitivity or photophobia. Bohnen et al. (1992) developed a computerized rating technique to assess tolerance to intense sound (95 dB) and light (1500 lux) stimuli. Forty-three adults with uncomplicated MTBI were tested 10 days and 5 weeks after injury and their responses were compared with 43 matched controls. Although most patients recovered from both visual and acoustic hyperesthesia, 25% of them were still not able to endure intense stimuli 5 weeks after injury. In addition, visual hyperesthesia (photophobia) was related to a postconcussive/cognitive complaints scale.

Another area of concern in the patient with history of cranial or cranial–adnexal trauma is that of direct or indirect injury to the eye. The patient may report subjective complaints of "floaters," which are typically a manifestation of vitreous matter insults secondary to acceleration/deceleration effects. Retinal injury can also occur as retinal detachment and/or hemorrhage. Pupillary changes associated with anterior cervical sympathetic insults should also be kept in mind during the patient assessment. Frequently, direct ocular trauma will result in subconjunctival hemorrhage that is typically of a transient nature (Cytowic et al., 1988). In cases of prolonged visual symptomatology, optometric/opthalmologic assessment is clearly warranted.

Posttraumatic Headache

Posttraumatic headache (PTH) is the most common somatic complaint following MTBI (Packard and Ham, 1994). Prolonged PTH can have a significant negative affect on family life, recreation, and employment (Parker, 1995). Possible causes include nerve fiber damage, abnormal cerebral circulation, and neurochemical abnormalities. Commonly, the origin is not related to brain injury per se but to extracerebral injury and dysfunction. Although most cases resolve within 6–12 months, many patients have protracted or even permanent headache complaints (Alves et al., 1993). In approximately 20% of cases, trauma-triggered migraine may account for PTH or at least be a contributing factor (Elkind, 1989; Horn, 1992).

Trauma-triggered migraine may be more frequent in pediatric populations. In adults, studies have shown that posttraumatic migraine is more common in patients who have previously had a history of migraine or who have a family history of this condition (Haas and Ross, 1986). Other intracranial origins of PTH that must be considered, although they are not particularly common following MTBI, include the presence of extraaxial collections, particularly of venous origin, subclinical seizure disorders, and posttraumatic pneumocephalus. Despite a common belief that PTH resolves at legal settlement, studies have shown that permanent PTH is usually still present several years after a legal settlement.

Seizure Disorders

Posttraumatic epilepsy is a relatively rare, albeit significant neurologic consequence of MTBI. Devinsky (1996) described 12 cases of new-onset epilepsy occurring less than 6 months after MTBI. None of the subjects had other risk factors for epilepsy. No loss of consciousness occurred in three of the cases, and in the remaining nine, the duration of LOC was less than 10 minutes. Nine of the subjects had epileptiform activity or electroencephalographic (EEG) documented seizures; two others had focal EEG slowing. Interestingly, the incidence of this phenomenon has been shown to be about the same as de novo epilepsy in the general population, i.e., 1.5%–2.0% (Dalmady-Israel and Zasler, 1993). The incidence of early seizures (seizures within the first week postinjury) is significantly higher in children than in adults. In MTBI, incidence of early seizures is not linked with a greater risk for posttraumatic epilepsy (more than one seizure following the first week of injury) (Annegers et al., 1980).

Verduyn et al. (1992) speculated that a substantial number of patients with MTBI may experience transient absence or partial seizures postinjury, which remit over the first 1–2 years postinjury. In a study he and his colleagues conducted (Roberts et al., 1996), 25 children and adolescents (aged 4–19) who had sustained MTBI and 25 who had sustained a severe TBI were administered a partial seizure symptom (PSS) inventory. All subjects (or their parents) commonly endorsed such symptoms as staring spells, memory gaps, and temper outbursts, and most of those treated with anticonvulsants demonstrated improved functioning.

Sleep Disturbances

Sleep–wake cycle disturbances are commonly reported by patients with MTBI (Kowatch, 1989). Sleep disturbances typically fall into two broad categories known as DIMS (disorders of initiation and maintenance of sleep) and DOES (disorders of excessive somnolence). Components of sleep–wake cycle alterations may include problems with sleep initiation and maintenance, decreased sleep efficiency, decreased ability to fall back to sleep when sleep is interrupted, fewer and less vivid dreams, and daytime fatigue.

Sexual Disorders

Patients with a history of MTBI may also have complaints of altered sexual function. Typically, postconcussive sexual complaints focus on problems with decreased libido (Kosteljanetz et al., 1981; Zasler, 1994b). Changes in sexual arousal may have multiple contributing factors, including physical ones such as neck and back pain, headache, and fatigue, substance abuse, side effects of medications, and emotional factors such as depression. A holistic assessment is appropriate and may include appropriate neuroendocrine work-up.

Psychiatric Disturbances

More severe types of psychiatric disturbance have also been reported following MTBI although these are relatively rare. Some psychiatric conditions reported following MTBI include mania, bipolar affective disorder (Zwil et al., 1993), major depression (Mobayed and Dinan, 1990), obsessive–compulsive disorder (Kant et al., 1997), and psychosis (Silver et al., 1994). Psychoemotional and psychiatric issues, secondary to the MTBI or unrelated, must always be given consideration as potential etiologies of an atypical recovery pattern involving late decline.

Related and Unrelated Medical Disorders

One must consider the possibility of concurrent medical and/or neurologic conditions that may occur in isolation or with MTBI that may complicate diagnosis and treatment. Neuroendocrine disorders, such as diabetes insipidus, have been reported following MTBI (Zasler, 1992). Other disorders that may complicate the diagnosis of MTBI include hypothyroidism, chronic fatigue syndrome, Lyme's disease, and reversible and nonreversible dementias (Zasler, 1995).

Cognitive Disturbances

Chronic pain, sensory disturbances, fatigue, depression, and anxiety may all impact negatively on cognitive capabilities and functional adaptation. Complications from medications and concurrent psychiatric diagnoses such as posttraumatic stress disorder must also be considered when assessing the origins of cognitive impairment in an individual status post MTBI (Zasler, 1996a). A brief mental exam will rarely capture the subtle deficits in complex attention and cognitive processing characteristic of this disorder, and referral for neuropsychological assessment should be made when problems persist.

Malingering

Physicians must also be sensitive to symptom embellishment and dissimulation [faking bad]. Malingering is one form of "faking bad" that is, by definition, consciously mediated and associated with some type of secondary gain that may or may not be financial in nature (Ruff et al., 1993; Weintraub, 1995; Zasler, 1994a ; Miller, 1996; Zasler et al., 1998).

Neuromedical and Rehabilitative Management

Diagnostic Issues

Regardless of whether MTBI is present alone or concurrently with cranial trauma and/or cervical injury, the clinician must elicit a comprehensive history from the patient and rely on this and the physical exam findings as a basis for the clinical diagnosis (Horn, 1992; Evans, 1992a; Teasell and Shapiro, 1993). Many diagnostic techniques may help the clinician establish or confirm a clinical impression of MTBI, cranial trauma and/or CAD injury (see Table 2.1). Testing may include: MRI, EEG, quantified electroencephalography (QEEG), SPECT, PET, electronnystagmography (ENG) with calorics, and posturography, among other studies (Zasler, 1993).

Standard neurologic assessment via CT and EEG will commonly not show any definitive abnormalities that are diagnostic or consistent with organic brain dysfunction secondary to MTBI. Recent research has shown that a variety of neurodiagnostic measures may have a higher yield relative to documentation of cerebral dysfunction following MTBI. Magnetic resonance imaging has been a much more sensitive modality for static brain imaging in comparison to CT in this population. Newer MRI technologies such as MRI spectroscopy and magnetic source imaging (MSI) are also being considered as adjuvants to the existing diagnostic armamentarium (Benzel et al., 1993). Use of functional imaging including SPECT and PET are also gaining acceptance as potentially significant neurodiagnostic measures in this population, even in the presence of normal static imaging (Stringer et al., 1991).

Electroencephalgram of the postconcussive patient may demonstrate subtle findings consistent with diffuse cerebral dysfunction or it may more rarely show focal abnormalities (even in the presence of a normal neurologic exam). There does not seem to be any clinical correlation between postconcussive symptoms and standard EEG findings. More recent literature suggests a greater role for a nonstandard EEG such as power spectral analysis/quantitative EEG in the neurodiagnosis of postconcussive individuals (Gevins et al., 1992; Tebano et al., 1988; Thatcher et al., 1989; Zasler, 1992).

Posturographic evaluation and ENG may be helpful in objectifying balance deficits and/or vestibular disturbances. Neurootologic testing is useful in identifying the nature and source of hearing impairments. Evoked potentials, including brain stem auditory evoked responses, may be of utility in select patients with specific posttraumatic complaints such as dizziness, but in general have not been correlated with outcome or magnitude of postconcussional symptoms. Cognitive event related potentials, including the P-300, appear to be a promising neurophysiologic marker

TABLE 2-1 Neurodiagnostic testing for specific posttraumatic sequelae

Posttraumatic Sequelae	Neurodiagnostic Procedure
Attentional deficits	Cognitive evoked potentials
Balance dysfunction	Posturographic assessment
Cerebral perfusion changes	Single photon emission computerized tomography
Cerebral metabolic changes	Positron emission tomography
Electroencephalographic abnormalities	Sleep deprived EEG, 24-hour holter EEG, video-EEG, BEAM, MEG
Erectile dysfunction	Nocturnal penile tumescence monitoring
Eye movement disorders	Electrooculography, rotary chair
Neuralgic scalp pain including cervical roots	Diagnostic/therapeutic local anesthetic block
Olfactory and gustatory dysfunction	Chemosensory evaluation for smell and taste
Perilymphatic fistula	Platform fistula test (?) on posturography, surgical exploration
Sensorineural and conductive hearing loss	Audiologic evaluation, BAERs electrocochleography
Sleep disturbance	Polysomnography with median sleep latency test
Structural parenchymal changes	MRI
Vascular injury	MRA
Vestibular dysfunction	Electronystagmography with calorics, BAERs
Vertebrobasilar insufficiency	TCD, angiography
Focal and/or diffuse brain dysfunction	MSI

?, questionable utility; EEG, electroencephalogram; BEAM, brain electrical activity mapping; MEG, magnetoencephalogram; BAER, brain stem auditory evoked response; MRA, magnetic resonance angiography; MRI, magnetic resonance imaging; TCD, transcranial color duplex/doppler; MSI, magnetic source imaging.
Modified from Zasler, N. (1993). *Journal of Head Trauma Rehabilitation, 8,* 20.

of disordered attentional processing; however, further research is necessary before advocating for its standard use. A polysomnogram (sleep study) may be beneficial in documenting sleep architecture and/or posttraumatic sleep disturbances such as sleep apnea, narcolepsy, nocturnal seizures, etc., and may help guide treatment of sleep disturbances that have been intractable to sleep hygiene education and/or pharmacologic intervention. Finally, objective evaluation of olfactory and gustatory function is also possible through a variety of valid, reliable chemosensory evaluation protocols (Zasler, 1993). Neuritic and neuralgic pain may be assessed further with diagnostic local anesthetic blocks.

Treatment and Related Issues

Referral for physical therapy treatment may be appropriate for a variety of cranial trauma and CAD injury-related sequelae. Treatment by a neurologically oriented physical therapist of higher level balance deficits with vestibular habituation training and functional balance retraining is often useful. Rehabilitative approaches to the patient with CAD injury are reviewed in more detail in Table 2.2. The physician should prescribe phar-

Table 2-2 Treatment interventions for mild traumatic brain injury

Treatment Intervention	Description
Cervical passive mobilization techniques	Massage, muscle stretching, traction, manipulation, and passive joint mobilization
Cervicothoracic muscular stabilization techniques	Stabilization training: mobility, stability flexibility, postural reeducation, exercise
Thermotherapy	Superficial heat, diathermy, cold (ice massage/ice packs), ultrasound, vapocoolant sprays
Intermittent cervical traction	30 degrees neck flexion: 15–30 pounds if evidence of radiculopathy
Medications	NSAIDs, muscle relaxants. Avoid narcotic analgesics except for brief period during acute post-injury phase
Trigger point injections	Sterile water, local anesthetic with or without steroids, dry needling
Bed rest	Early and only after severe injuries
Cervical zygapophyseal joint injections	Intra-articular local anesthetic or via blockade of the joint dorsal rami
Neural blockade	Occipital nerves and/or cervical epidural block
Correct any promulgating factors for myofascial pain	Postural issues, occlusal imbalance, leg length discrepancy, small hemipelvis, and short upper arms
Denervation and ablation procedures	Percutaneous denervation procedures, open neurectomy & disectomy fusion
Manual medicine techniques	High velocity, low amplitude
Massage	Temporary benefit for pain relief
Exercise	Emphasize stretching and progressive increase in endurance
Transcutaneous electrical stimulation	For pain management
Education	Regarding disease process, prognosis, and treatment goals
Cervical collars	Should not be prolonged and/or chronic; need to wean

Table 2-3 Pharmacologic interventions for common posttraumatic sequelae

Common Posttraumatic Sequelae	Pharmacologic Intervention
Anxiety	Serotonergic agonist: buspirone, sertraline, paroxetine, trazodone
BAM	Antimigraine regimens, psychotropic anticonvulsants
Depression	TCAs, SSRIs, venlafaxine, MAOIs, lithium, carbonate, carbamazepine
Emotional lability and/or irritability	SSRIs, psychotropic anticonvulsants, TCAs, lithium carbonate, trazodone
Libidinal alteration: decreased	Noradrenergic agonists, hormone replacement if low to borderline low
increased	SSRIs, trazodone, hormones - cyproterone or medroxyprogesterone acetate
Myofascial pain/ dysfunction	NSAIDs, TCAs, SSRIs, mild muscle relaxants, capsaicin
Neuralgic and neuritic pain	Capsaicin, TCAs, SSRIs (?), carbamazepine and other AEDs, NSAIDs, local anesthetic blockade
Posttraumatic stress disorder	Antidepressant medications, psychotropic anticonvulsants, propranolol, clonidine, MAOIs, lithium, benzodiazepines
Sleep initiation problems	Serotonergic agonists - trazodone, doxepin, amitriptyline
Sleep maintenance problems	Catecholaminergic agonists - nortriptyline
Tinnitus	Gingko biloba(?), tocainide(?), anti-migraine medications (?)
Vascular headache	Antimigraine regimens: • symptomatic • abortive • prophylactic Atypical agents: valproic acid
Fatigue	Catecholaminergic agonists: • Methylphenidate • Amantadine • Dextroamphetamine Caffeine
Cognitive dysfunction	Nootropes, catecholaminergic agonists, cholinergic agonists and/or precursors, neuropeptides (?), vasoactive agents (?)

?, questionable efficacy; BAM, basilar artery migraine; TCA, tricyclic antidepressants; SSRI, serotonin specific reuptake inhibitors; MAOI, monoamine oxidase inhibitors; NSAID, nonsteroidal antiinflammatory drugs; AED, antiepileptic drugs.

Modified from Zasler, N. (1993). *Journal of Head Trauma Rehabilitation, 8(3),* 21.

macologic agents in an appropriate manner to assist in facilitating neural, neuromusculoskeletal, and functional recovery, but should avoid drug prescriptions that might interfere with cognitive–behavioral recovery (Horn, 1992; Zasler, 1993). (See Table 2.3.)

Appropriate instruction should be given regarding avoidance of alcohol early after injury. During the early recovery stages, patients should be encouraged to optimize their diets, structure their daily activities, and minimize any "controllable" external stressors. Sleep promoting strategies should be emphasized to optimize sleep efficiency and duration. Staged reentry into preinjury activities, including driving and vocational and avocational pursuits, are critical and dictated by patient and family reports and assessment findings.

Patient and family education regarding MTBI and associated injuries, including basic pathophysiology, recovery course, and prognosis, should be an integral part of any comprehensive rehabilitation effort. Supportive counseling services should be provided to deal with expected emotional adjustment issues.

Referral for neuropsychological assessment is indicated if the patient continues to complain of cognitive and emotional symptoms, and has not returned to near preinjury levels of function at home, school, or work. Adequate assessment for nonorganic contributions to the presenting condition such as malingering, factitious disorders, somatoform disorders, and injury-related psychoemotional or psychiatric disorders such as PTSD and reactive depression should be thoroughly explored (Ruff et al., 1993).

Prognosis

Functional outcomes may be modified by a number of factors including but not limited to: age, socioeconomic status, quality of family system, degree of anxiety and depression, symptom magnification, preinjury personality, pre- and postinjury psychiatric status, presence of litigation issues, past or present use of drugs and alcohol, and/or chronic pain (Zasler, 1996b). Functional prognosis should be considered separately from neurologic prognoses. The presence of neurologic impairment following MTBI does not rule out the possibility of fully functional reentry into community, vocational, and avocational roles (Englander et al., 1992). A functional prognosis may not be appropriate in some patients with established MTBI until at least 18 to 24 months postinjury, given the long-term nature of impairment in at least a small, albeit significant, number of patients (Bohnen et al., 1992).

Many investigators have sought links between symptom persistence and ongoing litigation (Kay, 1992; McCaffrey et al., 1993). Kay has noted that persons in litigation compared with those not in litigation are more likely to: report more symptoms, have persistence of symptoms, and not return to work as quickly (Kay, 1992). Rutherford correctly points out that this may be related to negative effects of litigation or simply that people with more functional disability tend to be more likely to pursue litigation (Rutherford, 1989). The process of litigation, at least from an experiential standpoint, does tend to heighten symptoms and perpetuate them. Notably however, the incidence of gross malingering, a very different phenomena, is probably quite low (Kreutzer et al., 1991).

Conclusions

There is growing literature regarding diagnosis and treatment of MTBI and associated injuries. Many controversies remain to be studied including the most sensitive neurodiagnostic measures and the most efficacious interventions. It is important to be aware of and to continue to explore effective interventions for this special group of patients (Harrington et al., 1993) and their families to optimize their physical, emotional, and functional recovery.

References

Alves, W., Macciocchi, S.N., and Barth, J.T. (1993). Postconcussive symptoms after uncomplicated mild head injury. *Journal of Head Trauma Rehabilitation, 8*(3), 48–59.

Anderson, S.D. (1996). Postconcussional disorder and loss of consciousness. *Bulletin of the American Academy of Psychiatry and the Law, 24*(4), 493–504.

Annegers, J.F., Grabow, J.D., Groover, R.V., et al. (1980). Seizures after head trauma: A population study. *Neurology, 30*, 683–689.

Baker, R.S., and Epstein, A.D. (1991). Ocular motor abnormalities from head trauma. *Survey of Ophthalmology, 35*, 245–267.

Barnsley, L., Lord, S., and Bogduk, N. (1993). The pathophysiology of whiplash. In R.W. Teasell and A.P. Shapiro (Eds.), *Cervical Flexion-Extension/Whiplash Injuries*. Philadelphia, PA: Hanley & Belfus, pp. 329–354.

Benzel, E.C., Lewine, J.D., Bucholz, R.D., and Orrison, W.W. (1993). Magnetic Source Imaging: A review of the Magnes System of biomagnetic technologies incorporated. *Neurosurgery, 33*(2), 252–259.

Bohnen, N., Jolles, J., and Twijnstra, A. (1992). Neuropsychological deficits in patients with persistent symptoms six months after mild head injury. *Neurosurgery, 30*, 692–696.

Bohnen, N., Twijnstra, A., Wijnen, G., and Jolles, J. (1992). Recovery from visual and acoustic hyperaesthesia after mild head injury in relation to patters of behavioral dysfunction. *Journal of Neurology, Neurosurgery and Psychiatry, 55*(3), 222–224.

Brandt, T. (1991). *Vertigo: Its Multisensory Syndromes*. New York, NY: Springer-Verlag.

Costanzo, R.M., and Zasler, N.D. (1991). Head trauma—sensorineural disorders: Diagnosis and management. In T.V. Getchell, R.L. Doty, L.M. Bartoshuk, and J.B. Snow (Eds.), *Smell and Taste in Health and Disease*. New York, NY: Raven Press, pp. 711–730.

Cytowic, R., Stump, D.A., and Larned, D.C. (1988). Closed head trauma: Somatic, ophthalmic, and cognitive impairments in nonhospitalized patients. In H.A. Whitaker (Ed.), *Neuropsychological Studies of Nonfocal Brain Damage*. New York, NY: Springer-Verlag.

Dalmady-Israel, C., and Zasler, N.D. (1993). Posttraumatic seizures: A critical review. *Brain Injury, 7*(3), 263–273.

Devinsky, O. (1996). Epilepsy after minor head trauma. *Journal of Epilepsy, 9*(2), 94–97.

Elkind, A.H. (1989). Headache and head trauma. *The Clinical Journal of Pain, 5*, 77–87.

Englander, J., Hall, K., Stimpson,. T, and Chaffin, S.(1992). Mild traumatic brain injury in an insured population: Subjective complaints and return to employment. *Brain Injury, 6*(2), 161–166.

Evans, R.W. (1992a). Some observations on whiplash injuries. The Neurology of Trauma. *Neurologic Clinics, 10*(4), 975–997.

Evans, R.W. (1992b). The postconcussion syndrome and the sequelae of mild head injury. *Neurologic Clinics, 10*(4), 815–847.

Gevins, A., Le, J., Brickett, P., and Cutillo, B., et al. (1992). The future of high-resolution EEGs in assessing neurocognitive effects of mild head injury. *Journal of Head Trauma Rehabilitation, 7*(2), 78–90.

Gross, H., Kling, A., Henry, G., and Herndon, C., et.al. (1996). Local cerebral glucose metabolism in patients with long-term behavioral and cognitive deficits following mild traumatic brain injury. *Journal of Neuropsychiatry and Clinical Neurosciences, 8*(3), 324–334.

Gualtieri, T. (1991). *Neuropsychiatry and Behavioral Pharmacology*. New York, NY: Springer-Verlag.

Haas, D.C., and Ross, G.S. (1986). Transient global amnesia triggered by mild head injury. *Brain, 109*(pt.2), 251–257.

Harrington, D.E., Malec, J., Cicerone, K., and Katz, H.T. (1993). Current perceptions of rehabilitation professionals towards mild traumatic brain injury. *Archives of Physical Medicine and Rehabilitation, 74*, 579–586.

Hellerstein, L.F., Freed, S., and Maples, W.C. (1995). Vision profile of patients with mild brain injury. *Journal of the American Optometric Association, 66*(10), 634–639.

Horn, L. (1992). Post-concussive headache. In L. Horn and N.D. Zasler (Eds.), *Rehabilitation of Post-Concussive Disorders*. Philadelphia, PA: Hanley and Belfus, Inc.

Kant, R., Smith-Seemiller, L., Isaac, G., and Duffy, J. (1997). Tc-HMPAO SPECT in persistent post-concussion syndrome after mild head injury: Comparison with MRI/CT. *Brain Injury, 11*(2), 115–124.

Kay, T. (1992). Neuropsychological diagnosis: Disentangling the multiple determinants of functional disability after mild traumatic brain injury. In L. Horn and N.D. Zasler (Eds.), *Rehabilitation of Post-Concussive Disorders*. Philadelphia, PA: Hanley & Belfus, Inc., pp. 109–127.

Kosteljanetz, M., Jensen, T.S., and Norgard, B., et al. (1981). Sexual and hypothalamic dysfunction in the post-concussional syndrome. *Acta Neurologica Scandinavica, 63*, 169–180.

Kowal, L. (1992). Opthalmic manifestations of head injury. *Australian and New Zealand Journal of Ophthamology, 20*(1), 35–40.

Kowatch, R.A. (1989). Sleep and head injury. *Psychiatric Medicine, 7*(1), 37–41.

Kreutzer, J., Marwitz, J., and Myers, S. (1991). Neuropsyhologolical issues in litigation following brain injury. *Neuropsychology, 4*(4), 249–259.

McCaffrey, R.J., Williams, A.D., Fisher, J.M., and Laing, L.C. (1993). Forensic issues in mild head injury. *Journal of Head Trauma Rehabilitation, 8*(3), 38–47.

Miller, L. (1996). Malingering in mild head injury and the postconcussion syndrome: Clinical, neuropsychological, and forensic considerations. *Journal of Cognitive Rehabilitation, 14*(4), 6–17.

Mobayed, M., and Dinan, T.G. (1990). Buspirone/prolactin response in post head injury depression. *Journal of Affective Disorders, 19*(4), 237–241.

Packard, R.C., and Ham, L.P. (1994). Posttraumatic headache. *Journal of Neuropsychiatry and Clinical Neurosciences, 6*(3), 229–236.

Parker, R.S. (1995). The distracting effects of pain, headaches and hyperarousal upon employment after " minor head injury." *Journal of Cognitive Rehabilitation, 13*(3), 14–23.

Roberts, M.A., Verduyn, W.H., Manshadi, F.F., and Hines, M.E. (1996). Episodic symptoms in dysfunctioning children and adolescents following mild and severe traumatic brain injury. *Brain Injury, 10*(10), 739–747.

Ruff, R.M., Wylie, T., and Tennant, W. (1993). Malingering and malingering-like aspects of mild closed head injury. *Journal of Head Trauma Rehabilitation, 8*(3), 60–73.

Rutherford, W.H. (1989). Postconcussion symptoms: Relationship to acute neurological indices, individual differences, and circumstances of injury. In H.S. Levin, H.M. Eisenberg, and A.L. Benton (Eds.), *Mild Head Injury*. New York, NY: Oxford University Press, pp. 217–228.

Severy, D.M., Mathewson, J.H., and Bechtol, C.O. (1955). Controlled automobile rear end collisions: An investigation of related engineering and medical phenomena. *Canadian Journal of Medical Services, 11* , 727–759.

Shumway-Cook, A., and Horak, F.B. (1990). Rehabilitation strategies for patients with vestibular deficits. Diagnostic Neurotology. *Neurologic Clinics, 8*(2), 441–457.

Silver, J.M., Yudofsky, S.C., and Hales, R.E. (1994) (Eds.), *Psychiatric Aspects of Traumatic Brain Injury*. Washington, DC: American Psychiatric Press, Inc.

Stein, S.C., Spettell, C., Young, G., and Ross, S.E. (1993). Limitations in neurological assessment in mild injury. *Brain Injury, 7*(5), 425–430.

Stringer, W., Balseiro, J., and Fidler, R. (1991). Advances in traumatic brain injury neuroimaging techniques. *NeuroRehabilitation: An Interdisciplinary Journal, 1*(3), 11–30.

Teasell, R.W., and Shapiro, A.P. (1993).(Eds.) Cervical flexion- extension/ whiplash injuries. *State of the Art Reviews: Spine, 7*(3).

Tebano, M.T., Cameroni, M., and Gallozzi, G., et al. (1988). EEG spectral analysis after minor head injury in man. *Electroencephalography and Clinical Neurophysiology, 70*(2), 185–189.

Thatcher, R.W., Walker, R.A., Gerson, I., and Geisler, F.H. (1989). EEG discriminant analyses of mild head trauma. *Electorencephalography and Clinical Neurophysiology, 73*(2), 94–106.

Tollison, C.D., and Satterthwaite. (1992). *Painful Cervical Trauma: Diagnosis and Rehabilitative Treatment of Neuromusculoskeletal Injuries.* Baltimore, MD: Williams & Wilkins.

Verduyn W.H., Hilt J., Roberts M.A. and Roberts R.J. (1992). Multiple partial seizure-like symptoms following "minor" closed head injury. *Brain Injury, 6*(3), 245–260.

Weintraub, M.I. (1995). Malingering and conversion reactions. In M.I. Weintraub (Ed.), *Neurologic Clinics, 13*(2).

Williams, G.H., and Giordano, A.M. (1989). Temporal bone trauma. In Becker & Gudeman (Eds.), *Textbook of Head Injury.* Philadelphia, PA: W.B. Saunders, pp. 367–377.

Zasler, N.D. (1992). Neuromedical diagnosis and treatment of post-concussive disorders. In L.J. Horn and N.D. Zasler (Eds.), *Rehabilitation of Post-Concussive Disorders.* Philadelphia, PA: Hanley & Belfus, Inc, pp. 33–68.

Zasler, N.D. (1993). Mild traumatic brain injury medical assessment and intervention. *Journal of Head Trauma Rehabilitation, 8*(3), 13–29.

Zasler, N.D. (1994a). Mild traumatic brain injury and post-concussive disorders: neuromedical and medicolegal caveats. *Network: News for the Legal News Consultant, 5*(3), 3–5.

Zasler, N.D. (1994b). Sexual function in traumatic brain injury. In J.M. Silver, S.C. Yudofsky, and R.E. Hales (Eds.), *Psychiatric Aspects of Traumatic Brain Injury.* Washington, DC: American Psychiatric Press, Inc, pp. 443–470.

Zasler, N.D. (1995). Catastrophic traumatic brain injury. In D.R. Price and P. Lees-Haley (Eds.), *The Insurer's Handbook of Psychological Injury Claims.* Seattle, WA: Claims Books, pp. 213–238.

Zasler, N.D. (1996a). Neuromedical diagnosis and management of post-concussive disorders. In L. Horn and N.D. Zasler (Eds), *Medical Rehabilitation of Traumatic Brain Injury.* Philadelphia, PA: Hanley & Belfus, pp. 133–170.

Zasler, N.D. (1996b). Impairment and disability evaluation in post-concussive disorders. In M. Rizzo and D. Tranel (Eds), *Head Injury and Post-Concussive Syndrome.* New York, NY: Churchill Livingstone, pp. 351–374.

Zasler, N.D., and Martelli, M.F. Assessing mild traumatic brain injury. The Guides Newsletter. American Medical Association. Nov/Dec 1998, pp. 1–5.

Zasler, N.D., and Ochs, A. (1992). Oculovestibular dysfunction in symptomatic mild traumatic brain injury. *Archives of Physical Medicine and Rehabilitation, 73,* 963.

Zwil, A.S., McAllister, T.W., Cohen, I., and Halpern, L.R. (1993). Ultra-rapid cycling bipolar affective disorder following closed head injury. *Brain Injury, 7*(2), 147–152.

3

Assessment Issues

CATHERINE A. MATEER

The literature on the assessment of individuals with mild traumatic brain injury (MTBI) is mixed and the subject continues to be hotly debated. Many studies have shown deficits in attention, memory, and executive functions, particularly in the early stages following injury, although others have not. Prospective studies of consecutive admissions have demonstrated that most individuals who sustain uncomplicated MTBI return to preinjury levels of functioning within a year. However, it has also been documented that a significant minority (5%–10%) continues to report symptoms a year or more following injury (Alexander, 1995; Dikmen and Levin, 1993; Leininger et al., 1990). The patients with persistent symptoms and concerns will most commonly be seen for neuropsychological assessment.

The challenges of diagnosis in this population have historical roots. There has been a longstanding debate about whether postconcussive syndrome (PCS), a term sometimes used synonymously with MTBI, has an organic basis or is purely functional. Early physical and cognitive symptomatology are generally accepted to have a neurophysiological underpinning. However, persistent symptoms are frequently viewed as resulting from preexisting emotional or personality variables, current emotional difficulties, issues related to secondary gain, or from iatrogenic effects in the form of suggestions that the person is brain injured.

The task of sorting out these potential factors is often the responsibility of the clinical neuropsychologist or another rehabilitation professional. The process is commonly hampered by limited information about the person's functioning before the injury. Premorbid functioning can be gleaned from educational records, vocational history, and the reports of patients and their families. Typically, however, little if any information about preinjury mood or personality variables exists. In addition, current levels of emotional functioning are commonly affected by other variables such as pain, loss of employment, loss of self-confidence, financial losses, and litigation stresses. Finally, neurological examinations and imaging techniques are likely to be insensitive to subtle changes in neurological functioning and/or to microscopic or neuropharmacologic changes in the brain.

This chapter focuses on issues relevant to the differential diagnosis of MTBI. The goals of neuropsychological assessment include not only diagnosis, but the development of an accurate picture of patients' cognitive, emotional and adaptive functioning, their ability to carry out everyday activities, (including work or leisure pursuits), and their interpersonal functioning in home and society. What background information about the person and about MTBI is it important to have before undertaking the neurodiagnostic process? How can the evaluating professional best determine the source and nature of difficulties in everyday functioning? What information can be gathered to assist in the diagnosis and management of individuals with persistent complaints after MTBI? This chapter addresses these questions in a general way, as a detailed discussion of neuropsychological testing procedures is beyond the scope of the book.

Interpreting the Medical Record

Reviewing the Medical History

Typically, there is a limited medical history of the injury, per se, in cases of MTBI. Asking patients if they recall the events of the injury is important, and if they do not, examiners should inquire about their last recollections before the injury. Such questions shed light on the likelihood of even brief loss of consciousness and the existence of a brief retrograde amnesia. There may or may not be a specific reference to these factors in the medical record. In many cases of MTBI there seems to be at least a brief loss of awareness (e.g., not remembering how one ended up in the middle of the intersection). Even without such a report, however, it seems generally accepted that a loss of consciousness is *not* required in order for an MTBI to have occurred (Alexander, 1995; Anderson, 1996). Periods of retrograde memory loss following MTBI of more than 1 hour are uncommon.

It is also useful to question the patients' recollection of events immediately following the accident. Ask about their first awareness that an accident had taken place, and their recall of events at the scene following the accident, during the ambulance ride if one occurred, in the emergency room, and over the 24–hour period following injury. Corroborative information from family members or from the medical record regarding events and behaviors exhibited by the patient during the early posttraumatic period can be very helpful in establishing whether there was agitation, posttraumatic amnesia (PTA), confusion, and/or other posttraumatic sequelae. It is often useful to try to establish from the patient or family the point at which connected and continuous memory was established, as this has been a more accurate measure of the resolution of the amnesic condition than is specification of the first postaccident memory alone (Shores et al., 1985). In general, periods of PTA up to 5 minutes are considered very mild, 5 minutes to 60 minutes in the mild range, 1–24 hours in the moderate range, and more than 1 day in the severe range (Levin et al., 1987). There are inconsistent reports, however, regarding the importance of PTA. Although studies have suggested a strong relationship between PTA and degree of recovery in moderate to severe head trauma (Jennett, 1976), duration of PTA has not been reliably related to the subjective impact of MTBI symptoms (Karzmark et al., 1995).

Ambulance personnel and the medical record can also be used to gather information about areas of bruising or contusion about the face or head suggestive of a blow or impact. Besides focusing on possible head injury sequelae, gathering information about other injuries is important, including neck or back injuries, orthopedic injuries, and any injuries that might have resulted in lack of oxygen or reduced respiratory function. Some literature suggests that individuals who sustain additional physical injuries or complications may be more prone to development of persistent postconcussive symptoms. Headaches and dizziness, for example, have been shown to exacerbate the effects of neuropsychological problems (Conboy et al., 1986; Coonley-Hoganson et al., 1984; McLean et al., 1984).

In addition to reviewing medical records about the injury in question, reviewing the prior medical history and records is often useful. And, because of their potential impact on the current pattern of recovery, incidents of prior brain injury and/or neurological impairments or symptoms are of interest. The effects of a second brain injury following a prior injury have been described as exponential rather than additive (Gronwall, 1989). That is, the consequences of the second injury may be significantly more than that which would have occurred without the first.

Also of interest in the prior medical record are indications of other medical conditions that could lead to cognitive symptomatology (e.g., epilepsy, prior treatment for toxic exposure, thyroid disorders, long term substance abuse). In the presence of a positive history for such disorders, determining the onset of symptoms is important, and one should be aware of possible interactions between the conditions and their effects. The prior medical record may also indicate past emotional or psychiatric disorders, or a personality profile suggesting somatization, anxiety, or depression. Other risk factors for prolonged symptomatology include age over 40 years (discussed in Chapter 13), and involvement in a highly demanding occupation or training program (Lawler and Terregino, 1996).

The Relationship between Imaging Studies and Neuropsychological Outcome

Mild head trauma is only rarely associated with abnormal computed tomography (CT). In a study by Moran et al. (1994) which reviewed CT records of 200 individuals seen for MTBI, none of the patients who had not sustained LOC and who had an emergency room GCS of 13–15, had a positive scan. Of 93 patients with LOC, only 8 had a positive scan, and of 9 patients with skull fracture, only 5 had a positive scan. The authors suggested that patients without LOC and with a GCS of 13–15 do not require CT scanning unless clinically indicated.

Although magnetic resonance imaging (MRI) appears to yield abnormal results much more frequently (Levin et al., 1987), positive findings are often not judged to be related to the injury in question. Radiologists' reports will frequently indicate that small areas of focal abnormality are not clearly resultant from the injury and are of "unknown significance." This is in part related to the fact that base rates for high intensity lesions are quite high in the normal population. Further complicating this issue, some studies have demonstrated evidence of lesions on imaging studies early after injury, but not on later imaging studies. It is unclear whether "disappearing" MRI lesions following brain injury signal some underlying dysfunction that could have clinical significance.

Functional Imaging Studies

Since CT and even MRI scanning identify only areas of structural damage in the brain, and do not address the functioning of the brain, measures that address brain activity may be better suited to the analysis of MTBI. The arrival of more sophisticated functional imaging techniques, such as xenon computerized tomography and positron emission tomography (PET), has brought the promise of objectively evaluating subtle cerebral pathology.

Nedd et al. (1993) compared SPECT and CT scan results in 16 patients with mild to moderate TBI. Single photon emission computerized tomography showed differences in cerebral blood flow significantly more often than CT revealed structural lesions (87.5% vs. 37.5%). In patients with lesions in both modalities, the area of involvement was relatively larger on SPECT scans than on CT scans. Based on similar studies with SPECT, Jacobs et al. (1994) concluded that SPECT alterations correlated well with severity of trauma, and with subjective postconcussive symptomatology.

Additional evidence supporting the utility of functional imaging in individuals with poor outcome from MTBI comes from two studies. Varney et al. (1995) reported SPECT results in 14 patients with a history of MTBI, but who had normal CT and/or MRI scans. All of the patients had been unable to sustain any occupation despite multiple attempts over many years following injury. This group of subjects consistently showed anterior mesial temporal hypoperfusion, though very infrequent posterior temporal lobe abnormalities. The authors concluded that some "mild" head injuries with unusually catastrophic psychosocial consequences demonstrate regional abnormalities in cerebral perfusion that are consistent with the mechanisms of head trauma. In the second study, Ruff and his colleagues (1994) reported PET with neuropsychological examination in nine individuals who had sustained MTBI and who had little or no evidence of brain damage on CT or MRI. Positron emission tomography findings and neuropsychological assessment were corroborative, and the PET procedure documented frequent neuropathology in the frontal and anteriotemporo-frontal regions not evident with other imaging techniques. In addition, the authors reported no differences between cases with reported loss of consciousness and those without.

Electrophysiological Studies

Although standard clinical EEG analysis rarely provides indication of significant abnormality in individuals with MTBI, finer grained analyses of brain electrical activity through spectral or quantitative analyses have shown promise. Tebano et al. (1988) found a significant increase in the mean power of slow alpha, a reduction of fast alpha, and a reduction of fast beta in 18 patients who had sustained minor head injuries 3–10 days earlier, in comparison to age and sex-matched controls. This work suggested changes in brain function in the early stages following MTBI, consistent with many other reports of cognitive inefficiency during this period.

Obviously, more controversy surrounds the late symptoms of MTBI. Penkman (1994) compared results for 16 patients with mild head injury (MHI), 16 unipolar depressed patients, and 16 controls on the Continuous Performance Task (CPT) and on a quantitative encephalogram (QEEG). While both the MHI and depressed subjects exhibited slower reaction times than controls on the CPT task, the MHI group demonstrated enhanced slow wave (delta) activity compared with the depressed patients. Delta activity was positively correlated with clinical ratings of depression in MHI but not in the depressed group. These results suggest a different basis of brain involvement in MTBI than in unipolar depression.

Although of interest theoretically, it will be extremely uncommon for patients to have undergone more detailed and extensive examinations such as these outside of an experimental context. In some cases, however, it may be appropriate to refer the patient for more detailed assessment when diagnostic questions are of primary importance.

Interpreting Self-Reported Symptoms

The most commonly reported problems following MTBI include memory impairment, headache, dizziness, concentration difficulty, blurred vision, photophobia, ringing of the ears, irritability, fatigue, anxiety, and depression (World Health Organization, 1978; Youngjohn et al., 1995). Although not every symptom is reported in every case, the overall consistency of this cluster of symptoms following MTBI or concussion has been used to argue in support of an organic basis for the disorder (Alexander, in response to Peterson, 1996; Alves et al., 1986).

Alternatively, it has been argued that the common symptoms of PCS are not specific for brain injury. Gouvier et al. (1988) found that the base rate of complaints from the PCS constellation is very high in the normal, non brain-damaged population. There is also some indication of a "conventional wisdom" about the common effects of head injury. Mittenberg et al. (1992), for example, found that naive subjects with "imaginary" concussions endorsed a cluster of symptoms very similar to PCS. They also reported that actual patients consistently underestimated the premorbid prevalence of these symptoms compared with the base rates in the general population. It is not clear whether this "communal knowledge" results from personal experience, logical deduction, or messages received from others or from the media. Even cartoon characters commonly experience problems with dizziness, balance, headache, blurred vision, and confusion after a blow to the head. Although symptoms usually disappear quickly in such media images, the message about what one might expect is clear. Findings such as these have been interpreted as suggesting that a patient's expectations may play a substantial role in the emergence of PCS symptoms.

Measuring the occurrence of symptoms or the number of symptoms present may not provide a complete description of their effects on the individual. In this regard, assessing the frequency and severity of symptoms in cases of MTBI is important, as opposed to simply the *incidence* of symptoms. While it is certainly true that all normal individuals have occasional headaches, memory lapses, and difficulty with concentration, such symptoms have been reported to occur much more frequently in the MTBI population than in the non-MTBI population. In a series of studies involving more than 400 adults with MTBI and a large number of matched controls, Bohnen and his colleagues (1994, 1995) reported a three-factor model, containing dysthymic, vegetative/bodily complaints, and cognitive performance factors. Vague everyday complaints in different and distinct respects were more prevalent and severe in subjects with mild head injuries. It is important, therefore, to ask not just whether the person is experiencing symptoms but how often, with what degree of severity, and with what level of disruption in normal activities.

Bohnen and his colleagues (1992a,b) also reported that subjects with persistent PCS complained of more emotional symptoms, performed more poorly on attentional measures, and showed reduced tolerance to light and sound than subjects who sustained head injury but recovered. Persistent neurobehavioral deficits were correlated with scores on a PCS rating scale, but not with scores on an emotional/vegetative scale.

Use of a structured interview or a rating scale can help in identifying the frequency and severity of common PCS symptoms and can provide a better understanding of the real and subjective burden experienced by the patient (Ruff et al., 1986). Cicerone and Kalmar (1995) found that most of the subjects with MTBI who resumed productive activity clustered in groups with few or primarily cognitive–affective symptoms, whereas those who did not tended to cluster in groups with prominent somatic or severe global symptoms. These patient clusters were largely unrelated to neurological or neuropsychological functioning. The authors argued that subjective complaints provide clinically meaningful information and are strongly related to the nature and extent of disability after MTBI.

Appendix A provides the Postconcussion Symptom Checklist (Gouvier et al., 1992) and the Rivermead Postconcussion Symptom Questionnaire (King, 1996), which allow patients to rate the subjective severity of commonly reported somatic/physical, emotional, and cognitive complaints. Although such scales can be useful clinical and research tools, it is advisable initially to elicit a description of symptoms in a more open-ended interview before administering a symptom checklist, as reviewing the inventory of common symptoms may encourage symptom reporting or magnification by suggestion. This is particularly important in medicolegal cases or when working with individuals who may be suggestible, fearful, or somatically focused.

Another issue related to symptom reporting concerns the temporal onset of symptoms; that is, the distinction between early and late symptoms (Rutherford, 1989). It is common for physical symptoms (e.g., dizziness, nausea, blurred vision) to be focused on and documented in early medical records from the emergency room or a physician's office. Cognitive symptoms (e.g., attention and memory difficulty) are typically not documented early in the medical record, either because they are not specifically evaluated, or because the patient has not yet or has only recently begun to return to a pattern of normal activities. Just after an injury, both patients and family members may anticipate the need for a period of rest and recovery before the patient returns to domestic duties and work activities. It is often only after the person has attempted to return to former activities that problems with concentration, memory, efficiency, and stamina are recognized. Therefore, it is not unusual for there to be a lack of documentation of cognitive symptoms in the medical record for several weeks or even a few months following injury.

If, however, a few months or more had passed without any reference to such problems in the record, one might become suspect as to why such problems were not identified earlier in a client presenting with symptoms long after injury. In general, one should look for the gradual resolution of symptom severity rather than an increase in symptoms or the addition of many new symptoms. Such a pattern would suggest that nonorganic factors such as depression, somatization, or issues of secondary gain may be involved.

It is also important to monitor for symptoms that would be highly unusual as a consequence of MTBI or that would be highly improbable from a neurological perspective. Such symptoms might include, for example, monocular diplopia (double vision with one eye closed), triple vision, an extended period of total retrograde amnesia, greatly heightened sensitivity to smells, or tingling and numbness in the arms or legs. The report of such symptoms might suggest conscious malingering, exaggeration of symptoms, hysteria, underlying emotional factors contributing to functional symptomatology, and/or other comorbid or preexisting neurological disorders. In reference to coexisting disorders, the author is reminded of a patient with MTBI who reported unusual visual symptoms, and, upon further investigation, was found to have a brain tumor. In the absence of neurological disorder, bizarre symptoms may or may not reflect deliberate simulation, and classification along the conscious/unconscious dimension may be more useful than a contrast between psychogenic and organic bases (Barbarotto et al., 1996).

In cases of moderate to severe brain injury, patients often demonstrate a degree of unawareness or denial of changes in their physical, cognitive, and behavioral functioning. In individuals with MTBI the situation often seems to be reversed. That is, these individuals often seem to be most acutely aware of perceived changes in thinking, remembering, concentrating, and accomplishing goals (Mateer et al., 1987). To gather information regarding the likely existence and real impact of these deficiencies on functioning at home and at work, it is often useful to separately interview family members, employers, and/or co-workers (assuming a release by the patient for the professional to do so). Of importance is inquiring about specific instances of cognitive inefficiency or failure, and about productivity levels in general. Also, asking about changes in social behavior, emotional stability, and resilience in the face of work demands is beneficial. Speaking to ancillary parties can often assist in determining more accurately the nature, severity, and frequency of the problems, although these individuals may have no way of estimating levels of additional effort the patient may be making to complete activities.

Although information about adjustment to everyday school, work, and social demands is very important, gathering such information in a systematic fashion is often difficult. Most of the scales developed are applicable to moderately or severely injured patients, but have not been used systematically in MTBI. Such scales include the Brock Adaptive Functioning Questionnaire (Dywan and Segalowitz, 1996), the Portland Adaptability Inventory (Lezak, 1987), and the Patient Competency Rating Scale (Prigatano, 1986).

Neuropsychological Testing

Well-controlled prospective studies examining MTBI consistently have found the presence of cognitive deficits immediately after trauma (Barth

et al., 1989; Dikmen et al., 1986; Gronwall and Wrightson, 1974; Hugenholtz, Stuss et al., 1988; Levin et al., 1987). Impairments appear most commonly on measures that are sensitive to attention, speed of information
processing, verbal and visual memory, and executive functions. In general, these studies have found that most patients recover cognitive abilities within several months of injury, with little or no persisting disability. In every study, however, a proportion of individuals continued to be
symptomatic and described changes in everyday functioning 6 months
or more following injury. Appendix B provides a handout for patients
that explains what to expect after a mild traumatic brain injury. As each
chapter in this volume deals with specific diagnostic issues related to the
particular cognitive or emotional domain under discussion, a detailed listing of individual tests that might be used is not included here. Rather, issues in assessment that cut across many domains are reviewed.

Dealing with Issues of Test Selection and Interpretation

Neuropsychological testing typically involves the use of batteries of tests
that evaluate many different cognitive abilities (including attention, memory, language, visuoperceptual, and executive functions), and a variety
of perceptual and motor functions. They also commonly include assessments of intellectual functioning, academic achievement, and personality
and emotional functioning. One does not expect to see difficulties on all
or even most of the tests administered. Measured intellectual ability, expressive and receptive language skills, visuoperceptual functioning, and
academic achievement levels have all been quite robust in cases of MTBI.
Areas of difficulty tend to include performance on speeded measures,
tasks requiring complex attention and working memory, and efficiency
of new learning. Some more robust findings in MTBI have been observed
in impaired performances on the Paced Auditory Serial Addition Test
(Gronwall, 1977; Gronwall and Wrightson, 1974), a modified version of
the Stroop Test (Bohnen et al., 1992a), the Consonant Trigrams Test (Stuss
et al., 1989), and verbal learning tests (Mateer, 1992). Appendix C provides a useful handout for patients and significant others regarding commonly asked questions about neuropsychological evaluations.

Raskin et al. (1998) examined neuropsychological test results in a group
of 148 individuals (80 women, 68 men) who met the criteria for MTBI
adopted by the American Congress of Rehabilitation Medicine (Kay et al.,
1993). Consistent with previous studies (Kraus and Nourjah, 1988), this
group was somewhat older than the general brain injury population ($\bar{x}$ =
38.14). Mean educational level was 13.4 years. Subjects averaged 21.75
months post injury. Of the 126 individuals in this study employed at the
time of injury, 83 were employed at the time of testing. As in previous studies, there was no significant correlation between the duration of loss of consciousness and any neuropsychological or emotional variable. When impairment was defined as performance greater than one standard deviation

below the age-adjusted normative mean for that test, tests on which the greatest number of individuals were impaired were tests of time-dependent complex attention, working memory, and shifting mental set (Test of Reading Speed, Symbol-Digit Modalities Test, Trail Making B, Picture Rapid Naming, and the Alternating subtest of Attention Processs Training) and tests of verbal learning (Paired Associates and Logical Memory subtests of the Wechsler Memory Scale-Revised, and California Verbal Learning Test, Trial 1). Tests of general intellectual functioning were the least likely to demonstrate impairment. (See Table 3.1) These results are quite typical of what has been described in both the clinical and experimental literature.

Appreciating Base Rate Phenomena

Faced with a patient who is demonstrating problems on several above-mentioned tests, it is compelling to attribute problems to the incident or trauma in question. Being aware of the base rate phenomena is important, however. For example, among normal individuals with no neurological history and intellectual functioning in the average range of intelligence, Dodrill (1987) estimated that 15.6% of scores on an adaptation of the Halstead Reitan Neuropsychological Test Battery will fall in the mildly deficient range, 3.3% will fall in the moderately deficient range, and 0.5% will fall in the severely deficient range. These estimates decrease as the subject's intellectual level increases. These results suggest that obtaining a sufficiently large number of test scores is imperative and one must be aware of base rates for impairment on the tests selected. It is also important to obtain multiple indicators of impairment across separate tests tapping into the same kind of ability before deciding that an impairment in some aspect of cognitive ability is present. Convergence of evidence from different tests is an important principle in interpretation of tests of cognitive ability (Lezak, 1994).

Dealing with Problems Related to Sensitivity of Tests

The ability to detect impairments is only as powerful as the tools developed for this purpose. Recognize that few of the major neuropsychological tests and none of the major test batteries was designed specifically to identify the cognitive and adaptive problems experienced by individuals with MTBI. Indeed, the strongest and most obvious deficits in the MTBI literature are reported for experimental tests specifically designed to measure such areas as complex attention or working memory (Gronwall, 1987; Stuss et al., 1989). In some studies, for example, only a modified version of the Stroop Test that put greater demands on attentional control revealed impairments in subjects with MTBI (Bohnen et al., 1992a).

The difficulty in assessing executive functions through use of traditional psychometric tests is particularly well documented (Lezak, 1994). Although it is apparent from clinical experience that individuals with MTBI have particular difficulty managing multiple sources and kinds of

Table 3-1 Percent of MTBI sample impaired on each neuropsychological measure (Raskin, Mateer & Tweeten, 1998).

Test	Cutoff	Percent Impaired
TORS	< 27	51
WMS-R verbal paired associates I	< 18	48
Symbol digit modalities—written	< 46	35
WMS-R verbal paired associates II	< 7	32
Symbol digit modalities—Spoken	< 53	30
Trail making test part B	> 73	28
WMS-R logical memory II	< 13	26
PRN	> 76	26
Attention process test alternating	< 14	25
Stroop interference	> 159	25
CVLT I	< 6	22
WMS-R logical memory I	< 17	21
Rey-Osterreith immediate recall	< 25	20
WRAT-R2 arithmetic	< 29	20
CVLT free recall I	< 9	18
Controlled oral word association	< 28	17
Attention process test selective	< 16	16
WAIS-R information subtest	< 7	16
Trail making test part A	> 39	15
WMS-R digit span forwards	< 7	15
Wisconsin card sorting test categories	< 5	15
Rey-Osterreith copy	< 60	15
California free recall II	< 9	15
California cued recall II	< 10	15
Rey-Osterreith delayed recall	< 26	14
WMS-R visual reproductions II	< 24	13
California cued recall I	< 10	13
WMS-R digit span backwards	< 5	12
Attention process test sustained	< 15	12
Attention process test divided	< 25	12
California recognition	< 14	12
WAIS-R digit span	< 7	12
WAIS-R vocabulary	< 7	12
WMS-R visual reproductions I	< 28	10
California trial V	< 11	10
WAIS-R comprehension	< 7	10
WAIS-R similarities	< 7	10
WAIS-R arithmetic	< 7	7
WAIS-R picture completion	< 7	7
WAIS-R digit symbol	< 7	7
WAIS-R picture arrangement	< 7	6
WAIS-R object assembly	< 7	6
Attention process test simple	< 29	3

(continued)

Table 3-1 Percent of MTBI sample impaired on each neuropsychological measure (Raskin, Mateer & Tweeten, 1998). (*continued*)

Test	Cutoff	Percent Impaired
California false positive	> 4	3
WAIS-R block design	< 7	2

TORS, test of reading speed; WMS-R, Wechsler Memory Scale-Revised; PRN, picture rapid naming; CVLT, California Verbal Learning Trial; WRAT, wide range achievement test; WAIS-R, Wechsler Adult Intelligence Scale-Revised (age-corrected scores). From Raskin et al. (1998). *The Clinical Neuropsychologist, 12*, 21–30, with permission.

information and working in noisy or distracting environments, very few tools are available to evaluate these kinds of higher order abilities. A greater understanding of the nature of executive function disorders has come about primarily through the development of new experimental tasks that are theoretically based and designed specifically to evaluate discrete areas of ability. Shallice and Burgess (1991a,b) have demonstrated, for example that frontally impaired patients who demonstrate normal or above average intellectual ability and who perform normally on most standardized tests, may do very poorly on an open-ended task with multiple subgoals. They developed the Six Element Task in which subjects are asked to complete some portion of several different tasks within a specified time frame. Frontally impaired patients displayed difficulty with planning, self-monitoring, attention to the passage of time, and adherence to rules. This is discussed in more detail in Chapter 6.

A final concern about test sensitivity involves practice effects. Repeated test administrations are likely to reduce the sensitivity of a particular test. Many patients with TBI have undergone repeated testing with one or more practitioners on neuropsychological batteries that have not been modified to contain new items or material. The effectiveness of these tests after multiple exposures must be seriously questioned.

Dealing with Nonorganic Factors

One possible explanation for prolonged postconcussional symptoms is a previous neurotic condition or personality disorder that is intensified by the trauma or by other extrinsic factors. As yet, there is much speculation but little data to support this contention. Fenton et al. (1993) reported that chronic social difficulties and the number of adverse life events in the year preceding the injury were associated with the emergence and persistence of PCS, while other studies such as that by Karzmark et al. (1995) specifically refuted the impact of preinjury variables.

It is commonly believed that performance on neuropsychological tests may be influenced by a variety of affective states including depression and anxiety. Indeed, postconcussive symptoms often include anxiety and depression (Dinan and Mobayed, 1992; Uomoto and Esselman, 1993), consistent with the suggestion that emotional disturbance may contribute, at least in part, to cognitive inefficiency in the MTBI population. There is some general support for this notion. In the Karzmark et al. study (1995), for example, the number of elevated Minnesota Multiphasic Personality Inventory (MMPI) scales was strongly associated with subjective impact of PCS symptoms. However, there has been little or no indication of a clear relationship between neuropsychological test performance and self-report of depression and/or anxiety.

Raskin et al. (1998) examined the relationships between performance on neuropsychological measures and emotional and personality factors in 148 individuals with persistent symptoms following MTBI. No significant relationships were demonstrated between the MMPI scales and the neuropsychological measures using correlation coefficients. When the group was divided into two groups, one with a T-score on MMPI Scale 2 (depression) greater than 70, and one with a T-score less than 70, there were no significant differences between the two groups on any of the neuropsychological measures. These findings suggest that performance on neuropsychological tests cannot be explained solely based on depression.

A somewhat different perspective regarding the impact of emotional factors on persistent symptoms of MTBI argues that emotional changes occur in response to organic changes, which are, in turn, affected by emotional responses. This perspective views organic factors as responsible for early experience of cognitive symptoms after MTBI, and holds that it is the affected individual's personality style, beliefs, and self-perception that determine the individual's affective response to the difficulties experienced (Kay, 1992). When a task that was previously readily accomplished suddenly feels difficult or is done only with more effort and increased errors, anxiety and distress may result. This can lead to anticipatory anxiety so that the next time the person attempts the task or has difficulty on a related task, his/her anxiety response may increase. Now each time the person attempts particular tasks, the anxiety puts him or her at even higher risk for failure. Repeated associations between attempts to perform and a perception of either failure or fear of failure creates links that affect performance. This process can be particularly problematic for individuals who premorbidly have very high self-expectations, who are somewhat perfectionistic or rigid, or who derive a great deal of their self-concept and image from their ability to perform or to be in control. Ruff et al. (1996) provide an excellent framework for working with patients with MTBI who have premorbid personality disorders or traits such as grandiosity, narcissism, borderline features, overachievement, perfectionism, dependency, and depression. Such features will color an individual's response to injury, and interact with preexisting defenses, fears, needs, and coping styles.

Standard measures of emotional and personality functioning, such as the MMPI and MMPI-2, often are used to assess individuals with MTBI.

Cripe (1989, 1991) has argued that using such scales may be inappropriate, and that results need to be interpreted cautiously as many test items loading on different scales can be indicators of or found to be in association with neurologic disease or disorder. Items asking about headache, problems with sleep, dizziness, numbness, visual problems, concentration, and memory problems, for example, can be consistent with either psychiatric disorders or with underlying neurological problems.

With this caveat, MMPI profiles in patients with documented brain damage secondary to moderate to severe injuries have yielded fairly consistent findings. In general, mean scale score on the D scale (depression) is higher than the Hs (hysterical) or Hy (hypochondriacal) scales (Burke et al., 1990; Gass and Russell, 1991). In contrast, Youngjohn and his colleagues, (Youngjohn, et al., 1995) report higher mean Hs and Hy than D scale scores (MMPI- 2) in a group of patients with history of compensable MTBI. In another sample, MTBI patients demonstrated significant elevations on Hs, D, Hy and Pt (psychasthenia) over a group of patients with severe TBI (Youngjohn et al., 1997). These findings are consistent with other investigators who have reported that more severely brain-injured patients paradoxically have lower MMPI elevations than patients complaining of PCS after minor head trauma, particularly on scales Hs and Hy (Leininger et al., 1991; Novack et al., 1984). Mild traumatic brain injury patients often report seeing themselves as having more physical and emotional symptoms and being more disabled by those symptoms than do patients with moderate to severe brain damage. In part, this may reflect the blunting of awareness patients with severe TBI demonstrate concerning changes in their functioning. It also may reflect heightened level of anxiousness and concerns for physical and mental functioning in patients with MTBI. This might result from frustration about continuing physical, cognitive, or emotional problems for which they have received no clear diagnosis, or from factors related to secondary gain (litigation, off-work status, change in responsibilities), which are serving to support and reinforce disability.

The MMPI patterns characteristic of many individuals with MTBI are similar to those seen in chronic pain patients and suggests a focus on somatic concerns with potentially hysterical or exaggerated features. Similarities between chronic pain patients and individuals with MTBI have been drawn by other researchers (Uomoto and Esselman, 1993; Iverson and McCracken, 1997). Minnesota Multiphasic Personality Inventory test results suggest significant elements of somatization or functional overlay to the self-reports of many individuals with MTBI. It is possible that MTBI patients, as a group, do have a high rate of associated soft tissue injury and pain. Importantly, however, many intervention strategies used in the management of chronic pain may be appropriate for individuals with MTBI. Increasing work tolerance, providing self- management strategies (relaxation, pacing, self-talk, meditation), and use of thought stopping and mental distraction techniques are often useful. Cognitive–behavioral interventions can be used to modify distorted beliefs or black-and-white thinking.

Dealing with Issues Related to Motivation, Effort, and Symptom Validity

It is assumed by most practitioners that neuropsychological test results are valid to the extent that the client has put forward effort and is motivated to succeed on the tasks presented. Inability to expend effort can presumably result from a variety of factors that are essentially under the patient's control. It seems reasonable to assume that fatigue, lack of sleep in the previous 24 hours, pain, tinnitus, and other physical symptoms or states would make full effort and participation in the assessment process more difficult. Although there is little data bearing on this hypothesis, a couple of studies are pertinent. Tsushima and Newbill (1996) administered a cognitive battery and the MMPI to 37 patients with MTBI whose headaches were rated at the time of testing. No significant differences were found on any of the measures between subjects grouped by headache severity (none, mild, severe). Townsend and Mateer (1997) studied a group of patients with pain secondary to degenerative joint disease (rheumatoid arthritis). They also found no consistent relationship between level of reported pain and neuropsychological test results.

It has been proposed that a major factor underlying some, if not many, poor test performances by individuals with possible MTBI involves either a conscious or unconscious attempt to do worse than they are capable of so as to receive financial or other compensation for injury. It has been argued that patients involved in workers' compensation or personal injury cases are not motivated to do well on a neuropsychological assessment, in that some patients perceive they will be rewarded with financial compensation for poor performance. Others may believe that they must do poorly, if they are to persuade others of the problems they are convinced they experience. Estimates of malingering on neuropsychological tests by individuals being evaluated for MTBI in the medicolegal context range widely from as low as 5% to as high as 50% or more (Binder, 1993a; Kay, 1992; Snow, 1992; Youngjohn et al., 1995). Variations may be due to the setting in which the evaluation takes place (e.g., medical, medicolegal, forensic, rehabilitation, etc.), the nature of referral sources, the procedures used to define or determine malingering, or the expectations and perspective of the examiner.

It is also important to be aware of differences between malingering, somatization, and conversion disorders. The distinctions between these can be extremely difficult and overlaps are common. In each condition, clinicians are confronted with similar discrepancies between laboratory findings and self-report, and between objective signs and subjective symptoms (Resnick, 1988). Individuals with any of these disorders may avoid unpleasant activity and seek support or compensation. The critical element that has classically distinguished somatization and conversion disorders from malingering is that symptoms related to the former disorders are not under voluntary control. Patients with somatization and conversion disorders are said to "deceive themselves" as well as others, whereas malingerers consciously attempt to deceive others. The disability associated with these disorders may serve a variety of psychological needs for dependency, retaliation, or escape from an intolerable situation, although overt report of symptoms commonly associated with depression and anxiety are commonly denied.

I worked with a young man who had been a body builder. Two weeks before a high stakes international competition, he was involved in a motor vehicle accident associated with a mild head injury and whiplash. While not "severe," his injuries did not allow him to pursue the competition. Over the next 6 months he developed extremely disabling physical symptoms, including a functional gait disorder, and marked cognitive and behavioral symptoms such that he no longer cared for himself or worked. Inventories related to depression and anxiety were within normal limits. Conversion disorder, secondary to the loss of his "dream" of winning the competition he had intensively trained for over many years, was thought to be the most likely diagnosis.

The individual with conversion disorder is ill, and confrontation with the nonorganic nature of the illness is not necessarily beneficial or therapeutic. Rather, psychological assistance and support, coupled with gradual return to functional activities can provide relief and return of functioning for many individuals. Unfortunately, the differential diagnosis relies on the difficult and imprecise task of measuring consciousness. Researchers have suggested that patients with conversion disorders are likely to be cooperative, appealing, clinging, and somewhat dependent, while malingerers are more likely to present as sullen, ill-at-ease, suspicious, uncooperative, blaming, and resentful (Engel, 1970; Travin and Potter, 1984; Trimble, 1981). Tests for malingering that are valid with reference to organic diseases may not be valid with conversion disorders.

It is clearly important to assess for cooperation, effort, and motivation for success when evaluating persons who are being, or potentially could be, compensated for their injuries. This can be done in a variety of ways, including an examination of the history of injury and symptom evolution; an evaluation of the pattern and constellation of scores on the neuropsychological examination; and through the use of specialized symptom validity measures. Certain patterns of responses that occur very rarely or that don't make neuropsychological "sense" should be suspect. This might include unusual findings such as much better spontaneous recall than recognition, bizarre intrusions on verbal recall tasks or on reproductions of visual designs, inability to read, count, or recognize simple figures, erratic learning curves, failures on easy items as opposed to more difficult items, and changing a correct response to an incorrect one. Some of these have been specifically codified in the Symptom Index - Revised (Rawling, 1992, 1993; Rawling and Brooks, 1990). One must exert caution, however, as some of the items coded as possible indicators of malingering on this index can represent actual impairments in a variety of clinical neurologic populations (Milanovich and Axelrod, 1996). The examiner should also determine whether the nature and degree of difficulty demonstrated on formal tests is consistent with the client's daily activities and presentation, and with observations made in and out of the test environment.

There have been several recent reviews of existing methods for assessing cooperation with neuropsychological testing (Binder and Willis, 1991; Rogers et al., 1993). One of the better validated instruments is the Portland Digit Recognition Test (PDRT) (Binder, 1990, 1992, 1993a,b). It is based on a forced choice symptom validity methodology, whereby patients who choose significantly fewer correct answers than would be expected if they were responding randomly (i.e., by chance), are statistically demonstrated to be either consciously or unconsciously motivated to do poorly. It has the advantage of extensive validation data of groups of normals, patients with documented brain damage but no financial disincentives for doing well, uncompensated patients with emotional disturbances, and simulated malingerers.

Youngjohn et al. (1995) reported on a study of 55 patients with MTBI (less than 30 minutes loss of consciousness, less than 24 hours posttraumatic amnesia, and PCS persisting for at least 6 months), all of whom were involved in some form of litigation or compensation. Fifteen percent of the sample performed below chance on one or more of the PDRT trials or on the whole test, suggesting that they were consciously or unconsciously motivated to do poorly on at least part of the exam. These results are similar to those of compensated minor head trauma patients reported by Binder (1993a). In addition, approximately 30% of the patients performed more poorly than any of a group of 120 uncompensated patients with documented brain injury reported in the Binder study. When results from another symptom validity test were added (i.e., the Dot Counting Test), 26 patients out of the sample of 54 (48%) demonstrated poor performance on one or both measures of cooperation/motivation. These results suggested that motivational factors may have adversely affected the neuropsychological test performance in almost half of the cases.

The validity scales of the MMPI are often used clinically to determine the truthfulness or general attitude in responding displayed by the patient. Studies have generally failed to document an association between the MMPI-2 validity scales and measures of motivation during neuropsychological testing (Greiffenstein et al., 1994; Youngjohn et al., 1995). This would suggest that MMPI-2 validity scales sensitive to exaggeration of psychopathology are not necessarily sensitive to exaggeration of neuropsychological impairment. A comprehensive review of issues related to the assessment of malingering is beyond the scope of this chapter but several recent reviews of this issue are available (Miller, 1996).

SUMMARY

Guiding Principles in the Assessment of Individuals with Mild Traumatic Brain Injury

As can be seen from the previous discussion, many different factors need to be considered in the evaluation of individuals with MTBI. The examiner must be knowledgeable about the literature and controversies in this field, must be aware of instruments that will maximize sensitivity while maintaining specificity, must be well trained in the assessment of emotional function and personality, and must be mindful of the adaptive functioning of the client in the settings in which they must live and work (Stuss, 1995). A number of guiding principles should be kept in mind during this process.

Principle 1.
The effects of MTBI are multiply determined. Therefore, the assessment must be comprehensive, and include evaluation of both preinjury and postinjury health, cognitive, emotional, and personality status.

Principle 2.
The effects of MTBI should make sense from a pathophysiological, neurological, and neurophysiological perspective, and should be consistent with major findings in the literature. Performance far below the expected level for MTBI should suggest that nonneurologic issues are contributing and must be explored.

Principle 3.
The severity of TBI must be defined by the acute injury characteristics and not by the severity of symptoms at random points after trauma. When postacute symptoms far exceed the apparent severity of injury, the role of psychological factors in the genesis and maintenance of symptoms must be considered. An accepted reference point for severity provides a framework for both clinical practice and research. This does not mean that the long-term impact of a mild injury cannot be significant or that interventions should not be considered or withheld.

Principle 4.
The most common natural history is for symptoms of mild TBI to gradually improve. Although the course of recovery may be much longer in some patients, improvement over time should be anticipated. Significant

worsening of symptoms should suggest psychogenic or environmental factors that need to be considered in any treatment plan.

Principle 5.
Professionals involved in rehabilitation have a clinical responsibility to patients with MTBI. To the extent that symptoms are ever iatrogenic, we provide a disservice to patients. To the extent that symptoms are neurologically, emotionally, environmentally, or motivationally based, we have a responsibility to understand and address these issues clinically to the best of our ability.

With these guiding principles in mind, and with a solid knowledge of both neuropsychology and clinical psychology, the clinician should be prepared to undertake the assessment of individuals with MTBI. It is critical to remember that formal or psychometric assessments are only indications of what an individual can do at a particular time and in a particular context; these can serve as approximations to what is possible or likely in other settings or contexts. While useful and potentially revealing, they never tell the full story. It is critical not to reify any procedure or test, but rather to gather information from many sources in a truly investigative and diagnostic endeavour. The field needs competent, multidisciplinary, longitudinal research, and the benefit of clinical experience to understand how best to evaluate individuals with prolonged symptomatology after MTBI.

References

Alexander, M.P. (1995). Mild traumatic brain injury: Pathophysiology, natural history, and clinical management. *Neurology, 45*, 1253–1260.

Alves, W.M., Colohan, A.R., O'Leary, T.J., Rimel, R.W., and Jane, J.A. (1986). Understanding post-traumatic symptoms after minor head injury. *Journal of Head Trauma Rehabilitation, 1*, 1–12.

Anderson, S.D., (1996). Postconcussional disorder and loss of consciousness. *Bulletin of the American Academy of Psychiatry and the Law, 24*, 493–504.

Barbarotto, R., Laiacona, M., and Cocchini, G. (1996). A case of simulated, psychogenic or focal pure retrograde amnesia: Did an entire life become unconscious? *Neuropsychologia, 34*, 575–585.

Barth, J.T., Alves, W.M., Ryan, T.V., Macciocchi, S.N., Rimel, R.W., Jane, J.A., and Nelson, W.E. (1989). Mild head injury in sports: Neuropsychological sequelae and recovery of function. In H.S. Levin, H.M. Eisenberg, and A.L. Benton (Eds.), *Mild Head Injury*. New York, NY: Oxford, pp. 257–275.

Binder, L.M. (1990). Malingering following minor head trauma. *The Clinical Neuropsychologist, 4*, 25–36.

Binder, L.M. (1992). Malingering detected by forced choice testing of memory and tactile sensation: A case report. *Archives of Clinical Neuropsychology, 7*, 155–163.

Binder, L.M. (1993a). Assessment of malingering after mild head trauma with the Portland Digit Recognition Test. *The Clinical Neuropsychologist, 7,* 170–182.

Binder, L.M. (1993b). An abbreviated form of the Portland Digit Recognition Test. *The Clinical Neuropsychologist, 7,* 104–107.

Binder, L.M., and Willis, S.C. (1991). Assessment of motivation after financially compensable minor head trauma. *Psychological Assessment: A Journal of Consulting and Clinical Psychology, 3,* 175–181.

Bohnen, N.J., Jolles, J., and Twijnstra, A. (1992a). Modification of the Stroop Colour Word Test improves differentiation between patients with mild head injury and matched controls. *The Clinical Neuropsychologist, 6,* 178–188.

Bohnen, N.J., Twijnstra, A., and Jolles, J. (1992b). Post traumatic and emotional symptoms in different subgroups of patients with mild head injury. *Brain Injury, 6*(6), 481–487.

Bohnen, N.J., van-Zutphen, W., Twijnstra, A. and Wijnen, G., et al. (1994). Late outcome of mild head injury: Results from a controlled postal survey. *Brain Injury, 8,* 701–708.

Bohnen, N.J., Wijnen, G., Twijnstra, A., van-Zutphen, W., et al. (1995). The constellation of late post-traumatic symptoms of mild head injury patients. *Journal of Neurologic Rehabilitation, 9,* 33–39.

Burke, J.M., Imhoff, C.L., and Kerrigan, J.M. (1990). MMPI correlates among post-acute TBI patients. *Brain Injury, 4,* 223–231.

Cicerone, K.D., and Kalmar, K. (1995). Persistent postconcussion syndrome: The structure of subjective complaints after mild traumatic brain injury. *Journal of Head Trauma Rehabilitation, 10,* 1–17.

Conboy, T.J., Barth, J., and Boll, T. (1986). Treatment and rehabilitation of mild and moderate head trauma. *Rehabilitation Psychology, 31,* 203–215.

Coonley-Hoganson, R., Sachs, N., Desai, B.T., and Whitman, S. (1984). Sequelae associated with head injuries in patients who were not hospitalized: A follow-up survey. *Neurosurgery, 14,* 315–317.

Cripe, L.I. (1989). Neuropsychological and psychosocial assessment of the brain-injured person: Clinical concepts and guidelines. *Rehabilitation Psychology, 34,* 93–100.

Dikmen, S., and Levin, H. (1993). Methodological issues in the study of mild head injury. *Journal of Head Trauma Rehabilitation, 8*(3), 30–37.

Dikmen, S., McLean, A., and Temkin, N. (1986). Neuropsychological and psychosocial consequences of minor head injury. *Journal of Neurology, Neurosurgery and Psychiatry, 49,* 1227–1232.

Dinan, T.G., and Mobayed, M. (1992). Treatment resistance of depression after head injury: A preliminary study of amitryptyline response. *Acta Psychiatrica Scandinavica, 85,* 292–294.

Dodrill, C.B. (1987). What's Normal? Paper presented at the Pacific Northwest Neuropsychological Association, Seattle, WA.

Dywan, J., and Segalowitz, J. (1996). Self- and family ratings of adaptive behavior after traumatic brain injury: Psychometric scores, and frontally generated ERPs. *Journal of Head Trauma Rehabilitation, 11*(2), 79–95.

Engel, G.L. (1970). Conversion symptoms. In C.M. MacBryde and R.S. Blacklow (Eds.), *Sings and Symptoms.* Philadephia, PA: R.S. Lippencott.

Fenton, G., McClelland, R., Montgomery, A., and MacFlynn, G. (1993). The postconcussional syndrome: Social antecendents and psychological sequelae. *British Journal of Psychiatry, 162*, 493–497.

Gass, C.S., and Russell, E.W. (1991). MMPI profiles of closed head trauma patients: Impact of neurologic complaints. *Journal of Clinical Psychology, 47*, 253–260.

Gouvier, W., Cubic, B., Jones, G., Brantley, P., and Cutlip, Q. (1992). Postconcussion symptoms and daily stress in normal and head-injured college populations. *Archives of Clinical Neuropsychology, 7*, 193–211.

Gouvier, W.D., Uddo-Crane, M., and Brown, L.M. (1988). Base rates of postconcussional symptoms. *Archives of Clinical Neuropsychology, 3*, 273–278.

Greiffenstein, M.F., Baker, J., and Gola, T. (1994). *MMPI-2 vs. domain specific measures in detecting neuropsychological dissimulation.* Paper presented at the International Neuropsychological Society Annual Meeting, Cincinnati, OH.

Gronwall, D. (1977). Paced Auditory Serical Addition Task: A measure of recovery from concussion. *Perceptual and Motor Skills, 44*, 367–373.

Gronwall, D. (1987). Advances in assessment of attention and information processing after head injury. In H.S. Levin, J. Grafman, and H.M. Eisenberg (Eds.), *Neurobehavioral Recovery From Head Injury.* New York, NY: Oxford University Press, pp. 355–371.

Gronwall, D. (1989). Cumulative and persisting effects of concussion on attention and cognition. In H.S. Levin, H.M. Eisenberg, and A.L. Benton (Eds.), *Mild Head Injury.* New York, NY: Oxford University Press, pp. 153–162.

Gronwall, D., and Wrightson, P. (1974). Delayed recovery of intellectual function after mild head injury. *Lancet, ii*(7894), 1452.

Hugenholtz, H., Stuss, D.T., Stethem, L.L., and Richard, M.T. (1988). How long does it take to recover from a mild concussion? *Neurosurgery, 22*, 853–858.

Iverson, G.L., and McCraken, L.M. (1997). "Postconcussive" symptoms in persons with chronic pain. *Brain Injury, 11*, 783–790.

Jacobs, A., Put, E., Ingels, M., and Bossuy, A. (1994). Prospective evaluation of technetium-99m-HMPAO SPECT in mild to moderate traumatic brain injury. *Journal of Nuclear Medicine, 35*(6), 942–947.

Jennett, B. (1976). Assessment of the severity of head injury. *Journal of Neurology, Neurosurgery and Psychiatry, 39*, 647–655.

Karzmark, P., Hall, K., and Englander, J. (1995). Late-onset post-concussion symptoms after mild brain injury: the role of premorbid, injury related, environmental, and personality factors. *Brain Injury, 9*(1), 21–26.

Kay, T. (1992). Neuropsychological diagnosis: disentangling the multiple determinants of functional disability after mild traumatic brain injury. In L. Horn and N. Zasler (Eds.), *Rehabilitation of Post-Concussive Disorders.* Philadelphia, PA: Henley and Belfus, pp. 109–127.

Kay, T., Harrington, D., Adams, R., and Anderson, T., et al. (1993). Definition of mild traumatic brain injury. *Journal of Head Trauma Rehabilitation, 8*, 86–87.

King, N. (1996). Emotional, neuropsychological, and organic factors: Their use in the prediction of persisting postconcussion symptoms after mild head injuries. *Journal of Neurology, Neurosurgery, and Psychiatry, 61*, 75–81.

Kraus, J., and Nourjah, P. (1988). The epidemiology of mild traumatic brain injury. *Brain Injury, 3*, 177–186.

Lawler, K.A. and Terregino, C.A. (1996). Guidelines for evaluation and education of adult patients with mild traumatic brain injuries in an acute care hospital setting. *Journal of Head Trauma Rehabilitation, 11*, 18–28.

Leininger, B., Gramling, S., Farrell, A., Kreutzer, J., and Peck, E. (1990). Neuropsychological deficits in symptomatic minor head injury patients after concussion and mild concussion. *Journal of Neurology, Neurosurgery and Psychiatry, 53*, 293–296.

Leininger, B.E., Kreutzer, J.S., and Hill, M.R. (1991). Comparison of mild and severe head injury emotional sequelae using the MMPI. *Brain Injury, 5*, 199–205.

Levin, H., Amparo, E., and Eisenberg, H.M. (1987). Magnetic resonance imaging and computerized tomography in relation to the neurobehavioral sequelae of mild and moderate head injuries. *Journal of Neurosurgery, 66*, 706–713.

Levin, H.S., Mattis, S., and Ruff, R.M. (1987). Neurobehavioral outcome following mild head injury. *Journal of Neurosurgery, 66*, 234–243.

Lezak, M. (1987). Relationships between personality disorders, social disturbances, and physical disability following traumatic brain injury. *Journal of Head Trauma Rehabilitation, 2*, 57–69.

Lezak, M.D. (1994). *Neuropsychological Assessment* (3rd ed.). New York, NY: Oxford.

Mateer, C.A. (1992). Systems of care for post-concussive sundrome. In L.J. Horn and N.D. Zasler (Eds.), *Rehabilitation of Post-Concussive Disorders*. Philadelphia, PA: Henley and Belfus, pp. 145–160.

Mateer, C.A., Sohlberg, M.M., and Crinean, F. (1987). Perception of memory impairment in closed head injury. *Journal of Head Trauma Rehabilitation, 2*, 74–84.

McLean, A.J., Dikmen, S., and Temkin, N. (1984). Psychosocial functioning at one month after head injury. *Neurosurgery, 14*, 393–399.

Milanovich, J.R., and Axelrod, B.N. (1996). Validation of the simulation index-revised with a mixed clinical population. *Archives of Clinical Neuropsychology, 11*(1), 53–59.

Miller, L. (1996). Malingering in mild head injury and the postconcussion syndrome: Clinical, neuropsychological, and forensic considerations. *Journal of Cognitive Rehabilitation, 14*(4), 6–17.

Moran, S.G., McCarthy, M.C., Uddin, D.E., and Poelstra, R.J. (1994). *Predictors of positive CT scans in the trauma patient with minor head injury.* Paper presented at the Annual Meeting of the Midwest Surgical Association, Lincolnshire, IL.

Nedd, K., Sfakianakis, G., Ganz, W., Uricchio, B., Vernberg, D., Villanueva, P., Jabir, A.M., Bartlett, J., and Keena, J. (1993). TcHMPAO SPECT of the brain in mild to moderate traumatic brain injury patients: compared with CT—a prospective study. *Brain Injury, 7*(6), 469–479.

Novack, T.A., Daniel, M.S., and Long, C.J. (1984). Factors relating to emotional adjustment following head injury. *International Journal of Clinical Neuropsychology, 6*, 139–142.

Penkman, L. (1994). The role of depression in mild head injury: Attentional correlates and quantitative EEG. Unpublished manuscript. University of Ottawa.

Prigatano, G.P. (1986). *Neuropsychological Rehabilitation after Brain Injury*. Baltimore, MD: Johns Hopkins University Press.

Raskin, S., Mateer, C., and Tweeten, R. (1998). Neuropsychological evaluation of mild traumatic brain injury. *The Clinical Neuropsychologist, 12*, 21–30.

Rawling, P.J. (1992). The simulation index: A reliability study. *Brain Injury, 6*, 381–383.

Rawling, P.J. (1993). *Simulation Index—Revised Manual*. Balgowlah, Australia: Rawling and Associates.

Rawling, P.J., and Brooks, D.N. (1990). Simulation Index: A method for detecting factitious errors on the WAIS-R and WMS. *Neuropsychology, 4*, 223–238.

Resnick, P.J. (1988). Malingering of posttraumatic disorders. In R. Rogers (Ed.), *Clinical Assessment of Malingering and Deception*. New York, NY: Guilford Press, pp. 34–53.

Rogers, R., Harrell, E.H., and Liff, C.D. (1993). Feigning neuropsychological impairment: A critical review of methodological and clinical considerations. *Clinical Psychology Review, 13*, 255–274.

Ruff, R.M., Camenzuli, L., and Mueller, J. (1996) The miserable minority: Emotional risk factors that influence the outcome of a mild traumatic brain injury. *Brain Injury, 10*, 551–565.

Ruff, R.M., Crouch, J.A., and Troster, A.I., et al. (1994). Selected cases of poor outcome following a minor brain trauma: comparing neuropsychological and positron emission tomography assessment. *Brain Injury, 8*(4), 297–308.

Ruff, R.M., Levin, H.S., and Marshall, L.F. (1986). Neurobehavioral methods of assessment and the study of outcome in minor head injury. *Journal of Head Trauma Rehabilitation, 1*, 43–52.

Rutherford, W.H. (1989). Post-concussion symptoms: Relationship to acute neurological indices, individual differences, and circumstances of injury. In H.S. Levin, M. Eisenberg, and A.L. Benton (Eds.), *Mild Head Injury*. New York, NY: Oxford University Press, pp. 217–228.

Shallice, T., and Burgess, P.W. (1991a). Deficits in strategy application following frontal lobe damage in man. *Brain, 114*, 727–741.

Shallice, T., and Burgess, P.W. (1991b). Higher-order cognitive impairments and frontal-lobe lesions in man. In H. Levin, H.M. Eisenberg, and A.L. Benton (Eds.), *Frontal Lobe Function and Injury* . Oxford, England: Oxford University Press.

Shores, E.A., Marossezeky, J.E., Sandanam, J., and Batchelor, J. (1985). Preliminary validation of a clinical scale for measuring the duration of post-traumatic amnesia. *The Medical Journal of Australia, 144*, 569–572.

Snow, W.G. (1992). *Implications of base rates for the diagnosis of malingering*. Paper presented at the International Neuropsychological Society Annual Meeting, San Diego, CA.

Stuss, D.T. (1995). A sensible approach to mild traumatic brain injury. *Neurology, 45,* 1251–1252.

Stuss, D.T., Stethem, L.L., Hugenholtz, H., and Richard, M.T. (1989). Traumatic brain injury: A comparison of three clinical tests, and analysis of recovery. *Clinical Neuropsychologist, 3,* 145–156.

Tebano, M.T., Cameroni, M., Gallozzi, G., Loizzo, A., Palazzino, G., Pezzini, G., and Ricci, G.F. (1988). EEG spectral analysis after minor head injury in man. *Electroencephalography and Clinical Neurophysiology, 70,* 185–189.

Townsend, L., and Mateer, C.A. (1997). The effects of pain intensity on tasks of attention and memory. *Canadian Psychology, 28*(2a), 127.

Travin, S., and Potter, B. (1984). Malingering and malingering-like behavior: Some clinical and conceptual issues. *Psychiatric Quarterly, 56*(3), 189–197.

Trimble, M.R. (1981). *Post-Traumatic Neurosis from Railway Spine to the Whiplash.* New York, NY: John Wiley and Sons.

Tsushima, W.T., and Newbill, W. (1996). Effects of headaches during neuropsychological testing of mild head injury patients. *Headache, 36,* 613–615.

Uomoto, J.M., and Esselman, P.C. (1993). Traumatic brain injury and chronic pain: Differential types and rates by head injury severity. *Archives of Physical Medicine and Rehabilitation, 74,* 61–64.

Varney, N., Bushnell, D.L., Nathan, M., Kahn, D., Roberts, R., Rezani, K., Walker, W., and Kirchner, P. (1995). NeuroSPECT correlates of disabling mild head injury: Preliminary findings. *Journal of Head Trauma Rehabilitation, 10*(3), 18–28.

Youngjohn, J.R., Burrows, L., and Erdal, K. (1995). Brain damage or compensation neurosis? The controversial post-concussive syndrome. *The Clinical Neuropsychologist, 9*(2), 112–123.

Youngjohn, J.R., Davis, D., and Wolf, I. (1997). Head injury and the MMPI-2: Paradoxical severity effects and the influence of litigation. *Psychological Assessment, 9*(3), 177–184.

APPENDIX A

The Postconcussion Syndrome Checklist and the Rivermead Post Concussion Symptom Questionnaire are provided as examples of questionnaires used to gather information on subjective complaints.

<u>The Postconcussion Syndrome Checklist (PCSC)</u>

(Gouvier *et al*., 1992)

NAME_____   DATE_____

FREQUENCY	INTENSITY	DURATION
1 = Not at all	1 = Not at all	1 = Not at all
2 = Seldom	2 = Vaguely present	2 = A few seconds
3 = Often	3 = Clearly present	3 = A few minutes
4 = Very Often	4 = Interfering	4 = A few hours
5 = All the time	5 = Crippling	5 = Constant

POSTCONCUSSIVE SYMPTOM	FREQUENCY	INTENSITY	DURATION
Headache			
Dizziness			
Irritability			
Memory Problems			
Difficulty Concentrating			
Fatigue			
Visual Disturbances			
Aggravated by Noise			
Judgement Problems			
Anxiety			

The Rivermead Post Concussion Symptoms Questionnaire

After a head injury or accident some people experience symptoms which can cause worry or nuisance. We would like to know if you now suffer any of the symptoms given below. As many of these symptoms occur normally, we would like you to compare yourself now with before the accident. For each one please circle the number closest to your answer.

0 = Not experienced at all
1 = no more of a problem
2 = a mild problem
3 = a moderate problem
4 = a severe problem

Compared with before the accident, do you now (I.e. over the last 24 hours) suffer from:

Headaches	0	1	2	3	4
Feelings of dizziness	0	1	2	3	4
Nausea and/or vomiting	0	1	2	3	4
Noise sensitivity, easily upset by loud noise	0	1	2	3	4
Sleep disturbance	0	1	2	3	4
Fatigue, tiring more easily	0	1	2	3	4
Being irritable, easily angered	0	1	2	3	4
Feeling depressed or tearful	0	1	2	3	4
Feeling frustrated or impatient	0	1	2	3	4
Forgetfulness, poor memory	0	1	2	3	4
Poor concentration	0	1	2	3	4
Taking longer to think	0	1	2	3	4
Blurred vision	0	1	2	3	4
Light sensitivity easily upset by bright light	0	1	2	3	4
Double vision	0	1	2	3	4
Restlessness	0	1	2	3	4

Are you experiencing any other difficulties?
Please specify, and rate as above:

1. _____	0	1	2	3	4
2. _____	0	1	2	3	4

APPENDIX B

This flyer was prepared at the Good Samaritan Center for Continuing Rehabilitation in Puyallup, Washington, as an educational tool for persons with mild traumatic brain injury.

Mild Traumatic Brain Injury — What To Expect

Greater than 6.5 million people per year in the United States sustain "mild" head injuries.

Although neither loss of consciousness nor a direct blow to the head may have occurred, these individuals may still suffer subtle cognitive and behavioral deficits that seriously impair their ability to work and interact normally with family and friends. Such persons are truly the victims of what professionals are now calling the "Silent Epidemic."

What is Mild Traumatic Brain Injury?

An injury to the head resulting in brief loss of consciousness or a period of being dazed with no loss of consciousness, posttraumatic amnesia of less than 1 hour, a Glasgow Coma Scale score of greater than 13 (normal being 15), and a negative neuroimaging scan. An example might be the high school football player who is knocked unconscious for only a few seconds. He may be led off the field looking a little dazed and confused, but after a brief rest is back in the game.

What Causes MTBI?

Automobile accidents, sports-related injuries (particularly in activities such as football, cycling, boxing, hockey, and diving), and falls are common causes of MTBI. Brain injury, however, can occur even if there is no direct blow to the head. Examples include the child who is violently shaken by an angry parent, or a person thrust forward and backward in an automobile accident without striking the

How is MTBI Diagnosed?

Diagnosing a mild traumatic brain injury with standard neurological testing is difficult, if not impossible. Tests such as EEG (electroencephalography) and CAT (computerized axial tomography) scans are generally normal. Neuropsychological testing, however, can be a very effective method of diagnosing the subtle cognitive deficits of MTBI. A comprehensive neuropsychological battery generally takes from 4-6 hours and involves administration of a broad range of intellectual, cognitive, motor, sensory, and perceptual tests.

COMMON SYMPTOMS OF MILD TRAUMATIC BRAIN INJURY		
PHYSICAL	*COGNITIVE*	*PSYCHOSOCIAL*
Dizziness	Inability to concentrate	Depression
Fatigue	Memory problems	Anger outbursts
Headaches	Impulsivity, poor judgment	Irritability
Visual complaints	Slowed task performance	Personality changes
Sleep disturbances	Difficulty putting thoughts into words	Suspiciousness

What are the effects of MTBI?

The common symptoms of MTBI are shown above. When unrecognized and untreated, these symptoms often lead to disruption in the individual's work setting and family relationships. People frequently report feeling that they are "going crazy." Health care providers may further diagnose them as neurotic or overanxious, when what they are really experiencing are the intellectual and physical symptoms resulting from the head injury.

What are expectations for recovery from MTBI?

1. **Fatigue:** Most people with a concussion experience some degree of fatigue during their recovery. The need to sleep may be more than usual, and it may be harder to do things at the end of the day. It's a good idea to get extra sleep. An afternoon nap may be helpful if functioning later in the day is difficult.

2. **Return to Work**: It is a good idea to return to usual activities as soon as one feels able, but bit by bit rather than all at once. Returning to work on a part-time basis is optimal, then gradually increasing to full-time. The same is true for other activities. Return to household chores, bill-paying, exercise programs, hobbies, social activities, etc. soon, but at a lower level of involvement. Gradually increase involvement as tolerated. Fatigue, inefficiency, headaches, irritability, or increased stress and emotionality are signs that you are pushing too hard or too soon.

3. **Irritability and Emotions**: Some people are irritable and emotional for awhile after a concussion. They may yell or say things they wouldn't normally say. Some may even get violent. Getting emotional, frustrated, or tearful when you normally wouldn't are also common. If any of these episodes happen, it is usually a sign that it is time to take a rest from what you are doing and get away from it. Going some place quiet to calm down may be helpful. Definitely seek professional help if you find you become violent or others fear you may become violent.

4. **Uncertainty**: Many people feel uncertain, perplexed, or confused after a concussion. Their minds and feelings don't react in the ways they used to. They may fear they are going crazy. These feelings are normal reactions to head injury, and it is helpful to talk about them with someone you trust. Because your mind is not as reliable for a period of time, it is a good idea to check with someone you trust about important decisions to be made.

5. **Concentration and Memory**: You may experience a period of time when it is hard to concentrate or to remember recent events. Dealing with noisy or busy surroundings, keeping track of several things at once, switching from one thing to another, or doing complicated activities may be problematic. At first, avoiding noisy settings may be helpful, then return to them gradually. Write down important things you have to remember, or ask for reminders.

6. **Alcohol:** It is best not to drink alcohol or use any recreational drugs during the period of recovery post-MTBI.

Is there any treatment for MTBI?

Most people recover fully from a mild brain injury. Usually, they get better rapidly in the first few days, and problems that linger may clear up in a few weeks. Some problems may become more apparent as you return to your usual activities. For example, you may not realize you get tired easily until you try to work for 8 hours. Even so, people usually get better after a head injury, not worse. If problems like headaches, dizziness, double vision, ringing in your ears, or fatigue continue, you should see your doctor again.

Until recently, little more than acute medical treatment was provided for survivors of MTBI. People were often discharged from hospital emergency rooms without adequate follow-up. Today, however, rehabilitation programs are available that may address cognitive retraining, psychosocial adjustment, communication and leisure skills, and vocational issues. With appropriate support and therapy, individuals with difficulties related to MTBI can learn to overcome and compensate for their deficits, resulting in successful reintegration into their home and work environments

APPENDIX C

This brochure was developed by the Connecticut Neuropsychological Society to inform patients about the process of neuropsychological evaluations.

Answers to Questions About Neuropsychological Evaluation

WHAT IS NEUROPSYCHOLOGICAL EVALUATION ?

Neuropsychological evaluation is a comprehensive assessment of cognitive and behavioral functions using a set of standardized tests and clinical procedures. Various mental functions are systematically tested, including:

- Intelligence
- Problem solving and conceptualization
- Planning and organization
- Attention, memory, and learning
- Language
- Academic Skills
- Perceptual and motor abilities
- Emotions, behavior and personality

WHO IS QUALIFIED TO CONDUCT NEUROPSYCHOLOGICAL EVALUATIONS ?

A neuropsychological evaluation can only be done by a psychologist who has had specialized training and experience which includes:

- Predoctoral training in psychology and neuropsychology
- Formal postdoctoral training focusing on brain-behavior relationships and neuropsychological assessment
- Expertise in specialized techniques of assessment and clinical interpretation

WHEN IS A NEUROPSYCHOLOGICAL EVALUATION NEEDED ?

Neuropsychological evaluation is indicated for any case in which brain-based impairment in cognitive function or behavior is suspected. Typical referrals are made to diagnose or rule out the following conditions and/or to describe their impact on a person's cognitive functioning:

- Traumatic Brain Injury
- Strokes
- Developmental Learning Disabilities
- Attention Deficit Disorders
- Psychiatric or Neuropsychiatric Disorders
- Seizure Disorders
- Medical Illnesses or Treatments
- Effects of Toxic Chemicals or Chronic Substance Abuse
- Dementing Conditions (e.g. Alzheimer's)

Neuropsychological evaluation is particularly useful for systematically tracking progress in rehabilitation after brain injury or other neurological disease. Neuropsychological assessment can assist greatly in planning educational and vocational programs. It can also be invaluable for disability determination or for forensic (legal) purposes.

ARE ALL NEUROPSYCHOLOGICAL EVALUATIONS THE SAME ?

No. A neuropsychological evaluation should not be thought of as a fixed series of tests which anyone can give. Specialized training allows the neuropsychologist to select, administer, and interpret the particular tests and procedures which will yield the most comprehensive understanding of an individual's strengths and weaknesses. Further, all clients will not necessarily be given the same tests.

WHAT IS THE EXAM LIKE ?

- Involves a wide variety of tasks most of which are done sitting at a table. There are no invasive procedures, no pain, no needles or electrodes.
- Often takes 6 to 8 hours face to face contact; can vary widely, dependent on referral question.
- Can be scheduled in shorter segments depending on client's tolerance.

WHAT KINDS OF HELP OR OUTCOMES CAN RESULT FROM BEING EVALUATED ?

That depends on the reason for the evaluation. Neuropsychological evaluations may:

- Confirm or clarify diagnosis.
- Provide a profile of strengths and weaknesses to guide rehabilitation, educational, and vocational interventions or other treatment.
- Document changes in functioning since prior examinations, including effects of treatment.
- Result in a referral to other specialists, such as educational therapists, cognitive rehabilitation professionals, neurologists, psychiatrists, psychologists, special education teachers, or vocational counselors.
- Clarify what treatment options and compensatory strategies would help to maximize functioning.
- Assist both patient and family in understanding and dealing with the problems which led to the referral, and in accessing relevant services.

II

TREATMENT OF
COGNITIVE SEQUELAE

4

Attention

CATHERINE A. MATEER

Impairments in attention and concentration are among the most common neuropsychological problems following traumatic brain injury (Lezak, 1994). Although patients with moderate to severe injury have deficits in attention at the most basic levels, such as arousal and focusing of attention, those who sustain MTBI often complain of difficulties with higher or more complex aspects of attention. This chapter reviews some of the relevant literature on the attention-processing capacities of individuals with MTBI, suggests techniques for the evaluation of attention, and discusses a variety of rehabilitation strategies for alleviating or compensating for deficits in attention.

Disorders of Attention Following Mild Traumatic Brain Injury

Individuals with MTBI frequently report concentration problems, distractibility, forgetfulness, and difficulty doing more than one thing at a time (Ettlin et al., 1992; Hinkeldey and Corrigan, 1990). Common concerns voiced to clinicians include taking more time to complete tasks than in the past, having difficulty concentrating on tasks in noisy environments, and forgetting what one was about to say or do.

Mateer et al. (1987) used a self-report questionnaire to study the frequency of different kinds of forgetting failures. In all three groups sampled (a control group, an MTBI group, and a group with moderate to severe TBI) the most common forgetting experiences were those related to attention, mental control, and prospective memory. Items related to attention included such statements as, "I have difficulty remembering what I went into a room for," and, "It's hard to keep numbers in my head." The group with milder injuries reported more difficulty than both the control group and the group with more severe injuries, which may have reflected both actual difficulties and greater awareness and concern about the problems by the MTBI group.

Research focusing on the psychometric assessment of attentional capacities in individuals with MTBI has generally supported the presence of impaired attention and slower mental processing in the early stages following injury. However, the literature is mixed with regard to the nature of these attentional problems and particularly their persistence or permanence (Dikmen et al., 1986, 1995). In addition, the term "attention" has been used to refer to a very broad and varied set of states, processes, and abilities. This has made it difficult to develop a clear concept of attention that can serve to elucidate the nature of attentional impairments following MTBI and to inform both assessment and rehabilitation. The following sections review some of the literature on the attentional capacities of individuals who have suffered cerebral concussion or MTBI.

Problems Related to Speed of Information Processing

One of the most consistent findings in individuals with MTBI has been slowed reaction time and speed of information processing (Arcia and Gualtieri, 1994; Gronwall and Sampson, 1974; Gronwall and Wrightson, 1974; Hinton-Bayre et al., 1997; MacFlynn et al., 1984; Ponsford and Kinsella, 1992; Stuss et al., 1989a,b; Van Zomeren & Brouwer, 1994).

Gronwall and her colleagues conducted a pioneering series of studies of information processing capacity in patients with MTBI (Gronwall, 1976, 1987, 1991; Gronwall and Sampson, 1974) using the Paced Auditory Serial Addition Test (PASAT) (Gronwall, 1977). Patients who had sustained MTBI were asked to rate the severity of 10 common symptoms of postconcussional syndrome (PCS) on a 5–point scale. This rating and the PASAT were repeated at weekly intervals. Symptom ratings correlated significantly with PASAT scores, such that as the PASAT improved, the number of PCS symptoms decreased. Mildly concussed patients (posttraumatic amnesia under 24 hours) showed significantly depressed performance on the PASAT 1 week following concussion; most, though not all patients, attained a normal performance on the PASAT by 1 month after injury. However, in follow-up assessment (1–3 years postinjury), in an air pressure chamber simulating a high altitude condition, patients who had sustained MTBI demonstrated a "latent" deficit on the PASAT that became apparent when the individual was faced with an environmental stressor (Ewing et al., 1980). Finally, Gronwall found that recovery on the PASAT was correlated with fitness for work and suggested that a "cognitive stress test" such as the PASAT be included in neuropsychological assessments of this population.

Many other studies of patients with MTBI have corroborated these findings. In most studies in which there are multiple assessments, improvements in speed of information processing are seen in the weeks and months following injury (Gentilini et al., 1985, 1989), with recovery to normal or near normal levels of performance by 6 months post injury (e.g., MacFlynn, et al., 1984). Jakobsen et al. (1987) also found that those MTBI patients who demonstrated slowing of RT shortly after injury were more likely to report postconcussional sequelae after 1 month, than those who did not. The reasons for this generalized reduction in processing speed early in recovery from MTBI are unclear. Although depression is often cited as a possible contributor to slowed processing in MTBI, the very early demonstration of these problems after injury argues for a biological rather than a functional etiology. Hypotheses about cognitive slowing in the early stages following MTBI invoke mechanisms such as slowing of synaptic transmission, information loss at each transmission, or disturbance of the norepinephrine (NE) system (Birren, 1974). This system arises in the locus coeruleus and projects widely through the brain, but in particular to the prefrontal cortex. It appears to be a critical component of cortically mediated attentional processes.

Distractibility
Despite frequent reports of poor concentration and over-sensitivity to noise or distraction in MTBI patients (Gronwall and Sampson, 1974), research regarding this aspect of attention has also been mixed. Stuss and his colleagues (1989a, 1989b) reported that MTBI subjects appeared to engage in unnecessary processing of redundant information, which might be interpreted as a kind of distractibility. Other investigators have reported a generalized slowing of performance as a function of increasing information load, but no direct impact of distraction per se (Miller and Cruzat, 1980; Ponsford and Kinsella, 1992).

Cicerone (1996) compared the performances of 15 MTBI subjects and 9 controls on a dual task paradigm in the presence of noise. The dual task demands produced a significant slowing in processing speed as compared with a single task for both groups, but the relative decline in processing speed was much greater for the MTBI Subjects, and they differed from controls only in the noise condition.

Overall, results are mixed with regard to the impact of distracting stimuli during task performance in individuals with MTBI. Clinically, however, many report difficulty working in noisy conditions or when there are distractions.

Focused attention
In addition to sustaining attention (vigilance) and dealing with distraction (selective attention), it is necessary to inhibit responding to some stimuli, and redirect attention to different stimuli (or different aspects of stimuli) as needed. Deficits have been consistently reported in TBI subjects when distracting stimuli elicit strong response tendencies that conflict with task requirements. On such tasks, accurate responding presumably requires a greater degree of top-down attentional control. The Stroop Test (Stroop, 1935), which requires individuals to ignore the au-

tomatic response of reading a printed word and instead name the color ink in which the word is printed, has been widely used to evaluate focused attention following TBI. Unfortunately, in its standard form, the Stroop test has not differentiated head injured from control subjects reliably (McClean et al., 1983; Stuss et al., 1985; Van Zomeren and Brouwer, 1987).

Bohnen and his colleagues (1992a & b), however, hypothesized that the Stroop Test may not be sufficiently challenging to elicit the deficit in focused attention resulting from closed head injury. Bohnen et al. (1992a) modified the Stroop Test so that rectangular lines were drawn around $^1/_5$ of the items comprising the color-word subtest. With the boxed items, subjects were asked to read the word rather than give the name of the color in which it is printed. The authors hypothesized that this task would require more flexibility in the naming and reading of the items. Subjects with a history of MTBI that occurred 3 months before were significantly slower on this modified task than controls, whereas there was no significant difference between the two groups with the original Stroop Test.

In subsequent studies, this group of investigators reported on the performance of MTBI patients divided into subgroups according to the persistence of postconcussive symptoms (Bohnen et al., 1992b, 1993). Interference scores on the original and the modified version of the Stroop Test discriminated between the two groups of MTBI patients.

Batchelor et al. (1995) replicated and extended these findings in a group of 35 MTBI patients and matched controls. In addition to poor performance on the modified Stroop Task, but not on the original version of the test, the MTBI group was significantly poorer than controls.

Divided attention

Complaints about difficulty dividing attention are also common and persistent in patients with TBI. The capacity to divide attention is required for many day-to-day living and work activities. In addition to the cognitive and motor skills demanded by the basic cognitive tasks themselves, divided attention requires allocation of attentional resources, switching between tasks that cannot be executed simultaneously, and time-sharing of processing resources.

Stablum and colleagues (1994) have posited a deficit in attentional control mechanisms in patients with TBI, based in part on lower performances on divided attention paradigms. Stablum et al. (1996) studied 26 mild head injury (MHI) subjects and 26 controls, matched for age, sex, and education, in a dual task paradigm. The double task–single task difference was greater for the mild closed head injury (CHI) group, but only for patients older than 30 years and/or with loss of consciousness. However, on retesting some patients 2 years later, the authors noted that the deficit was still present, suggesting that when deficits are seen, they may be persistent.

Summary

Experimental studies in individuals who have sustained MTBI have further refined our understanding of attentional problems in this population. There is overwhelming support for a slowing of cognitive processing and response time, particularly in the early postinjury period. Although speed of processing does appear to improve, a number of experimental studies have demonstrated persisting deficits in response to complex tasks or ambiguous stimuli. The results of investigations have been quite consistent in demonstrating difficulties with aspects of divided attention, attentional control, and anticipatory behavior. These aspects of attention merge with abilities that are often discussed under the rubric of executive functions or cognitive control capabilities. Individuals with MTBI typically demonstrate relatively subtle attentional deficits that are apparent primarily under conditions requiring effortful or controlled cognitive processing. Unfortunately, many of these deficits have been elicited in experimental paradigms, almost none of which are routinely included in a clinical assessment.

Models for Assessment of Attention

The assessment of attention is usually one part of a neuropsychological evaluation that looks at a broad range of cognitive, psychological, and behavioral factors. In cases of MTBI, however, it is important to recognize that attentional problems may be the primary and unifying impairments these individuals exhibit. Unfortunately, the systematic evaluation of attention has not traditionally been emphasized in clinical neuropsychological assessment, particularly at the level that might be predicted in individuals with MTBI. Clinical evaluation of attention has often been based on the "Freedom from Distractibility" subtests (Digit Span, Arithmetic, Coding/Digit Symbol) of the Wechsler intelligence scales, on attention- demanding tasks from the Halstead-Reitan Neuropsychological Battery, (e.g., Speech-Sounds Perception Test, Seashore Rhythm Test), or on specially developed measures derived from the experimental research (e.g., PASAT, Stroop Test, Consonant Trigrams Test). Cicerone (1997) evaluated the sensitivity of several commonly used clinical measures of attention in a sample of 57 patients with MTBI. Patients were more likely to demonstrate impairments on the PASAT and an auditory Continuous Performance Test of Attention, than on Digit Span and the Trail Making Test. He reasoned this was probably due to the interaction of task demands upon information processing speed and the capacity to respond to externally paced stimuli.

Although many other measures have been found to be sensitive to disorders of attention (Lezak, 1994), models to guide assessment of the attentional system have been rare. Most clinical tests were not developed within a particular theory of attention, and clinicians have disagreed about which attentional processes are measured by different tests. In addition, despite a long history of attentional research among cognitive and experimental psychologists, there has been little crossover between the clinical and cognitive–experimental psychological literatures (Butters, 1993; Cooley and Morris, 1990).

Several models of attention have been proposed. Each of them views attention as multidimensional, rather than as a unitary function. Components of some models are organized hierarchically, but in others no hierarchical organization is hypothesized. Mirsky proposed a model of attention derived from an exploratory factor analytic study of standard clinical and experimental measures of attention (Mirsky, 1987; Mirsky et al., 1991, 1995). Four components comprising the model include Sustain, Focus/Execute, Shift, and Encode. Shum and his colleagues (1990) have used principal components analysis to examine the factor structure among measures of attention administered to normal control subjects and TBI patients. They found that a three-component model best explained the data for both groups. This model includes a sustained selective attention factor (Serial 7s, Stroop Test), a factor related to visual–auditory span (Digit Span, Knox Cube Test), and a visuomotor scanning factor (Digit Symbol, Symbol Digit Modalities Test, Trail Making Tests, Letter Cancellation Test).

Clinical Model of Attention

Sohlberg and Mateer (1987, 1989b) described a model of attention, based on experimental attention research, clinical observation of brain-injured patients at different recovery stages, and the observations of patients themselves. Components of the model are shown in Table 4.1. The model is hierarchical; each level is viewed as more complex and as requiring effective functioning of the previous level. The model has been applied to the assessment and treatment of attentional disorders following brain injury and has served as the theoretical framework for materials used in the rehabilitation of attentional disorders (Attention Process Training I [Sohlberg and Mateer, 1989a] and Attention Process Training II [Sohlberg et al., 1993]).

Although additional empirical support is needed for the models discussed, they have several features in common. Each divides attention into a number of components, and each recognizes the presence of a sustained attention or vigilance component, a focused or selective attention component, and shifting or divided attention component. Working memory, the capacity to hold and manipulate information in mind is also commonly included. Most clinical measures of attention are multifaceted and cannot be classified easily into one of these more theoretical components. Research in MTBI would suggest that attentional measures with high demands for fast processing speed, rapid and flexible shifting of attention,

Table 4-1 Clinical model of attention

Focused attention	Ability to respond discretely to specific visual, auditory, or tactile stimuli. Does not imply purposefulness of response.
Sustained attention	Ability to maintain a consistent behavioral response during continuous and repetitive activity. Incorporates concepts of vigilance and, at perhaps a higher level, the concepts of mental control or working memory.
Selective attention	Ability to maintain a behavioral or cognitive set in the face of distracting or competing stimuli. Incorporates concept of "freedom from distractibility."
Alternating attention	Capacity for mental flexibility that allows individuals to shift their focus of attention and move between tasks having different cognitive requirements or requiring different behavioral responses, thus controlling which information will be selectively attended to. Incorporates concept of shifting an established "set" easily.
Divided attention	Ability to respond simultaneously to multiple tasks or multiple task demands. Two or more behavioral responses may be required, or two or more kinds of stimuli may need to be monitored.

From Sohlberg and Mateer (1989a). *Attention Process Training.* Association for Neuropsychological Research and Development, pp. 120–122.

divided attention, prepotent response inhibition, and working memory ability will be most sensitive to the effects of MTBI (e.g., PASAT, Consonant Trigrams, Trail Making Part B, Modified Stroop Test).

Evaluation of Everday Aspects of Attention

In addition to administration of standardized psychometric measures of attention, the initial evaluation should include an assessment of how attention deficits may be interfering with functioning in naturalistic contexts. An understanding of the patient's attentional abilities in real-world context allows the clinician to design intervention strategies that can actively facilitate the transfer of improvements in therapy to functional activities. In addition to interviewing the patient and significant others about attentional abilities, the clinician may ask the patient or family to record performance data on specified activities using individually designed record sheets, and/or may observe the patient themselves in naturalistic settings.

There are also a number of questionnaires that have been designed investigate the nature of everyday failures in cognitive ability. Ponsford and

Kinsella (1991) designed a self-report measure using a list of common attentional problems that conform to a hierarchical view of attention. Information about the patient's perception of his/her attentional abilities may provide valuable information for counseling during therapy as well as guide efforts for designing a treatment program.

Martin (1983) devised the *Everyday Attention Questionnaire* (*EAQ*) and the *Everyday Memory Questionnaire* (*EMQ*) to provide differentiated measures of these two components of cognitive activity. The *EAQ* consists of 18 probes designed to assess how easy people find it to pay attention in different everyday activities (e.g., "Imagine that you are carrying out some task you find easy [perhaps peeling potatoes or knitting]. What is the effect of humming or whistling to yourself on your ability to do this sort of task?"). Responses were scaled from "very distracting" to "very helpful." The *EMQ* consists of 37 relatively simple memory probes for different kinds of information (e.g., "The words of songs or poems"). Individuals judge how good they are at remembering such information relative to other people on a five-point response scale from "very poor" to "very good." Martin and Jones (1983) reported that a high self-reported susceptibility to cognitive failures was associated with relatively poor objective performance on tasks that make strong demands on the ability to distribute attention.

In summary, a comprehensive neuropsychological evaluation should include a thorough assessment of the attentional system. This can be done by using a balanced set of psychometric measures that evaluate different components of attention, by careful interview, clinical observation, and the use of a number of rating scales which focus on everyday attentional functioning.

Management of Attentional Problems

Various approaches to the management of attentional difficulties can be conceptualized in two broad domains. The first involves education about the nature of the difficulties, the various factors that contribute to difficulties, and ways in which these factors can be modified. This may include modifications of the environment or a variety of self-regulatory strategies. The second involves cognitively based interventions that are designed to improve various aspects of attention.

Attentional failures are frequent in daily life. Everyone experiences episodes in which they lose their train of thought, have a lapse in concentration during driving, forget something they intended to do, or get distracted by competing stimuli. The literature would suggest that individuals with MTBI experience such difficulties more frequently, and have more limited resources available for rapid and efficient processing of information.

Individuals with MTBI often report feeling frustrated and overwhelmed by these limitations. An initial step in the rehabilitation process often involves explaining some of the reasons why they may be experiencing more frequent attention failures. After exploring situations in which attention failures are common, a variety of strategies or environmental manipulations can be suggested. Appendix A contains a handout that we provided to individuals presenting with attention difficulties following TBI. Strategies include reducing distractions, avoiding fatigue, reducing interruptions, managing frustration, breaking down tasks into smaller steps, getting exercise, and asking for help.

Clinically, I have found such suggestions useful in working with individuals with MTBI in several respects. First, they serve as an acknowledgment to the patient of his/her subjective experience. Recognition of the person's feelings of frustration and perception of changed mental abilities often increases a sense of trust and being understood. Second, the suggestions assist the individual who is feeling overwhelmed and "victimized" by their cognitive difficulties in gaining a sense of control and self-efficacy. Use of such techniques can improve the individual's ability to manage both his/her external environment and internal emotional state. Third, the approaches are often reported anecdotally to increase efficiency of functioning.

More controversial, although actually more rigorously investigated, are the "direct intervention" techniques for working with individuals with attentional impairments. There is substantial literature on the rehabilitation of attention following traumatic brain injury, although the bulk of this research has focused on moderately to severely injured individuals (See Mateer and Mapou, 1996, for review).

The major premise of direct intervention or process specific approaches to the treatment of attentional impairments is that attentional abilities can be improved by providing opportunities for exercising a particular aspect of attention. Treatment usually involves having patients engage in a series of repetitive drills or exercises, designed to provide opportunities for practice on tasks with increasingly greater attentional demands. Repeated activation and stimulation of attentional systems are hypothesized to facilitate changes in cognitive capacity. Effects of training can be measured at several levels including (1) the task, (2) task-related psychometric tests of either attention or another cognitive ability dependent on attention, and (3) daily functioning.

Attention Process Training

Attention process training (APT) materials are a group of hierarchically organized tasks designed to exercise sustained, selective, alternating, and divided attention (Sohlberg and Mateer, 1987). Tasks make increasingly greater demands on complex attentional control and working memory. Examples of tasks include listening for descending number sequences, shifting set on calculation tasks and a series of Stroop-like activities, alphabetizing words in sentences, detecting targets under noise conditions, and dividing attention between tasks (e.g., card sorting by suit and letter; combined auditory target detection and visual cancellation).

My colleagues and I (Mateer, 1992; Mateer et al., 1990) have reported on the efficacy of a postacute program designed specifically for individuals with mild traumatic brain injury. The program provided cognitive rehabilitation, psychosocial counseling, and vocational services. Results were reported for five individuals who had suffered MTBI at least 1 year earlier and who were still symptomatic. All had been employed prior to injury but were unemployed or underemployed at the time of program entry. They participated in a part-time outpatient program for between 20 and 28 weeks. Each participant received approximately 3 hours per week of cognitively oriented therapy that focused on use of the APT training materials, consistent use of a memory/organizer system, and gradual resumption of daily activities. As a group, these individuals demonstrated significant improvement on measures of general intellectual function, speed of information processing, complex attention, and new learning and memory. All of the subjects returned to prior employment levels.

Attention Process Training-2

The attention process training-2 (APT-2) was developed as an upper extension of the APT by Sohlberg and her colleagues (Sohlberg et al., 1993) to address more specifically the attentional deficits in individuals with milder range cognitive dysfunction. It is based on the same treatment principles as those described for the APT, but incorporates additional training materials for working on self-regulation of attention and generalization.

Generalization Activities

A major addition to the attention training materials has been the development of a generalization program. Simply engaging an individual in a "naturalistic" activity may not be sufficient to address the specific higher level cognitive deficits that are disrupting performance, particularly in individuals with more subtle deficits secondary to MTBI. Most naturalistic activities (e.g., cooking, money management, driving, etc.) are multidimensional and depend on many different cognitive processes (e.g., reasoning, visuoperceptual processing, executive functions and attention), and hence may not directly target the underlying impairments in attentional control.

One aspect of the APT-II (e.g., Appendix B) generalization program makes use of two attention "logs," the Attention Lapse Log and the Attention Success Log. The purpose of these protocols is to provide an organized way of recording both breakdowns and successes in attention in naturalistic settings throughout the person's day. Although use of these logs must take the individual profile into account, clinically we have found it useful to focus initially on attention lapses. This increases the person's awareness of the situations and times in which attention is difficult and helps in focusing treatment. After a few sessions, the focus shifts so that successful activities that were demanding of attention can be monitored and recorded. Not only the nature of the lapse or the success is recorded, but how the individual responded to the lapse or failure is recorded. This often yields insights about ways in which the individual responds emotionally to situations. Reasons for successes and failures become more apparent and an assessment of the frequency and importance of the attentional problems may become clearer.

This use of a success log also provides a focus for discussing how the patients can take a more active role in managing and controlling both attentionally demanding situations and their own responses to cognitive successes or failures. It can become a focus for discussing and evaluating the effectiveness of stress management techniques. The individual can be assisted to feel a greater sense of self-control and control over the environment. This "empowerment" phase often leads to a redefinition of self in relation to cognitive inefficiency.

Another aspect of treatment involves the design and implementation of a generalization regime, which actually begins before treatment is initiated. For example, under the area of sustained attention, the clinician might measure the number of minutes the patient can read or the number of pages that can be typed in a $1/2$-hour period. Several probes are taken in naturalistic settings to obtain the range of baseline performance. When it becomes time to begin implementing generalization activities on a regular schedule, performance is again probed and generalization goals decided upon along with a schedule for measuring performance. A sample goal might be, "The patient will be able to sit at a desk in his/her living room for at least 25 minutes while paying bills or balancing a checkbook without feeling the need to get up and take a break." A sustained attention generalization sheet is filled out with the patient writing the goals, the schedule, and any other relevant information or instructions. It is important to make sure that the patient understands the rationale, the schedule, and the logistics for collecting performance data. Following return of the performance data, entries logged are reviewed with the clinician. At this point, either new generalization activities and strategies, modification of goals for previous activities, or changes in measurement parameters or settings can be implemented as is appropriate for the individual patient. A sample generalization program for a divided attention activity is provided in Appendix B. In addition, the reader is referred to a more extensive discussion of generalization issues in a paper by Sohlberg and Raskin (1996).

It is not possible to prescribe an exact regimen of attention therapy that will be applicable or appropriate across a large group of patients. Rather, the literature supports the importance of individualized programming in working with individuals with TBI. Individualization depends on a careful psychometric assessment, and an analysis of when and where attentional lapses are occurring or are most problematic. It also depends on matching the treatment with the client's home and work situation, awareness level, emotional response to difficulties, and motivation for working on the difficulties. Helping the person to develop more realistic perceptions and expectations about his/her performance can often relieve anxiety, tension, and frustration that can exacerbate attentional difficulties.

Brain Bases for Attention Training

Despite growing support for the efficacy of various interventions for attentional impairment, it is by no means clear what may be happening in the brain itself as a function of attention training. Is the brain reorganized in some way, are new connections formed, are connections made more efficient, or does the individual learn to consciously or unconsciously compensate for attentional limitations? Evoked potential measures, particularly the P300 response, have been used extensively to study the nature of attention and attentional impairments. One component of the P300, the P3b response, is believed to index target detection in an oddball task and is hypothesized to be related to controlled as opposed to automatic processing. The P3b has been shown to be delayed and of reduced amplitude in the TBI population. Baribeau et al. (1989) measured the P300 response in TBI subjects before and after a period of cognitive rehabilitation that included training of attentional skills. The researchers reported a decrease in the latency of the P3b component, and hypothesized a change in some aspect of controlled processing as a consequence of the training. In the future, electrophysiological markers may assume greater importance not only as indicators of impairment and of recovery, but of response to therapeutic intervention.

Case Study

The client was a 36-year-old man, who had been involved in a head-on collision. Bruising suggested that he had hit his head on the steering wheel or windshield. His wife reported that he lost consciousness momentarily and appeared dazed, but was able to talk with officials at the scene and drove home. No medical attention was sought until the following day, when he saw his family physician because of a severe headache and dizziness. He had been working as a bank officer and attempted to return to work 1 week after the accident. However, he experienced a variety of cognitive and emotional difficulties including decreased attention and memory, increased fatigue, and irritability. He had difficulty accessing previously well-known computer codes, made multiple errors in paper work and had difficulty finishing tasks at work. He was placed on medical leave. Several months later, he was referred for a neu-ropsychological evaluation upon his own insistence that "something was wrong." Neuropsychological assessment revealed inefficiencies and mildly impaired scores on measures requiring speed of pro-cessing, verbal learning, working memory, and mental control. A brief course of outpatient treatment focusing on attentional skills, compensatory memory management strategies, and organizational skills was recommended. Psychological consultation to focus on anx-iety, increasing depression, and emotional instability (primarily manifest as irritability) was also recommended.

The patient underwent outpatient therapy, three times per week.

Weeks 1–2: The Attention Questionnaire and interviews with the client's spouse and with his employer were completed to sup-plement the neuropsychological assessment. The following at-tention tasks were selected to begin the therapy program: Al-phabet Sentence Exercise, Mental Math, Attention Tapes, and Serial Numbers.

Weeks 3–6: Therapy consisted of continued administration of these tasks increasing the difficulty level for each task over time (it also focused on continued practice using the organizational notebook system). Feedback during therapy sessions focused on adjusting performance expectations and accepting slight decre-ments in information processing ability.

Weeks 6–8: Therapy included the addition of alternating attention tasks such as the Alternating Alphabet and Number Change Ex-ercise. Additionally, the therapist and client initiated General-ization Activities which were practiced in the clinic and then carried out both in the home and at a job try-out at his former place of employment. Generalization exercises were tailored to those areas that client, spouse, and employer had indicated were difficult after injury. For example, he completed home repairs while listening to distractor tapes, and carried out alternating attention tasks in his work setting using set time intervals for switching between different paperwork tasks. Data collection protocols from the generalization activities were used to docu-ment performance.

Weeks 8–10: Efforts involved continuing the regimen prescribed for the previous 2 weeks with advancement to increasingly difficult levels. Vocational counseling focused on developing a part-time return to work plan at his place of employment.

Weeks 10–12: Therapy continued to focus on Attention Generaliza-tion Activities at home and at work. An appropriate break sched-ule was established in addition to training the use of relaxation strategies when the client reported feeling overwhelmed.

Outcome: The client returned to full-time work at his previous place of employment with no substantial modification in job duties. He continued to report that managing home and work felt more effortful than previous to the injury and that his capacity to engage in extra activities during the evenings and weekends was significantly decreased.

Summary and Conclusions

Over the last decade there has been increasing appreciation of the importance of attentional processing in all aspects of cognitive functioning. Although some aspects of arousal and sustained attention appear to be quite resilient to the effects of all but the most severe traumatic brain injuries, many individuals with MTBI clearly describe and demonstrate a wide variety of problems with efficient allocation and utilization of attentional resources. These impairments in attention have been shown to have significant impact on everyday functioning as indicated by both patient report and functional outcomes.

Although the attentional system does appear quite vulnerable to disruption, this system also appears to be one that can be modified with targeted intervention. Indeed, among those areas of cognitive processing that have been addressed in the cognitive rehabilitation literature, perhaps the most compelling findings are those that pertain to the improvement of attentional impairments. This appears to hold for individuals who have sustained MTBI as well as more moderate to severe traumatic brain injuries. A concerted focus on these problems can often lead to increased satisfaction on the part of patients and demonstrable functional improvements.

Although there seems to be substantial evidence that performance of tasks can change over time, important issues of generalizability to other tasks and situations will need to be further evaluated and addressed. Practitioners and increasingly researchers are adopting multifaceted approaches that include not only direct training through practice, but educational approaches to increase awareness, cognitive–behavioral approaches to alter feelings and attitudes as well as behaviors, and structured generalization approaches at home and in the workplace. Direct training approaches need not be office-bound or sterile and should incorporate techniques that reflect real-life situations and demands.

References

Arcia, E., and Gualtieri, C.T. (1994). Neurobehavioural performance of adults with closed-head injury, adults with attention deficit, and controls. *Brain Injury, 8*(5), 395–404.

Baribeau, J., Ethier, M., and Braun, C. (1989). A neurophysiological assessment of selective attention before and after cognitive remediation in patients with severe closed head injury. *Journal of Neurological Rehabilitation,* *3,* 71–92.

Batchelor, J., Harvey, A.G., and Bryant, R.A. (1995). Stroop Colour Word Test as a measure of attentional deficit following mild head trauma. *The Clinical Neuropsychologist, 9*(2), 180–186.

Birren, J.E. (1974). Translations in gerontology—From lab to life: Psychophysiology and speed of response. *American Psychologist, 29,* 808–815.

Bohnen, N., Jolles, J., and Twijnstra, A. (1992a). Modification of the Strop Colour Word Test improves differentiation between patients with mild head injury and matched controls. *The Clinical Neuropsychologist, 6,* 178–188.

Bohnen, N., Twijnstra, A., and Jolles, J. (1992b). Performance in the Strop Colour Word Test in relationship to the persistence of symptoms following mild head injury. *Acta Neurologica Scandinavica, 85,* 116–121.

Bohnen, N., Twijnstra, A., and Jolles, J. (1993). Persistence of postconcussional symptoms in uncomplicated mildly head-injured patients: A prospective cohort study. *Neuropsychiatry, Neuropsychology and Behavioural Neurology, 6,* 193–200.

Butters, N. (1993). Some comments on the goals and direction of Neuropsychology. *Neuropsychology, 7,* 3–4.

Cicerone, K.D. (1996). Attention deficits and dual task demands after mild traumatic brain injury. *Brain Injury, 10,* 79–89.

Cicerone, K.D. (1997). Clinical sensitivity of four measures of attention to mild traumatic brain injury. *The Clinical Neuropsychologist, 11*(3), 266–272.

Cooley, E.L., and Morris, R.D. (1990). Attention in children: A neuropsychologically based model for assessment. *Developmental Neuropsychology, 6,* 239–274.

Dikmen, S., McLean, A., and Temkin, N. (1986). Neuropsychological and psychosocial consequences of minor head injury. *Journal of Neurology, Neurosurgery and Psychiatry, 49,* 1227–1232.

Dikmen, S.S., Machamer, J.E., Winn, H.R., and Temkin, N.R. (1995). Neuropsychological outcome at 1–year post head injury. *Neuropsychology, 9,* 80–90.

Ettlin, T.M., Kischka, U., Reichmann, S., and Radii, E.W. (1992). Cerebral symptoms after whiplash injury of the neck: A prospective clinical and neuropsychological study of whiplash injury. *Journal of Neurology, Neurosurgery and Psychiatry, 55,* 943–948.

Ewing, R., McCarthy, D., Gronwall, D., and Wrightson, P. (1980). Persisting effects of minor head injury observable during hypoxic stress. *Journal of Clinical Neuropsychology, 2,* 147–155.

Gentilini, M., Nichelli, P., and Schoenhuber, R., et al. (1985). Neuropsychological evaluation of mild head injury. *Journal of Neurology, Neurosurgery, and Psychiatry, 48,* 137–140.

Gentilini, N., Nichelli, P., and Schoenhuber, R. (1989). *Assessment of Attention in Mild Head Injury.* New York, NY: Oxford University Press.

Gronwall, D. (1976). Performance changes during recovery from closed head injury. *Proceedings of the Australian Association of Neurology, 13,* 143–147.

Gronwall, D. (1977). Paced Auditory Serial Addition Task: A measure of recovery from concussion. *Perceptual and Motor Skills, 44*, 367–373.

Gronwall, D. (1987). Advances in assessment of attention and information processing after head injury. In H.S. Levin, J. Grafman, and H.M. Eisenberg (Eds.), *Neurobehavioral Recovery From Head Injury*. New York, NY: Oxford University Press, pp. 355–371.

Gronwall, D. (1991). Minor head injury. *Neuropsychology, 5*, 235–265.

Gronwall, D., and Sampson, H. (1974). *The Psychological Effects of Concussion*. Aukland, New Zealand: Aukland University Press.

Gronwall, D., and Wrightson, P. (1974). Delayed recovery of intellectual function after mild head injury. *Lancet, ii*, 1452.

Hinkeldey, N.S., and Corrigan, J.D. (1990). The structure of head injured patients' neurobehavioral complaints: A preliminary study. *Brain Injury, 4*, 115–134.

Hinton-Bayre, A., Geffen, G., and McFarland, K. (1997). Mild head injury and speed of information processing: A prospective study of professional rugby league players. *Journal of Clinical and Experimental Neuropsychology. 19*, 275–289.

Jakobsen, J., Baadsaard, S.E., Thomsen, S., and Henrikson, P.B. (1987). Prediction of post-concussional sequelae by reaction time test. *Acta Nerologica Scandinavica, 75*, 341–345.

Lezak, M.D. (1994). *Neuropsychological Assessment*. New York, NY: Oxford University Press.

MacFlynn, G., Montgomery, E.A., Fenton, G.W., and Rutherford, W. (1984). Measurement of reaction time following minor head injury. *Journal of Neurology, Neurosurgery and Psychiatry, 47*(12), 1326–1331.

Martin, M. (1983). Cognitive failure: Everyday and laboratory performance. *Bulletin of the Psychonomic Society, 21*, 97–100.

Martin, M., and Jones, G.V. (1983). Distribution of attention in cognitive failure. *Human Learning, 2*, 221–226.

Mateer, C.A. (1992). Systems of care for post-concussive syndrome. In L.J. Horn and N.D. Zasler (Eds.), *Rehabilitation of Post-Concussive Disorders*. Philadelphia, PA: Henley and Belfus, pp. 143–160.

Mateer, C.A., and Mapou, R. (1996). Understanding, evaluating and managing attention disorders following traumatic brain injury. *Journal of Head Trauma Rehabilitation, 11*(2), 1–16.

Mateer, C.A., Sohlberg, M.M., and Crinean, F. (1987). Perception of memory impairment in closed head injury. *Journal of Head Trauma Rehabilitation, 2*, 74–84.

Mateer, C.A., Sohlberg, M.M., and Yougman, P. (1990). *The Management of Acquired Attention and Memory Disorders Following Mild Closed Head Injury*. London: Taylor and Francis.

McClean, A., Temkin, N.R., Dikmen, N., and Wyler, A. (1983). The behavioral sequelae of head injury. *Journal of Clinical Neuropsychology, 5*, 361–376.

Miller, E., and Cruzat, A. (1980). A note on the effects of irrelevant information on task performance after mild and severe head injury. *British Journal of Social and Clinical Psychology, 20*, 69–70.

Mirsky, A.F. (1987). Behavioral and psychophysiological markers of disordered attention. *Environmental Health Perspectives, 74*, 191–199.

Mirsky, A.F., Anthony, B.J., Duncan, C.C., Ahearn, M.B., and Kellam, S.G. (1991). Analysis of the elements of attention: A neuropsychological approach. *Neuropsychology Review, 2*, 109–145.

Mirsky, A.F., Fantie, B.D., and Tatman, J.E. (1995). Assessment of attention across the lifespan. In R.L. Mapou and J. Spector (Eds.), *Clinical Neuropsychological Assessment: A Cognitive Approach*. New York, NY: Plenum Press, pp. 17–48.

Ponsford, J.L., and Kinsella, G. (1991). The use of a rating scale of attentional behavior. *Neuropsychological Rehabilitation, 1*, 241–257.

Ponsford, J.L., and Kinsella, G. (1992). Attentional deficits following closed head injury. *Journal of Clinical and Experimental Neuropsychology, 14*, 822–838.

Raskin, S., Mateer, C., and Tweeten, R. (1998). Neuropsychological evaluation of mild traumatic brain injury. *The Clinical Neuropsychologist, 12*, 21–30.

Shum, D. H.K., McFarland, K.A., and Bain, J.D. (1990). Construct validity of eight tests of attention: Comparison of normal and closed head injured subjects. *The Clinical Neuropsychologist, 4*, 151–162.

Sohlberg, M.M., Johnson, L., Paule, L., Raskin, S.A., and Mateer, C.A. (1993). *Attention Process Training-II: A Program to Address Attentional Deficits for Persons with Mild Cognitive Dysfunction*. Puyallup, WA: Association for Neuropsychological Research and Development.

Sohlberg, M.M., and Mateer, C.A. (1987). Effectiveness of an attention training program. *Journal of Clinical and Experimental Neuropsychology, 19*, 117–130.

Sohlberg, M.M., and Mateer, C.A. (1989a). *Attention Process Training*. Puyallup, WA: Association for Neuropsychological Research and Development.

Sohlberg, M.M., and Mateer, C.A. (1989b). *Introduction to Cognitive Rehabilitation: Theory and Practice*. New York, NY: Guilford Press.

Sohlberg, M.M., and Raskin, S.A. (1996). Principles of generalization applied to attention and memory interventions. *Journal of Head Trauma Rehabilitation, 11*(2), 65–78.

Stablum, F., Leonardi, G., Mazzoldi, M., Umilta, C., and Morra, S. (1994). Attention and control deficits following closed head injury. *Cortex, 30*, 603–618.

Stablum, F., Mogentale, C., and Umilta, C. (1996). Executive functioning following mild closed head injury. *Cortex, 32*, 261–278.

Stroop, J. (1935). Studies of interference in serial verbal reactions. *Journal of Experimental Psychology, 18*, 643–662.

Stuss, D., Ely, B.A., Hugenholtz, H., Richard, M.T., LaRochelle, S., Poirer, C.A., and Bell, I. (1985). Subtle neuropsychological deficits in patients with good recovery after closed-head injury. *Neurosurgery, 17*, 41–47.

Stuss, D.T., Stethem, L.L., Hugenholtz, H., Picton, T., Pivik, J., and Richard, M.T. (1989a). Reaction time after head injury: fatigue, divided and focused attention, and consistency of performance. *Journal of Neurology, Neurosurgery, and Psychiatry, 52*, 742–748.

Stuss, D.T., Stethem, L.L., Hugenholtz, H., and Richard, M.T. (1989b). Traumatic brain injury: A comparison of three clinical tests, and analysis of recovery. *The Clinical Neuropsychologist, 3*, 145–156.

Van Zomeren, A.H., and Brouwer, W.H. (1987). Head injury and concepts of attention. In H.J. Levin, J. Grafman, and H.M. Eisenberg (Eds.), *Neurobehavioral Recovery from Head Injury*. New York, NY: Oxford University Press, pp. 398–416.

APPENDIX A

This handout was developed at Good Samaritan Neuropsychological Services in Puyallup, Washington, to provide individuals with mild traumatic brain injury with information on attention difficulties and strategies for alleviating these difficulties.

Attention Compensation Techniques

Attention and concentration difficulties are very common following brain injury. The problems often get better on their own, usually rapidly at first and later more slowly. People with attentional difficulties often have to learn how to deal with those problems while they are recovering. There are many ways of adapting to these problems and compensating for them to make life easier.

Reduce distractions. Turn off radios, televisions and loud machinery when you are not actively using them or when you need to concentrate or have a conversation. Close the curtains or close your eyes if you need to. If noise can't be avoided, use earplugs.

Avoid crowds. Shop and drive on the off-hours and in the smaller stores and streets. Visit with people in small numbers. Sit at the edge of large gatherings, or visit with the people you really want to see a few at a time away from the main crowd. If you must (or if you want) to be in a crowd, don't try to do anything that requires concentration. Consider taking someone with you who can act as a guide or assist if necessary.

Watch out for fatigue. As soon as you feel yourself starting to get overwhelmed or hit information overload, take a break. The sooner you take the break, the faster you will be able to get back to what you were doing and be effective. If you are an achiever, used to pushing yourself to get something done, you have a habit that worked well before but may defeat you now. If you have to push yourself you will probably push yourself into frustration and confusion. Take a break, instead. This is NOT an excuse to be lazy. You need to be persistent and keep coming back to what you were working on, but you also need to take breaks to stay efficient.

Avoid interruptions. Unplug the phone or use an answering machine. Use a "Do Not Disturb" sign. Ask others not to interrupt when you are trying to do something that requires concentration. Do not try to do two things at once.

Get enough sleep. You probably need more sleep now than you used to. Be sure to get enough, including a nap, if necessary. If you have a persistent problem getting to sleep or staying asleep, talk to your doctor about it.

Get some exercise. We're not sure why, but regular physical exercise seems to help with attention problems.

Ask for help. Tell those closest to you that you trust about your problems (or show them this). Ask them to help you remember to do the things written here. For those who are not as close to you it's still OK to ask someone to turn off a radio, or go to a quieter place to talk, or wait a few minutes while you take a break.

(REPRINTED WITH PERMISSION OF TEDD JUDD)

APPENDIX B

An example from the Attention Process Training—II to aid in ensuring that the treatment protocals generalize to daily life.

APT-II
DIVIDED ATTENTION GENERALIZATION SHEET

Examples of Generalization Activities:

–increase the complexity of everyday task by choosing activities which require doing two or more things at the same time (e.g., prepare 2- dish meal; navigate and converse while riding as a passenger in the car; talk on the phone while making recipe list; work at computer while monitoring printout etc.)

Generalization Goal: *K. L. will formulate a discussion question directly related to the 50 min lecture class she is attending. The question must integrate topics discussed in each 10 min segment. Assignment: one question every 10 min.*

DATE	DESCRIBE TASK 1 *	DESCRIBE TASK 2 *	PERFORMANCE TASK 1	PERFORMANCE TASK 2	COMMENTS
4/3/96	Follow 50 min lecture class (taking notes not necessary)	Formulate one question pertaining to lecture topic— every 10 min	Was unable to follow lecture after writing first question. Had to borrow friend's notes.	Completed first question. Others were incomplete.	Felt frustrated when I could not keep up lecture material.
4/10/96			I could not catch up with the lecture. Had to look at neighbor's notes.	Wrote something for each question but not conclusive.	I stopped writing complete questions because I couldn't follow lecture.
4/17/96			Understood segments of the lecture about half.	Successfully completed some questions.	I wanted to discontinue question writing because I lost track of lecture.
4/24/96			Missed a few minutes of lecture following each question.	Wrote 2 thoughtful questions. But other questions missed several lecture topics.	Easier time understanding lecture and I was less frustrated.
5/1/96			Missed some lecture - had to ask a friend.	The questions only included last 5 min. of lecture material.	Less overwhelmed. Understood class as a whole.
5/8/96	↓	↓	Understood most of the lecture - missed about 15 min.	Completed each question but with same problem as before.	My questions seemed more thoughtful.

*Note performance when tasks performed alone

© Association For Neuropsychological Research & Development

5

Memory

SARAH A. RASKIN

Perhaps the most widely voiced complaint of survivors with mild traumatic brain injury (MTBI) is that of poor memory (Mateer, 1992), and
memory complaints following MTBI are maintained virtually unchanged
up to 1 year after the injury (Alves et al., 1986). Most studies, however,
have suggested that objective memory findings encountered by this population are due more to prefrontal memory systems, or to underlying difficulties with attention and organization (discussed in Chapter 4), rather
than deficits in traditional notions of learning and memory. In addition,
other factors may exacerbate memory deficits, such as depression and fatigue. Evaluation and management of memory difficulties must consider
each of these issues.

Models of Memory

Findings in cognitive psychology, neuropsychology, and neurobiology
have shaped current understanding of memory. In large part, this has involved models that are componential and reflect findings of disparate dis-
turbed and spared functions after various brain insults.

Retrospective memory has been divided into declarative and procedural memory. Declarative memory refers to memory that is directly ac-
cessible to conscious recollection, and includes facts and data acquired
through learning, both of general facts and of specific events from one's
own life.

Procedural memory, in contrast to declarative, is acquired through
learned skills. For example, when a motor task is practiced repeatedly,
one tends to improve in performance, although there is no consciously
gained knowledge. It is suggested that procedural learning is based on
subcortical structures, and spared in cases of cortically based memory disturbance. This finding has been used to guide rehabilitation techniques,
which we discuss later in this chapter.

Frontal Memory Systems

Memory systems presumed to be based on anterior cerebral structures include working memory, temporal organization of memory, and source memory (Milner, 1995). Working memory has been defined as the ability to hold information in mind, to internalize information, and to use that information to guide behavior without the aid of external cues (e.g., Goldman-Rakic, 1987). Individuals with MTBI have demonstrated deficits on tests of attention that require working memory, including the Paced Auditory Serial Addition Task (Gronwall, 1977; Kay, 1992) and the Consonant Trigrams Test (Stuss and Gow, 1992).

Temporal organization of memory includes the ability to judge which stimuli were seen most recently or to recreate the order in which stimuli were presented. It has been suggested that a breakdown in this system leads to an inability to order actions in appropriate temporal sequence. This leads to trouble with planning, goal-directed behavior, and sequencing. Source memory refers to the ability to recall the time and place when a piece of information was learned. In normal subjects, it has been demonstrated that good source recall improves recall for the information learned.

On 10 tasks of frontal memory functioning, we compared a group with MTBI, a group with severe TBI and a normal control group (NC) before a trial of cognitive rehabilitation (Raskin, 1997). The individuals with severe TBI performed significantly more poorly than the NC subjects or MTBI subjects before training. The subjects with MTBI did not differ from the NC subjects before training. It is noteworthy, however, that the subjects with MTBI did show significant improvement on these tasks following training. Given the literature demonstrating lack of improvement with practice for normal subjects on these tasks, explaining this finding is difficult. It is possible that the MTBI subjects did show an effect of training, but were at too high a level to show impairment on the tasks compared with NC subjects.

Traditional Memory and Mild Traumatic Brain Injury

Individuals with MTBI may experience a brief posttraumatic amnesia (PTA), defined as any disturbance of memory for events that occur in the period immediately following the brain injury (Ruff et al., 1989). During PTA, there is an inability to store information in memory, continuously causing the person to be disoriented and confused. No studies have demonstrated significant retrograde amnesia in MTBI, and retrograde memory loss is rarely for more than 30 minutes before impact (Ruff et al., 1989).

The literature on learning and memory functions following MTBI is somewhat mixed. Dikmen et al. (1986) compared 20 individuals with

MTBI to matched controls 1 month post injury. No differences were observed on most measures of memory, but the subjects with MTBI were impaired in recall of a 12–word list after 4 hours. This suggests that tests that measure retention only up to 1 hour may not be adequate.

Ruff et al. (1989) performed a three-center study with MTBI (defined as unconsciousness of 20 minutes or less, Glasgow Coma Scale score of 13–15 at admission, no focal neurological deficits, and no hemiparesis or impaired eye movements). One hundred fifty-five patients were administered baseline tests at 7 days post MTBI, 57 were administered follow-up tests at 30 days post MTBI, and 32 were administered follow-up tests at 3 months post injury. On baseline assessment, patients with MTBI were significantly worse on total recall of words on the Mattis-Kovner Verbal Learning and Memory Test and made more errors on the Benton Visual Retention Test. All three groups showed significant gains at 1 month follow-up with virtually no significant differences between any MTBI group and their respective controls except on digit span. At the 3 month follow-up, additional gains were exhibited on the memory tests but not digit span. In sum, individuals with single uncomplicated MTBI showed compromised memory functions at 1 week post injury, specifically for verbal and visual information, but by 1 month they had recovered to the level of controls. This was not true of digit span, but judged to be mostly due to attentional demands. Interestingly, when the same patients were asked in interviews about their memory functions, their subjective judgments of their memory at 1 month did not reflect the improvement demonstrated on testing, but rather they continued to complain of the same or worse memory deficits as at 1 week.

Like Ruff et al. (1989), Gentilini et al. (1989) reported that individuals with MTBI did not differ from normal controls on standard measures of memory functioning (Buschke Selective Reminding Test), but did perform significantly more poorly on tests specifically designed to evaluate complex attention processes.

Finally, Mateer (1992) conducted attention and memory testing in two groups of individuals ($n = 39$) referred for evaluation following TBI and a control group. Twenty of the subjects had sustained moderate to severe TBI; 19 had sustained what had seemed mild injuries but were reporting persistent postconcussion symptoms, including memory difficulty, 12 months or more post injury. Moderately to severely injured subjects performed more poorly than both the MTBI group and controls on the immediate recall portion of the Logical Memory subtest of the Wechsler Memory Scale-Revised (WMS-R). The same pattern was seen on several aspects of the Rey Auditory Verbal Learning Test, including recall after the fourth and fifth presentations of the word list, retention of the word list after distraction, and the recognition trial. The MTBI group did not differ from controls on these measures of memory. In contrast, the MTBI group performed more poorly than controls (and not significantly different from the moderate to severe TBI group) on the Digit Symbol subtest of the Wechsler Adult Intelligence Scale-Revised (WAIS-R), the Loss of Set score on the Wisconsin Card Sorting Test, the oral portion of the Symbol Digit Modalities Test, and the Visual Speed and Accuracy Test. These tests have the same requirements of speed of processing and attentional control. The data were interpreted to suggest that some individuals with MTBI, even a year or more post injury, demonstrate difficulty with timed measures requiring attention and concentration, although memory capacity as measured by psychometric tests may be intact. It was suggested that attentional problems may have been contributing to perceived memory failures.

Assessment

Squire (1986) suggested using a time line to measure the course of recovery of memory functions after brain injury. This is particularly sound advice in a rehabilitation setting and can provide an idea of the temporal dimensions of the memory deficit.

Many standard neuropsychological tests of memory functioning may not be sensitive to the memory deficits observed in MTBI. The Randt Memory Test (Randt et al., 1981) is useful because it contains sensitive tests, such as paired associate learning and incidental learning, and also a 24–hour delay, and it is repeatable, which is useful for cases in treatment. However, the only visual memory subtest is a relatively simple recognition test. Thus, it would be helpful to augment this with visual paired associate learning from the WMS-R (Wechsler, 1987) or the Rey Osterrieth Complex Figure (Rey, 1941). The California Verbal Learning Test (Delis et al., 1987) provides data on the individual's ability to organize information in memory by semantic category and to benefit from semantic cues and from a recognition format. The Bushke Selective Reminding Test (Bushke and Fuld, 1974) measures the ability to consistently retrieve information stored in memory. Both poor organization of material in memory and inconsistent storage and retrieval are frequently observed after MTBI. Including measures of delayed recall is especially important, preferably for longer than $1/2$ hour.

Tests of working memory deficits include the Consonant Trigrams Test (Peterson and Peterson, 1959) and the Paced Auditory Serial Addition Test (Gronwall, 1977). To our knowledge, no standardized tests of other prefrontal memory functions exist. We have created our own tests of temporal order that involve a list of 12 words read to the subject. The subject is then given the list of words out of order and asked to recreate the original order. Our test of recency discrimination involves again reading a list of 12 words. Then pairs of words are presented and the subject must indicate which word in each pair was presented most recently. For spatial memory, a group of pictures is presented on a large grid. The pictures are then removed and handed to the individual. The cards must then be replaced in their original position. For frequency of occurrence a list of words is read. Some words occur once, some twice, some three times. Then each word is presented and the person must indicate the number of times it was presented. To test source memory we read one list of 12 words. This list is presented several times. Then a second list of 12 words is read. Finally, words are presented one at a time and the subject must indicate if the word was from the first list or the second list.

We have used the Prospective Memory Screen (PROMS) (Sohlberg and Mateer, 1990) with individuals who have MTBI and have found the 24–hour delay item to be the most sensitive. Therefore, we would suggest using a modified version of the PROMS that includes items only to be completed outside the testing situation. For example, one might include items such as:

"There is a phone message for you. The person said to call at 1:00." and
    give the number of a telephone line in the clinic.
"Please call me at 2:00 tomorrow and confirm your next appointment."
"When you get home, please call and let us know."
"When you come in next week, remind me to give you something."

An example of a scoring sheet is provided in Appendix A.

Subjective rating scales are very important in the rehabilitation setting for many reasons. First and foremost, they provide documentation of the experience of the survivor. This experience should be validated and carefully incorporated into any feedback sessions provided. Any discrepancies between subjective report and objective test findings should also be explored and carefully explained. For example, an individual who expresses far greater memory impairment than observed on testing may be interpreting attention deficits as memory problems, may be experiencing depression that interferes with daily functioning, may be sensitive to even minor losses compared to premorbid functioning, or may be focused on minor losses because of people constantly remarking that she or he seems "fine." However, he/she may also be sensitive to declines from very high premorbid levels that standard tests are not able to measure. The reason for the discrepancy must be carefully considered and discussed with the individual over several sessions.

Some useful memory questionnaires include Sunderland et al.'s (1983) Everyday Memory Questionnaire and Mateer et al.'s (1987) Memory Questionnaire, which separates complaints into four factors. Questionnaires can also be given simultaneously to friends or family to determine the degree to which the survivor and the people in his/her life agree. This can be used to aid in education and counseling of all parties. Of course, significant others should not be incorporated into the treatment plan without the consent of the person with TBI.

Other factors, such as fatigue and current level of psychosocial stressors, should also be evaluated. The need for increased sleep, for example, has been demonstrated in MTBI (Wrightson and Gronwall, 1981). If this is not explained, individuals with MTBI are likely to attempt to sleep the same amount of time as premorbidly thereby feeling a constant sense of fatigue and exacerbating their memory deficits. Mild traumatic brain injury can also bring with it a number of psychosocial stressors. Changing family roles, problems at work or loss of work, the strain of litigation, going to medical appointments and paying medical bills are all added to whatever stressor were already present. These stressors can be distracting and anxiety provoking, thereby reducing overall memory abilities.

Rehabilitation

Rehabilitation approaches to memory changes after MTBI can be divided roughly into direct retraining, substitution, compensation, and facilitation. These are discussed below. In addition, attention training has been shown to improve memory functioning, since adequate attention processes are necessary to encode new information consistently. Approaches to attention deficits are discussed in Chapter 4. Finally, some early attempts at treatment of memory deficits with medication have been attempted, but have not been successful.

Direct Retraining

Direct retraining involves a set of exercises whereby an individual practices memory skills. This approach has been tried extensively and is based on the idea that repeated exposure and practice can facilitate learning. As Wilson et al. (1985) point out, there is little evidence to suggest that this approach is helpful for memory remediation (for a review see Franzen and Haut, 1991).

Skills training involves rote repetition of tasks to be performed in a job situation. For example, in one case, an individual in our program did not wish to take the time to participate in a full treatment program because of a strong desire to return to gainful employment immediately. With some assistance he found a job he wanted: assembling mailings and then delivering them. He frequently had trouble recalling which items to put in which envelopes and where to deliver them. By arranging all of the materials systematically in order and taping samples to his desk that he could match, these problems were relatively easily overcome. It should be noted that these methods did not "cure" his difficulties. He still would have difficulty deciding what to do if he ran out of an item or had other difficulties that broke from the routine. Thus, in specific situations, skills training can be useful. In general, however, skills training leads to very little generalization to daily life. As a result, if the memory deficit is influencing many aspects of the individual's life, skills training may be limited in its usefulness.

One particularly encouraging approach to direct retraining has been prospective memory training. Prospective memory has been defined as the ability to remember future events or the ability to "remember to remember." Early studies suggest its importance in people's daily lives and its susceptibility to subtle brain dysfunction (e.g., Sohlberg et al., 1992). However, there have been extremely few studies to date investigating the treatment of prospective memory deficits.

Substitution

Substitution refers to the use of functioning systems to bypass damaged memory systems. For example, visual imagery has been used in many studies to compensate for poor verbal memory (Crovitz, 1979; Moffat, 1984). However, usually studies have not shown these strategies to be useful for more than a few discrete pieces of information, nor has long-term retention been demonstrated (Schacter and Crovitz, 1977; Schacter and Glisky, 1986).

Compensation

Environmental modification can be used in some instances so that retrieval of information from memory is not necessary. For example, in a case of a man with MTBI who frequently turned on the wrong burner on his stove, colored burner covers and coordinated stickers were used to make it easier to select the correct knob and, simultaneously, to cue him to be aware of which burner he was turning on. Similarly, many individuals have reported benefits from having a list of important reminders inside their front door, so that they are sure to have the right things with them, to check that burners are off or doors are locked, and to be aware of where they need to be, as they leave the house in the morning.

Prosthetic memory aids serve as compensatory strategies to circumvent a dysfunctional memory system. These systems are most often in the form of a notebook or a datebook where all important information is written down, and individuals are trained in techniques of organizing the information to be written and cues to remind them to look in the book. Many individuals find it helpful to use electronic datebooks, electronic signaling devices for keys, pill boxes with alarms, or cassette recorders for important conversations or lectures.

Sohlberg and Mateer (1989) described a three-stage approach for learning to use a memory notebook in individuals with more severe brain damage. Much of their discussion, however, is also relevant to learning memory systems for individuals with MTBI. Foremost is that the act of using the notebook in an organized fashion must be made automatic through structured training and repetition.

In individuals with MTBI, it is perhaps even more important to be sure that the sections of the notebook coincide with the needs of the individual and that the system used is one that is comfortable for the person.

Many commercial systems are available and the individual can choose the size and style with which she or he feels most comfortable. The sections we have found most useful for individuals with MTBI are:

1. Datebook/calendar. This section is used to record the activities and appointments for each day. Most individuals are not resistant to this, as most of them used one premorbidly. Often included in this section, however, are specific times to perform activities that premorbidly they would have relied solely on their memory, such as going grocery shopping. We have found it helpful to schedule activities, such as shopping and paying bills, in a specific time on a specific day. Individuals with MTBI frequently have difficulty remembering to do these activities, planning their day, and managing time. Therefore, if a specific block of time is set aside, they regain more efficacy. Typically, in the treatment session, time is spent reviewing the activities of the past week and the percentage of scheduled tasks that were successfully completed. Then, a list of activities that need to be done in the next week is generated (or reviewed if the individual can generate this for homework). Specific times are set aside to do each task, with input from the therapist about realistic amounts of time required and the number of activities to do in 1 day. In this section, bills that need to be paid the same day each month (rent, loans) can be scheduled in for the year.

Many survivors also find it helpful to set aside the same time every day for certain daily activities. For example, for people who are unhappy and less productive because their desks are constantly covered with papers, setting aside 1 hour (e.g., 2:00PM–3:00PM) each day to clean and organize the papers on their desk establishes a routine that reduces the demands on planning and memory.

If the individual is experiencing depression, it may also be helpful to include time set aside for pleasurable activities in this section, or relaxation practice for anxiety. These can then be reviewed each week, as well. This is described in more detail in Chapter 8.

2. List of things-to-do. This is an ongoing list to which items are continually added. Once or twice per day (at a specified time, such as during meals), each item is then scheduled into a specific, realistic time. As tasks are completed, they are crossed off to ensure they are not repeated and to provide the reinforcement of seeing how much has been accomplished.

3. Journal or feelings log. In cases of MTBI, emotional changes are often predominant symptoms. Having a section in the notebook that is always with them where they can record their feelings can help provide a safe outlet and provide greater clarity. Reviewing this log throughout the treatment period can also help reinforce gains made in relief of emotional symptoms that might not otherwise be noticed.

4. Telephone numbers, addresses, etc. Most people find it helpful to have a place to record telephone numbers and addresses of people that are important in their personal and professional lives. This can also include information such as birthdays and anniversaries. Finally, this section can include emergency information about medical needs or babysitters for children, etc.

5. Things I forgot. We have found that people can benefit from keeping an ongoing list of items that were forgotten that caused problems in their lives. First, this serves in the early stages of therapy to tease out what types of material are forgotten to aid in designing the appropriate treatment protocol (for example, is verbal information forgotten but not visual information, is information only forgotten when presented in a distracting/busy environment, is information only forgotten when in a stressful environment, such as the boss's office, is information only forgotten when presented at the end of the day, etc.).

6. Memory successes. Individuals with MTBI often experience sadness at memory losses and may not be aware of improvement over time. Therefore, a section of the book devoted to memory success can be helpful. We often use a simple numerical chart to record the number of items from the things-to-do list completed each week, so that individuals become aware of the number of things they can accomplish.

Another form of compensation is the application of organizational tools. Often, one aspect of memory difficulties is poor organization of material to be remembered. Some people benefit from creating a specific place in the home for all-important material. For example, a large calendar in the kitchen can be used by all members of the household. This way, for example, the parent with MTBI is not forced to rely on memory to know where children are and when they need to be picked up. This can reduce the frustration level of all family members and help he/she retain a parental role without always feeling at a loss and flustered. A telephone message board in the same location and places for keys and wallet can aid in keeping track of these items.

Facilitation

One facilitation technique is derived from studies of distributed practice. Learning is facilitated by having review occur over a longer period; for example, 1 hour every day for a week, rather than 7 hours in 1 day. This seems to allow time for memory consolidation. Landauer and Bjork (1978) suggest starting with a short delay between presentation of the material and testing, and then slowly increasing the delay period.

Mnemonics have been tried extensively and, in general, have not been helpful for remembering more than a short list of material or names. Wilson (1989) stresses that these techniques should not be expected to generalize, but should rather be employed only in assisting people to learn limited pieces of information. Mnemonic strategy has been criticized for the high demand placed on encoding processes (Schacter and Glisky, 1986), attention, planning, and vigilance, all of which may be impaired.

Most strategies are based, in part, on using repetition and spared procedural learning. One important finding in this area is the demonstration of improved performance with errorless learning (Baddely, 1992; Wilson, 1992). In a series of studies, these authors demonstrated that people with severe amnesia learned more quickly and accurately when they were not permitted to make incorrect guesses. Thus, for rehabilitation profession-als, it may not be advisable to allow survivors to "go ahead and guess" during the learning phase of any treatment. Instead, if a response is not given within a prescribed time frame, the correct answer should be pro-vided and then another trial attempted.

Academic therapy, such as the PQRST technique, is also essentially a form of aiding encoding and storage. This acronym stands for: Preview, Question, Read, State, Test. That is, the individual is taught to first pre-view or skim the material. Then a series of questions are generated about the main theme and important points. The reading material is then read with a focus on finding the answers to the questions. At this point the an-swers are stated. Finally, an important aspect of this procedure is frequent testing and probing of retention of the material. This has been demon-strated to be effective in increasing retention of written material in a se-ries of case studies of individuals with moderate to severe brain injury (Wilson, 1987). I have used this technique clinically with individuals with MTBI, and it appears anecdotally to be a useful, structured approach to using repetition and organization to help with reading (Raskin, 1997).

The method of vanishing cues was designed to take advantage of prim-ing effects (Glisky et al., 1986). Using this method, maximum cuing is used initially, and then cuing is slowly reduced over repeated trials. Al-ternately, the cues can be less specific, such as an alarm watch set to go off at a time when a task needs to be done. This requires the individual to be able to recall the task at the sound of the alarm, or remember where to look up the information.

Multimodal Approaches

Mateer and Sohlberg (1988) suggested a three-pronged approach to treat-ing memory. This involved attention training, prospective memory train-ing and the use of memory notebooks simultaneously. They stress the need to tailor these systems to the individual's needs.

In a case study of an individual with MTBI, Crosson and Buenning (1984) used a combination of strategies including providing feedback on performance, visual imagery, and periodic questioning to help the per-son improve in reading retention. Unfortunately, 9 months following training, performance had dropped due to the individual not maintain-ing the use of the strategies.

Schacter & Glisky (1986) also describe a multimodal program for treat-ment of memory deficits after MTBI. This MTBI group was defined as having no skull fracture, no evidence of neurologic deficit, and no long period of posttraumatic amnesia. In the program they describe there are three stages. Stage 1 was described as an individual session consisting of reassurance and counseling as well as assessment with a battery of tests of attention and memory. Individuals are asked open-ended questions about what problems have been noted since the injury and then subsequently questioned about specific deficits. If the individual displays neuropsychological deficits she or he then enters Stage 2 of the program. This consists of 3 hours per day, 3 days per week of treatment. The treatment consists of 2 hours of some combination of individual and group activities, stress management, assessment, and cognitive rehabilitation as well as group support and discussion. This continues until a criterion of performance on the PASAT is obtained. At that point Stage 3 is initiated, which is a slow return to work.

Generalization

Parente and DiCesare (1991) stress the importance of designing studies that will ensure generalization, using transfer of learning models and avoiding models that require the individual to learn new response sets after training or to reorganize what she or he has learned.

Franzen and Haut (1991) discuss the various ways in which generalization of memory training must occur. Generalization can occur across time, settings, tasks, modalities, and types of memory. They conclude that the procedure used and the measure of generalization must be appropriate to the memory impairment and to the individual.

We have found that generalization is maximized when problems that are real in the person's daily life are targeted as the goals of treatment. Remediation takes an individually tailored and multimodal approach to combine the use of retraining (such as attention training), compensation training, and where appropriate, skills training. By targeting the memory complaints that the person experiences in his/her daily life and being flexible in combining techniques as necessary, we have had many successes. Frequent probes of daily memory functioning, such as the prospective memory screen (PROMS), can guide ongoing treatment and help increase awareness by discussing problems that occur and generating strategies for them together.

Case Study

LH is a 47–year-old attorney. He was driving an automobile and was hit head-on by another driver. His head hit the windshield and was bruised. He believes that he lost consciousness briefly and was taken to the emergency room. The following day, LH experienced a severe headache and nausea and presented to a nearby hospital, where he was given a prescription for pain medication. He was followed by his physician for the next month, who documented continued headache and memory problems. Computerized tomography scan of the head was performed and was negative.

Approximately 1 month after the accident, he was seen for a neuropsychological evaluation. His cognitive abilities were noted to be extremely variable with inconsistencies noted on measures of executive functions, concentration, and verbal abilities. Significant reductions were noted on measures of memory and new learning. It was assumed that with time, many of these abilities would recover and LH was referred for a brief course of cognitive remediation (1 hour per week) focused on improving attention skills and teaching organizational strategies.

While developing treatment goals and strategies, it was determined that his prospective memory span was extremely short (approximately 2 minutes) and that his attention deficits were interfering with his memory processes. Therefore, treatment focused on attention training and prospective memory training. He also developed compensation strategies, such as cues shown in Appendix B.

Six months after the initiation of treatment and 7 months after the accident, a reevaluation was done. At that time, LH showed improvement in both his attention and his memory processes. See Table 5.1 for a listing of his test scores. However, he continued to exhibit deficits in divided attention and visual organization. These deficits were severe enough that he was essentially unable to continue as an attorney. He slowly disbanded his practice and, at the end of treatment, was in process of applying for other jobs. This created significant loss of self-esteem, financial and marital strain.

Table 5-1 Scores on select tests prior to and following treatment

	9/6/91	3/12/92
Wechsler Memory Scale-Revised		
Logical Memory I	17	24
Logical Memory II	16	25
Visual Reproduction I	21	34
Visual Reproduction II	21	27
Verbal Pairs I	12	21
Verbal Pairs II	6	8
Rey-Osterrieth Figure	<10	25
Verbal Fluency	29	40
Digit Span		
Forwards	4	7
Backwards	5	7

References

Alves, W.M., Colohan, A.R.T., O'Leary, T.S., et al. (1986). Understanding post-traumatic symptoms after minor head injury. *Journal of Head Trauma Rehabilitation, 1*, 1–12.

Baddeley, A. (1992). Implicit memory and errorless learning: A link between cognitive theory and neuropsychological rehabilitation? In L. Squires and N. Butters (Eds.). *Neuropsychology of Memory, 2nd Ed*. New York, NY: The Guilford Press, pp. 309–314.

Buschke, H., and Fuld, P.A. (1974). Evaluation of storage, retention, and retrieval in disordered memory and learning. *Neurology, 11*, 1019–1025.

Crosson, B., and Buenning, W. (1984). An individualized memory retraining program after closed-head injury: A single-case study. *Journal of Clinical Neuropsychology, 6*, 287–301.

Crovitz, H.F. (1979). Memory retraining in brain-damaged patients: the airplane list. *Cortex, 15*(1), 131–134.

Delis, D.C., Kramer, J.H., Kaplan, E., and Ober, B.A. (1987). California Verbal Learning Test: Adult Version. San Antonio, TX: The Psychological Corporation.

Dikmen, S., McLean, A., Temkin, N. (1986). Neuropsychological and psychosocial consequences of minor head injury. *Journal of Neurology, Neurosurgery, and Psychiatry, 49*, 1227–1232.

Franzen, M., and Haut, M. (1991). The psychological treatment of memory impairment: A review of empirical studies. *Neuropsychology Review, 2*, 29–63.

Gentilini, M., Nichelli, P., and Shoenhuber, T. (1989). Assessment of attention in mild head injury. In H. Levin, H. Eisenberg, and A. Benton (Eds.), *Mild Head Injury*. New York, NY: Oxford University Press, pp. 163–175.

Glisky, E., Schacter, D., and Tulving, E. (1986). Learning and retention of computer-related vocabulary in memory-impaired patients: Method of vanishing cues. *Journal of Clinical and Experimental Neuropsychology, 8*, 292–312.

Goldman-Rakic, P.S. (1987). Development of cortical circuitry and cognitive function. *Child Development, 58*(3), 601–622.

Gronwall, D. (1977). Paced auditory serial addition task: A measure of recovery from concussion. *Perceptual and Motor Skills, 44*, 367–374.

Kay, T. (1992). Neuropsychological diagnosis: disentangling the multiple determinants of functional disability after mild traumatic brain injury. In L. Horn and N. Zasler (Eds.), *Rehabilitation of Post-Concussive Disorders. Physical Medicine and Rehabilitation: State of the Art Reviews, 6*, 109–127.

Landauer, T., and Bjork, R. (1978). Optimum rehearsal patterns and name learning. In M. Gruneberg, P. Morris, and R. Sykes (Eds.), *Practical Aspects of Memory*. London: Academic Press.

Mateer, C. (1992). Systems of care for post-concussive syndrome. In L. J. Horn and N. D. Zasler (Eds.), *Rehabilitation of Post-Concussive Disorders*. Philadelphia, PA: Henley and Belfus, pp. 143–160.

Mateer, C.A., Sohlberg, M.M., and Crinean, J. (1987). Perceptions of memory function in individuals with closed-head injury. *Journal of Head Trauma Rehabilitation, 2,* 74–84.

Milner, B. (1995). Aspects of human frontal lobe function. *Advanced Neurology, 66,* 67–81.

Moffat, N. (1984). In B.A. Wilson and N. Moffat (Eds.), *Clinical Management of Memory Problems.* London: Croom Helm, pp. 86–119.

Parente, R., and DiCesare, A. (1991). Retraining memory: Theory, evaluation, and applications. In J. Kreutzer and P. Wehman (Eds.), *Cognitive Rehabilitation for Persons with Traumatic Brain Injury: A Functional Approach.* Baltimore, MD: Paul Brookes Publishing Company, pp. 147–162.

Peterson, L., and Peterson, M. (1959). Short-term retention of individual verbal items. *Journal of Experimental Psychology, 58,* 193–198.

Randt, C.T., Brown, E.R., and Osborne, D.P. (1981). A memory test for longitudinal measurement of mild to moderate deficits. *Clinical Neuropsychology, 2*(4), 184–194.

Raskin, S. (1997). Rehabilitation of cognitive deficits (abstract). Cognitive Neuroscience Society. Boston, MA.

Rey, A. (1941). Psychological examination of traumatic encephalopathy. *Archives de Psychologie, 28,* 286–340; sections translated by J. Corwin and F.W. Byysma, *The Clinical Neuropsychologist,* 1993, 4–9.

Ruff, R., Levin, H., Mattis, S., High, W., Marshall, L., Eisenberg, H., and Tabaddor, K. (1989). Recovery of memory after mild head injury: a three-center study. In H. Levin, H. Eisenberg, and A. Benton (Eds.), *Mild Head Injury.* New York, NY: Oxford University Press, pp. 176–188.

Schacter, D.L., and Crovitz, H.F. (1977). Memory function after closed head injury: A review of the quantitative research. *Cortex, 13,* 150–176.

Schacter, D.A., and Glisky, E.L. (1986). Memory remediation: Restoration, alleviation and the acquisition of domain specific knowledge. In B. Uzzell and Y. Gross (Eds.), *Clinical Neuropsychology of Intervention.* Boston, MA: Martinus Nijhoff.

Sohlberg, M., and Mateer, C. (1989). Training use of compensatory memory books: A three-stage behavioral approach. *Journal of Clinical and Experimental Neuropsychology, 11,* 871–891.

Sohlberg, M., and Mateer, C. (1990). *Prospective Memory Screening.* Puyallup, WA: Association for Neuropsychological Research and Development.

Sohlberg, M., White, O., Evans, E., and Mateer, C. (1992). An investigation of the effects of prospective memory training. *Brain Injury, 6,* 139–154.

Squire, L. (1986). The neuropsychology of memory dysfunction and its assessment. In I. Grant and K. Adams (Eds.), *Neuropsychological Assessment of Neuropsychiatric Disorders.* New York, NY: Oxford University Press, pp. 218–299.

Stuss, D., and Gow, C. (1992). "Frontal dysfunction" after traumatic brain injury. *Neuropsychiatry, Neuropsychology, and Behavioral Neurology, 5,* 272–282.

Sunderland, A., Harris, J., and Baddeley, A. (1983). Do laboratory tests predict everyday memory? A neuropsychological study. *Journal of Verbal Learning and Verbal Behavior, 22,* 341–357.

Wechsler, D. (1987). Wechsler Memory Scale-Revised manual. San Antonio, TX: The Psychological Corporation.

Wilson, B. (1987). *Rehabilitation of Memory*. New York, NY: The Guilford Press.

Wilson, B. (1989). Coping strategies for memory dysfunction. In E. Perecman (Ed.), *Integrating Theory and Practice in Clinical Neuropsychology*. Hillsdale, NJ: Lawrence Erlbaum Associates, pp. 155–174.

Wilson, B. (1992). Rehabilitation and memory disorders. In L. Squire and N. Butter (Eds.), *Neuropsychology of Memory, 2nd Ed*. New York, NY: The Guilford Press, pp. 315–322.

Wilson, B., Cockburn, J., and Baddeley, A. (1985). *The Rivermead Behavioural Memory Test*. Bury St Edmunds, Suffolk: Thames Valley Test Company.

Wrightson, P., and Gronwall, D. (1981). Time off work and symptoms after minor head injury. *Injury, 12*, 445–454.

APPENDIX A

The score sheet used for the Prospective Memory Screening test (PROMS) and the method by which generalization of prospective memory treatment was measured. This latter form was completed first by the therapist, person with brain injury, and significant other. Then the significant other measured prospective memory success for one week outside the clinic.

PROMS

Name_____

Date_____

Distractor Used_____

For each task, score as follows:
3 points for correct response at correct time (± 10%)
2 points for incorrect or no response but recognition
    that it was time to make a response at correct
    time(time cue tasks only)
1 point for incorrect response to associative cue
    (e.g., at end of session remembers to do task)
½ point for correct response but at incorrect time

Associative Cue Task	3 Correct	1 Wrong Response	0 No Response
1 hour			
4 hours			
24 hours			

Time Cue Task	3 Correct	2 Wrong Response	½ Wrong Time	0 No Response
1 hour				
4 hours				
24 hours				
1 week				

Measuring Memory Functioning Outside the Clinic

Client Name_____

Significant Other_____

Date Plan Made with Therapist/Trial #_____

INTRODUCTION: As we talked about, I need to have an idea of how _____'s memory is working outside the clinic. I will need your help in planning the measurement activities and making notes about how well he/she is able to complete them.

I. Select Setting and Corresponding Memory Tasks: We want to choose setting/activities that will span at least several hours and that are familiar to the person. We should try and choose a day when things are on a "regular" schedule (e.g., you do not have out of town guests and there is not something newly stressful like beginning remodeling project). Listed below are some examples.

SETTING	TYPES OF MEMORY TASKS
Errands in the Community	1. Remembering to get specific items in the grocery store; 2. Remembering to go different places to do errands (e.g., post office, fill car with gas);

Home Projects	1. Remembering to do certain cleaning or garden chores;
	2. Remembering to make phone calls, take pills, do certain correspondence;
	3. Remembering to take something out of the oven, to move wash to dryer, to tape t.v. show on VCR;
Hobbies	1. Remembering to do next step in a project after a waiting period (e.g., after glue dries can put on decals);

Using the above list as examples, let's select the setting and tasks you will plan to measure and fill out the form on the following page. Today we will fill out the first two columns and then when you actually do the measurement, you will fill out the last three columns.

Setting Date	Tasks	Approx. how long did s/he need to remember the task before doing it?	How well did s/he perform the task?	Did s/he do anything special (e.g., write reminder notes) to help remember each task?

APPENDIX B

An example of a daily checklist used by a person with mild traumatic brain injury.

Daily Priority

1. Look at Daytimer
2. Review normal daily chore list
3. Select household project
4. Select community outing
5. Write plan in Daytimer
6. Check items off
7. Write in daily diary (p.m.)

NORMAL DAILY CHORES

1. Make bed
2. Garbage (burning/trash)
3. Feed pets
4. Paper/mail
5. Sweep patio
6. Yard
7. Wood for wood stove
8. Defrost meat/start dinner
9. Dishwasher

6

Executive Functions

SARAH A. RASKIN

Problems related to executive functions are common following TBI. Difficulties such as failing to accomplish goals, problems performing multiple tasks, or trouble with sequencing steps in a task can occur in the presence of average or above average intelligence and adequate recall of information.

The term executive functions refers to many disparate functions. These functions are all presumed to be mediated by neuronal systems that include prefrontal cortex. This chapter presents a current model of executive functions and will use this model to conceptualize the treatment needs of individuals with MTBI.

A thorough review of the neuroanatomy of prefrontal cortex is beyond the scope of this text. However, it is worth noting that this is a vast region encompassing several subdivisions, and with afferent and efferent connections with other neocortical structures, subcortical structures, and projections within the frontal lobes. Thus, it is impossible to describe a single set of deficits associated with prefrontal dysfunction.

As reviewed in Chapter 1, prefrontal cortex is especially vulnerable to the mechanical effects of MTBI. Goldberg and Bilder (1986) argue that prefrontal cortex is, by its nature, the region most susceptible to dysfunction following diffuse brain injury for three reasons. The first is based on the extensive interconnections between prefrontal cortex and other regions, such that damage in many areas will lead to a disconnection of prefrontal cortex. Secondly, prefrontal cortex is the most phylogenetically and ontogenetically recent part of the brain. Thirdly, general structural damage is most likely to first affect the least overlearned functions, which are subserved by prefrontal cortex.

Some functions that are presumed to depend on prefrontal integrity are described elsewhere in this text. Included are frontal memory functions (e.g., working memory), which are described in Chapter 5, and personality changes, which are described in this chapter. Appendix A provides a handout for patients and families that describes sequelae of frontal lobe injury.

Theoretical Descriptions of Executive Functions

Numerous theories have been proposed to explain executive functioning (Lezak, 1993; Norman and Shallice, 1980; Shallice, 1982). Most theories describe functions that become necessary when nonroutine behavior is involved. Thus, executive functions come into play when the situation requires flexible problem-solving, planning, or shifting of mental set.

Sohlberg et al. (1992) provide a model of executive functions with a systematic hierarchy of functions and interconnections between each level of the hierarchy. The first level is sensory/perceptual information, which is domain specific, relatively automatic, and subserved by nonfrontal brain regions.

The second level is executive control, which receives input from the first level and serves to adjust and direct behaviors based on this input. The functional systems at this level are drive and sequencing (including maintaining and shifting mental set, thinking abstractly, and planning) (Stuss and Benson, 1986). Deficits in basic drive and motivation may present as an inability to initiate goal-directed activities or to direct attention appropriately. Individuals are able to carry out activities with prompting or cues but do not initiate activities themselves. Mental set can be defined as a state of brain activity that predisposes a subject to respond in a particular way when several alternatives are present (Flowers and Robertson, 1985). The ability to think abstractly includes translating knowledge of specific facts into appropriate action, grasping the totality rather than responding to specific parts, integrating details, and handling simultaneous sources of information (Stuss and Benson, 1986). To plan, one must have a prior conceptual scheme of the plan, preparation of each step to implement it, and the anticipation of its consequences. The third level in the model is self-reflectiveness or the ability to be aware of oneself and reflect on ongoing processes (Stuss, 1991). It is unusual for an individual with MTBI to present with poor awareness of deficits. However, they may have poor awareness of their own behavior, social cues, or affective presentation (Cicerone and Giacino, 1992).

Assessment of Executive Functions

Many authors have described the difficulty in assessing functions of the frontal lobes using standard neuropsychological techniques (Lezak, 1982; Stuss and Benson, 1986). Standard tests typically structure and organize the material for the individual, an explicit task is at hand, and initiation is cued by the examiner (Shallice and Burgess, 1991). Because executive function deficits may not affect routine, well-structured tasks, these deficits may not be apparent immediately after the injury and may never be apparent on formal testing. Varney and Menefee (1993) noted that individuals with MTBI may appear normal on most neuropsychological tests but be impaired in independent self-directed behaviors.

In addition, deficits on tests of attention that require working memory, like the delayed response task, have been documented. Examples include the Paced Auditory Serial Addition Task (Gronwall, 1977; Kay, 1992) and the Consonant Trigrams Test (Stuss and Gow, 1992).

Other tasks that were designed to minimize structure and cuing include Self-Ordered Pointing (Milner, 1982), Cognitive Estimation (Shallice and Evans, 1978), the Six Elements task, which requires the individual to carry out six open-ended tasks (Shallice and Burgess, 1991), and the Multiple Errands Task (Shallice and Burgess, 1991), but to our knowledge none have been used in this population.

To measure productivity and self-regulation, several fluency tests have been developed. The Design Fluency Test (Jones-Gotman and Milner, 1977) requires the individual to produce as many novel designs as possible in a specified amount of time. The Ruff Figural Fluency Test (Ruff et al., 1987) provides individual squares, each containing an array of points. The goal is to connect any two or more points within each square to make as many novel designs as possible in 1 minute. Verbal fluency tasks include the Controlled Oral Word Association Test (Benton et al., 1983) and the Animal Naming Subtest of the Boston Diagnostic Aphasia Examination (Goodglass and Kaplan, 1972). Individuals with MTBI have been shown to be impaired on both semantic and phonemic tasks of verbal fluency and to make more errors on these tasks than matched normal controls, despite a normal ability to retrieve information by semantic and phonemic clusters (Raskin and Rearick, 1996).

The Wisconsin Card Sorting Test (Grant and Berg, 1948) is probably the most widely used test to measure the ability to shift mental set. In particular, this test can be used to measure perseverative tendencies and the ability to use feedback to alter performance. Deficits on the Wisconsin Card Sorting Test (Stuss and Gow, 1992), and the Symbol Digit Modalities Test (Kay, 1992) have been noted after MTBI.

A more abstract version of set-shifting is measured with the Uses of Objects Test (Getzels and Jackson, 1962). On this test, the subject is required to provide unusual uses for common objects, such as using a brick as a bookend. Shifting from the most common association of the object is required.

The Similarities Subtest of the WAIS-R is probably the most widely used test of thinking abstractly. This test requires the individual to provide superordinate category names when given category members. Gorham's (1956) Test of Proverbs also provides an indication of the ability to think abstractly. Tests of reasoning and hypothesis testing have also demonstrated deficits in individuals with MTBI (Barth et al., 1983; Leninger et al., 1990; Yarnell and Rossie, 1988).

To assess planning, Lezak (1982) suggests analyzing the layout of designs on the Bender-Gestalt (Bender, 1938) or the approach to the Block Design Subtest of the WAIS-R. Maze tests are often also useful. The Porteus Mazes (Porteus, 1965) are probably the most widely used, although the Wechsler Intelligence Scale for Children-Revised (WISC-R) Mazes (Wechsler, 1974) are faster and have greater ease of administration. The Tower of Hanoi (Cohen and Corkin, 1981) and Tower of London (Shallice, 1982) both require planning in order to solve the puzzle in the minimum number of moves.

Lezak (1982, 1993) has suggested the Tinkertoy Test as a good test of purposeful behavior. The examiner provides 50 pieces of a standard Tinkertoy Test and requires the patient to "Make whatever you want with these. You will have at least 5 minutes and as much more time as you wish to make something." Scoring is based on the number of pieces used and the quality of the construction. In particular the construction is rated on whether there was a goal in mind, whether the construction resembles the goal, whether it has moving parts and is free standing, and whether the pieces are fitted together properly.

The Tinkertoy Test has been demonstrated to be sensitive to deficits following MTBI, whereas many of the same patients performed within normal limits on the Porteus Mazes and Wisconsin Card Sorting Test (Martzke et al., 1991). Performance on the Tinkertoy Test was also shown to correlate with ability of MTBI subjects to return to work (Bayless et al., 1989).

To assess awareness, Lezak (1993) suggests parts of the Cognitive Competency Test, which can demonstrate awareness of the patient's own needs, Verbal Reasoning to examine responses to practical problems, such as getting to an appointment on time, and Picture Interpretation, which requires awareness of background features to interpret the scene.

Finally, the Frontal Lobe Personality Scale may be helpful in measuring awareness of changes such as disinhibition, apathy, and executive dysfunction, and has been administered to a group of individuals with MTBI (Drake et al., 1998).

Although individuals with MTBI who seek treatment are often quite aware of the existence of deficits, they may not be fully aware of the exact nature of their difficulty, or may exaggerate the severity. Thus, it is important to include interviews from significant others who know the person well. The Iowa Collateral Head Injury Interview (Varney, 1991) has been used in subjects with MTBI (Varney and Menefee, 1993). Questions about common cognitive and psychosocial TBI symptoms are included. Collaterals of individuals with MTBI reported symptoms such as poor empathy, poor judgment, absentmindedness, indecisiveness, immaturity, and poor insight.

Treatment of Executive Function Deficits

A number of researchers have grappled with defining a model for treatment of executive system dysfunction (for reviews see: Cicerone and Wood, 1987; Sohlberg et al., 1992). One consideration is when to use a bottom-up approach, in which cues are provided for schemas or a top-down approach, in which preserved higher-level intellectual functions are used to train increased self-monitoring. Some of the approaches used to date are training of specific compensatory skills and strategies, remediation of underlying cognitive processes (e.g., attention), behavior modification, and the direct retraining of executive functions and awareness/metacognitive skills.

Compensation Strategies

Environmental modification is a compensation strategy that, for example, may remove dangerous situations that can result from impulsivity. Prosthetic devices, either people or otherwise, have also been employed (Hart and Jacobs, 1993). For example, someone with a deficit in initiation can be given an alarm watch programmed to go off at the appropriate time to initiate an activity, such as preparing meals. Cuing systems might involve training the person to use a watch with an alarm, a calendar system, or cue card with a list of daily activities. Developing a daily routine so that certain routine tasks are performed at the same time and in the same order is often helpful. Using lists and cue cards has also been suggested to help individuals with poor insight evaluate their own performance and compare it to their therapist's evaluation of them.

Many individuals with MTBI can benefit from more complex computer-based or interactive scheduling systems that allow for greater flexibility. Many inexpensive versions are available commercially, which include functions for daily schedules, important telephone numbers, planning lists and an alarm setting for important meetings or activities. Active and systematic training is required for the use of such compensatory strategies.

Training Underlying Cognitive Processes

An initial treatment intervention for an individual with executive function deficits might include maximizing attentional capacity through formal attention training (see Chapter 4).

Behavioral Techniques

The frontal lobes are essential for the effective initiation and sequencing of action programs. These action programs could be disrupted by problems with initiation or lack of drive, manifesting as apparent disinterest or inactivity. Generally, such people respond quite well to external cues or prompts to initiate activity, and their behavior can be modified through traditional behavior modification techniques (Cicerone and Giacino, 1992). Thus, treating executive function deficits may involve reestablishing conscious links between the social and environmental demands the person encounters and the responses of the individual. Self-observation is involved for anticipation deficits, self-instructional training for planning deficits, and self-monitoring for verification and error recognition deficits.

Successful behavior modification requires that the individual be amenable to that plan, that the reinforcement be meaningful without punitive withholding, and that the antecedents of any inappropriate behavior be carefully identified when developing the treatment plan (Hart and Jacobs, 1993). Individuals with MTBI who have preserved high levels of intellectual functioning can design and carry-out their own behavior modification plan. One woman in our program was extremely upset about frequently forgetting to return important work-related telephone calls. She tried to schedule 1 hour each day to do so, but found that she would always find some way to waste the time in other activities. She decided on a two-part plan. First, she would perform a brief relaxation exercise before initiating the calls to reduce her anxiety about the activity. Then, for each successful call made, she rewarded herself with 10 minutes of riding her horse. Eventually, she was able to move to rewarding herself with 1 hour for completing all the calls of the day, and finally, she no longer needed a reward to complete the calls.

Direct Retraining of Executive Systems

Certain aspects of executive functioning can be systematically retrained. In general, this involves breaking the function into component steps and working through a hierarchy of difficulty. Raskin and Gordon (1992b) demonstrated that set-shifting could be retrained by breaking the task into underlying components. A woman with MTBI was trained to shift mental set in complex situations. Presented with tasks such as lists of nouns, she was required to put a check next to the words that were vegetables and an "x" next to words that were not. She then practiced thinking abstractly and creating alternatives using a modification of the Uses of Objects Test. Next, she recorded problems encountered in her daily life and generated as many solutions as possible. Finally, she was observed while performing an activity of daily life (i.e., cooking) during which different "problems" were presented and she needed to problem-solve in order to deal with each of them. She showed the ability to work successfully through this hierarchy of tasks, improvement on neuropsychological measures of set-shifting, and improvement in set-shifting in her daily life using a rating scale and a daily log of activities.

Another approach was used with more severely impaired individuals. Patients were trained to break complex problems into their component parts (von Cramon and Mattes-von Cramon, 1990). The first stage of training was to learn to analyze problems. The second stage was to divide a multistage task into smaller steps, with immediate feedback given. Then four modules were initiated. The first involved generating goal-directed ideas in the form of possible solutions to a problem. The second involved systematic comparisons to allow for analyzing the possible solutions. The third module consisted of problems where multiple pieces of information needed to be processed simultaneously. The fourth module required drawing inferences. All training was performed in a group setting. The authors point out that work in a group facilitates the ability to take another person's point of view. Recognizing problem-solving deficits in others can help reinforce awareness of one's own problems. An example of an exercise given was, "Please prepare, in cooperation with your partners in the problem-solving training group, a visit by the ward to a museum in the city center of Munich. Wheelchair users should be able to participate."

The treatment session itself is an excellent opportunity for using this strategy. Generally, treatment sessions are carefully planned in advance by the therapist. Like most tests of executive functioning, this eliminates any need for the individuals to use executive functions themselves. Therefore, we have found it helpful to begin with the traditional model. Next, individuals are given the task of sequencing and monitoring the tasks to be completed within the session. This includes keeping track of the time spent on each task so that everything is accomplished in the time allotted. Finally they are given full responsibility for planning and carrying out the full treatment session. This provides a structured model for other tasks in their daily life and allows for feedback from the therapist on the progress of their executive skills (Good Samaritan Hospital, 1989).

The tasks at each stage may be pencil-and-paper tasks, commercial products, or computer programs. There are many commercially available computer programs that can be useful. Rattock (1990, Medisoft Software) has programmed the game Mastermind on computer so that the level of difficulty and type of stimuli can be tailored to the individual and made progressively more difficult. This game requires problem-solving and using feedback to guide performance with no memory component. We have used Where in the World Is Carmen Sandiego (Broderbund Software, Inc., 1990) with individuals who have difficulty integrating information from many sources to reach a goal. Thinking Skills (Top Class, Compedia, 1992) trains sequencing and sorting ability. Factory (Wings for Learning, Scotts Valley, CA, 1990) requires planning using visual–perceptual material.

Metacognitive Training Approaches

Functioning with awareness and self-regulatory capacity may, more than any other area, define the essence of frontal lobe activity. Treatment in this area presents a tremendous challenge for the rehabilitation professional.

Barco et al. (1991) discuss facilitation of intellectual, emergent, and anticipatory awareness using repetitive education of the survivors and their significant others. This education takes the form of teaching the person about any deficits and about their implications for daily living. Materials, workbooks, diagrams, and visual models are used. In addition, feedback is provided as the individual is performing tasks as to the quality of their own performance. In many cases, videotaping is also extremely helpful, as it is sometimes easier for people to understand the problem when viewing it themselves.

Eventually, the method of vanishing cues can be applied. Maximum cues as to impaired performance are provided as it occurs (or in advance if increased anticipatory awareness is the goal). Slowly, the amount of active cuing is withdrawn until individuals develop their own ability to monitor performance.

One approach to improving self-regulation that has been used is verbal mediation. This technique uses external cues to guide the organization and expression of thoughts (Luria, 1963). In one preliminary study, three subjects with executive function deficits were trained to use verbal mediation (Nicol and Raskin, 1997). One had severe brain injury, one moderate, and the third had mild traumatic brain injury. Although the individual with MTBI did not demonstrate improvement on standard test scores of executive functioning, he did demonstrate improvement on measures of functioning in his daily life. The technique used was to provide subjects with specific overt cues such as, "What is the problem I need to solve?" Once subjects were able to use these cues, they were instructed to say them very softly to themselves. Finally, they were instructed to think them without vocalization.

Generalization of Training

Given the complexity and range of executive functions and the limitations of formal psychometric assessment for these functions, it is a challenge to adequately capture their impact on everyday functioning. The Pro-Ex (Braswell et al., 1992) was designed to assess executive functions in the individual's daily life. It provides a structured method for the clinician to rate the individual's behavior in interview or in naturalistic settings on a number of scales. The scales included in this measure are Goal Selection, Planning/Sequencing, Initiation, Execution, Timesense, Awareness of Deficits, and Self-Monitoring. Individuals are measured in each of these areas on a seven point Likert-type scale, which serves to focus and make more explicit observations about different aspects of executive functioning in everyday contexts. It can be used by different clinicians in different settings, where behavioral demands and environmental controls and cues are quite different. These measurements can then be used to plan appropriate treatment strategies, educate the individual and significant others about the ways in which the brain injury is affecting functioning, and measure the efficacy of treatment. One example of a Pro-Ex scale is provided in Appendix B (Braswell et al., 1992).

Once training has been completed, there are generally two approaches to generalization training. The first is to apply the newly trained skills in the individual's own environment. If planning has been the focus of the session, the person is given specific tasks from their daily life to plan and carry out. Careful data is taken by significant others or by home-based therapists and feedback provided that is analogous to that given in the clinic. The second approach is to train the concept of generalization as an executive function skill. Individuals are first taught to recognize similarities and differences between simple objects and then work through a hierarchy until they are able to recognize similarities and differences in activities of daily life. In this way, they are able to recognize those activities that require the remediation strategies they have learned. An example of such a hierarchy is presented in Appendix C.

Case Studies

Case 1.

This case is one of poor impulse control. MN is a 43-year old right-handed woman. She was in a motor vehicle accident when the car turning left in front of her struck her car. She struck her head on the windshield and sustained a bruise to her right frontal forehead. She did not lose consciousness but was slightly dazed and disoriented for approximately $1^1/_2$ hours. She reported that for approximately 1 month after the accident she felt easily overwhelmed, and had difficulty dealing with more than one thing at a time. She was self-employed as a massage therapist and had to cut back the number of clients she was able to see. Her prior medical history was unremarkable. She presented for neuropsychological evaluation approximately 6 months following the motor vehicle accident. On testing, she exhibited superior range intellectual functioning. However, she demonstrated inconsistencies in her scores on tests of complex attention and concentration. She was noted to be easily distracted by nonsalient interfering information. In addition, she was experiencing symptoms of a severely anxious depression.

Cognitive remediation was initiated shortly after the neuropsychological evaluation. Her initial goals of treatment were focused on providing support and counsel in dealing with her profile of cognitive strengths and difficulties, and interpreting difficulties that arose each week. This tactic was chosen given the large amount of emotional distress she was experiencing. It is not unusual to need to spend some initial time on validation and support. Sessions were conducted for 1 hour each week.

At approximately 1 year following the MTBI, MN was reporting considerably less emotional distress. She continued to be able to see only approximately one-half of the clients she had seen premorbidly, but she was beginning to feel more in control of her difficulties and more able to predict problematic situations. At this time, the focus of treatment turned to reducing the frequency of impulsive behaviors, as she found these particularly distressing. For example, on one occasion, she noticed some furniture on the street. She assumed that it was being discarded, and began to collect pieces that she liked. At that point, the owners arrived, as they were merely in the midst of moving. This demonstrates her lack of ability to adequately evaluate a situation and generate a series of hypotheses before acting.

Treatment then consisted of presenting her with a series of ambiguous situations and asking her to provide three possible interpretations that matched all of the facts of the situation. Her time to complete these tasks was also measured and she was instructed to be sure to take sufficient time to be able to consider all of the facts provided. Data on her accuracy is provided in Figure 6.1. Time series analysis revealed that her improvement on this task was significant.

Case 2.

NO is a 34-year-old, right-handed man. He has a B.A. degree and worked for the Park Service. He was a pedestrian crossing the street when he was struck by a delivery van. He lost consciousness for ap-

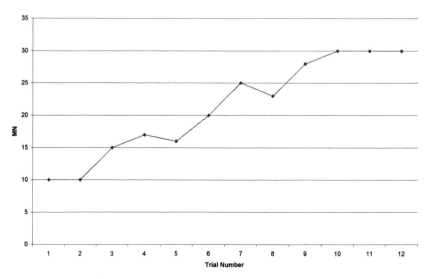

Figure 6-1 Improvement on problem-solving task.

proximately 5 minutes and then experienced posttraumatic confusion for approximately 2 hours. He received a left forehead laceration. Computerized tomography scan of the brain was normal. He was seen for neuropsychological evaluation approximately 6 months after the accident. At that time he complained of headache, concentration and memory deficits, and word-finding difficulties. On formal testing he was found to have cognitive abilities within normal limits in all functions, except for deficits in memory and learning. He was referred for cognitive remediation.

The initial cognitive remediation session occurred approximately 9 months after the accident. He was initially asked to keep a log for 1 week of difficulties encountered with his memory in his daily life. Analysis of the log revealed that his difficulties were due not solely to memory, but to difficulty with planning. He would often make lists of things to do, but then become overwhelmed when faced with the task itself and not know where to begin. He was an extremely active person and often had a list of several projects at his home to complete.

The first phase of treatment involved use of the Tower of Hanoi on a computer program. The task was initially set at five rings and he was unable to do this task in less than 200 moves. Verbal mediation strategies were attempted. These data are shown in Figure 6.2. As can be seen, despite repeated sessions of telling himself what to do with the task and how to analyze it, he was unable to improve

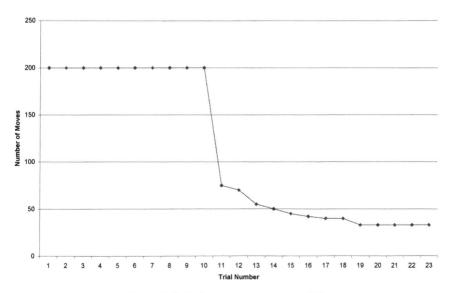

Figure 6-2 Performance on tower of Hanoi.

his performance. At this point, treatment was changed to present him with the same task but with three rings. He was able to solve this quickly and accurately. Next he was presented with four rings and again was able to solve this. He stated that with only four rings, he could "see" the steps at once, without having to hold information in his mind. Next, he performed the task at four rings and five rings alternatively. In this way he was able to use what he had done with four rings to guide his performance with five rings. After 12 sessions of this, he was able to solve the task consistently in 31 moves.

The final phase involved picking one task to complete at home each week. The tasks were first broken into their component steps in session. The steps were then arranged into their appropriate order and materials required listed with each step. In this way he was able to successfully complete one task each week for 4 weeks (e.g., make jam, smoke salmon, build a lamp). During the final 4 weeks of treatment he was merely told to perform one task each week and keep a log of his errors. These tasks were all successfully completed with two or fewer errors.

Conclusions

A variety of approaches have been discussed with reference to the treatment of individuals with executive deficits. In general, they involve moving from simple structured activities with significant external cuing and support to more complex, multistep activities in which external support is gradually reduced and internal support or self-direction is enhanced. Although a variety of articles have suggested success in using these techniques, there are as yet a very small number of cases and a limited number of studies in which such techniques have been experimentally manipulated. Clearly, more work in this area is needed. In addition to the more formal intervention procedures, some generic interventions should not be forgotten. Certainly, education of the family and significant others in how to respond to a person with such injuries is important. Often, an appreciation for the organic or nonvolitional nature of the behavior is helpful in alleviating fears and misconceptions. For example, poor initiation is often confused with poor motivation. As many different terms can be used to describe these behaviors and capacities, it is important to use consistent language and understandable terminology. Repetition will be a key factor and no matter what kind of intervention is utilized, whether it be restorative or compensatory, multiple opportunities for practice must be incorporated into the treatment program. Finally, it is vital that clinicians actively train for generalization.

Individuals with executive function compromise pose one of the greatest challenges to clinicians and to the rehabilitation system. In the last decade, we have made great strides in understanding at least some of the many multifaceted functions of the frontal lobes. With greater knowledge and understanding, we should be able to identify, develop, apply, and test specific interventions to mediate the effect of frontal system impairments. More so than physical limitations, or even many other cognitive impairments, executive function compromise has the potential to disrupt and limit an individual's capacity for independent, meaningful, and socially integrated functioning. Strides that we make in the understanding and treatment of the impairments will be valuable and rewarding to individuals with brain injury, their families, and society.

References

Barco, P., Crosson, B., Bolesta, M., Werts, D., and Stout, R. (1991). Training awareness and compensation in postacute head injury rehabilitation. In J. Kreutzer and P. Wehman (Eds.), *Cognitive Rehabilitation for Persons with Traumatic Brain Injury: A Functional Approach*. Baltimore, MD: Paul H. Brookes Publishing Co., pp. 129–146.

Barth, J., Macciocchi, and Giordani, B. (1983). Neuropsychological sequelae of minor head injury. *Neurosurgery, 13*, 529–532.

Bayless, J., Varney, N., and Roberts, R. (1989). Tinker Toy Test performance and vocational outcome in patients with closed head injuries. *Journal of Clinical and Experimental Neuropsychology, 11*, 913–917.

Bender, L. (1938). A visual motor gestalt test and its clinical use. *American Orthopsychiatric Association Research Monographs, No. 3*.

Benton, A., Hamsher, K., Varney, N., and Spreen, O. (1983). *Contributions to Neuropsychological Assessment*. New York, NY: Oxford University Press.

Braswell, D., Hartry, A., Hoornbeek, S., Johansen, A., Johnson, L., Schultz, J., and Sohlberg, M. (1992). *Profile of Executive Control System*. Puyallup, WA: Association for Neuropsychological Research and Development.

Broderbund Software Inc. (1990). Where in the World Is Carmen Sandiego? San Rafael, CA.

Cicerone, K., and Wood, J. (1987). Planning disorder after closed head injury: A case study. *Archives of Physical Medicine and Rehabilitation, 68*, 111–115.

Cicerone, K., and Giacino, J. (1992). Remediation of executive function deficits after traumatic brain injury. *NeuroRehabilitation, 2*(3), 12–22.

Cohen, N., and Corkin, S. (1981). The amnesic patient. H.M.: Learning and retention of cognitive skill. *Society for Neuroscience Abstracts, 7*, 517–518.

Compedia Inc. (1992). Advanced Thinking Games. Top Class.

Drake, A., Yoder, S., Gramling, L., and Bloom, J. (1998). Patient versus family ratings of behavioral and emotional changes associated with frontal lobe damage following mild traumatic brain injury. Paper presented at the International Neuropsychological Society, Honolulu, HI.

Flowers, K.A., and Robertson, C. (1985). The effect of Parkinson's disease on the ability to maintain a mental set. *Journal of Neurosurgical Psychiatry, 48*(6), 517–529.

Getzels, J.W., and Jackson, P.W. (1962). *Creativity and Intelligence*. New York, NY: John Wiley and Sons.

Goldberg, E., and Bilder, R.M. (1986). Neuropsychological perspectives: Retrograde amnesia and executive deficits, In L.W. Poon (Ed.), *Handbook for Clinical Memory Assessment of Older Adults*. Washington DC: American Psychological Association, pp. 55–68.

Good Samaritan Hospital (1989). *Executive functions: Model and Management*. Unpublished handbook.

Goodglass, H., and Kaplan, E. (1972). *Assessment of Aphasia and Related Disorders*. Philadelphia, PA: Lea and Febiger.

Gorham, D. (1956) A Proverbs Test for clinical and experimental use. *Psychological Reports, Monograph Supplement No. 1, 2*, 1–12.

Grant, D., and Berg, E. (1948). A behavioral analysis of degree of reinforcement and ease of shifting to new responses in a Weigl-type card-sorting problem. *Journal of Experimental Psychology, 38*, 404–411.

Hart, T., and Jacobs, H. (1993). Rehabilitation and management of behavioral disturbances following frontal lobe injury. *Journal of Head Trauma Rehabilitation, 8*, 1–12.

Jones-Gotman, M., and Milner, B. (1977). Design fluency: The invention of nonsense drawings after focal cortical lesions. *Neuropsychologia, 15*(4–5), 653–674.

Kay, T. (1992). Neuropsychological diagnosis: Disentangling the multiple determinants of functional disability after mild traumatic brain injury. In L. Horn and N. Zasler (Eds.), *Rehabilitation of Post-Concussive Disorders. Physical Medicine and Rehabilitation: State of the Art Reviews, 6*, 109–127.

Leninger, B., Gramling, S., and Farrell, A. (1990). Neuropsychological deficits in symptomatic minor head injury patients after concussion and mild concussion. *Journal of Neurology, Neurosurgery, and Psychiatry, 53*, 293–296.

Lezak, M. (1982). The problem of assessing executive function. *International Journal of Psychology, 17*, 281–297.

Lezak, M. (1993). Newer contributions to the neuropsychological assessment of executive functions. *Journal of Head Trauma Rehabilitation, 8*, 24–31.

Luria, A. (1963). *Restoration of Function after Brain Injury*. New York, NY: Pergamon Press.

Martzke, J., Swan, C., and Varney, N. (1991). Post traumatic anosmia and orbital frontal damage: Neuropsychological and neuropsychiatric correlates. *Neuropsychology, 5*, 213–225.

Milner, B. (1982). Some cognitive effects of frontal lobe lesions in man. *Philosophic Transactions of the Royal Society of London, B298*, 211–226.

Nicol, T., and Raskin, S. (1997). Use of verbal mediation in individuals with executive function deficits. Poster presented at the Cognitive Neuroscience Society, Boston, MA.

Norman, D., and Shallice, T. (1980). Attention to action: Willed and automatic control of behavior. *Center for Human Information Processing Technical Report, 99*.

Porteus, S.D. (1965). Porteus Maze Test. Fifty years' application. New York, NY: Psychological Corporation.

Raskin, S., and Gordon, W. (1992a). Implications of various disorders of awareness for memory and remediation. Presented at the International Neuropsychological Society meeting, San Diego, CA.

Raskin, S., and Gordon, W. (1992b). The impact of different approaches to cognitive remediation on generalization. *NeuroRehabilitation, 2*(3), 38–45.

Raskin, S., and Rearick, E. (1996). Verbal Fluency in Individuals with Mild Traumatic Brain Injury. *Neuropsychology, 10*, 416–422.

Rattock (1990). Master Thinking. Medisoft, New York.

Ruff, R.M., Light, R.H., and Evans, R.W. (1987). The Ruff Figural Fluency Test: A normative study with adults. *Developmental Neuropsychology, 3*, 37–52.

Shallice, T. (1982). Specific impairments in planning. *Philosophic transactions of the Royal Society of London, 298*, 199–209.

Shallice, T., and Burgess, P. (1991). Deficits in strategy application following frontal lobe damage in man. *Brain, 114*, 727–741.

Shallice, T., and Evans, M. (1978). The involvement of the frontal lobes in cognitive estimation. *Cortex, 14*, 294–303.

Sohlberg, M., Mateer, C., and Stuss, D. (1992). Contemporary approaches to the management of executive control dysfunction. *Journal of Head Trauma Rehabilitation, 8*(1), 45–58.

Stuss, D. (1991). Disturbance of self-awareness after frontal system damage. In G. Prigatano and D. Schacter. (Eds.), *Awareness of Deficit After Brain Injury*. New York, NY: Oxford University Press.

Stuss, D.T., and Benson, D.F. (1986). *The Frontal Lobes*. New York, NY: Raven Press.

Stuss, D., and Gow, C. (1992). "Frontal dysfunction" after traumatic brain injury. *Neuropsychiatry, Neuropsychology, and Behavioral Neurology, 5*, 272–282.

Varney, N. (1991). Iowa Collateral Head Injury Interview 1989. *Neuropsychology, 5*, 223–225.

Varney, N., and Menefee, L. (1993). Psychosocial and executive deficits following closed head injury: Implications for orbital frontal cortex. *Journal of Head Trauma Rehabilitation, 8*, 32–44.

von Cramon, D., and Mattes-von Cramon, G. (1990). Frontal lobe dysfunction in patients-Therapeutical approaches. In R. Wood and I. Fussey (Eds.), *Cognitive Rehabilitation in Perspective*. London: Taylor and Francis.

Wechsler, D. (1974). Wechsler Memory Scale Manual. San Antonio, TX: The Psychological Corporation.

Yarnell, P., and Rossie, G. (1988). Minor whiplash head injury with major debilitation. *Brain Injury, 2*, 255–258.

APPENDIX A

This handout was prepared at Good Samaritan Center for Continuing Rehabilitation in Puyallup, Washington, to provide education on the effects of frontal lobe injury.

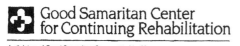 Good Samaritan Center for Continuing Rehabilitation

A division of Good Samaritan Community Healthcare

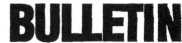 **BULLETIN**

Frontal Lobe Injury

Catherine A. Mateer, PhD, ABPP,
Diplomate in Clinical Neuropsychology

The frontal lobes, constituting large portions of the cerebral cortex just behind the forehead, are the most recently developed part of the brain in an evolutionary sense and are the latest to develop in the maturing individual. It has been well established that this region has rich connections to many other parts of the brain, but only in recent years has their importance begun to be appreciated. The frontal lobes function to organize and regulate behavior necessary to accomplishment. They are critical to the so-called "executive functions" of anticipation, goal selection, planning, self-monitoring, use of feedback, and completion of purposeful activities. The frontal lobes are also critical to the selection and control of socially relevant behavior.

Impairment of any or all of these abilities may be present in spite of strong intellectual skills and apparently unaffected language function. As a result, individuals with frontal lobe deficits presents a perplexing and frustrating paradox to professional and layperson alike. In very severe cases, individuals with frontal injury may appear to lose all ambition, even failing to begin or complete activities associated with grooming and hygiene. In less severe cases, they may have trouble getting started on routine tasks, preparing a simple meal, keeping appointments, managing finances, following a sequence of directions, and maintain-

ing attention to tasks or situations which involve judgement, social reasoning and inventive problem solving. They may engage in repeated activities which are seemingly irrelevant to the situation at hand, failing to notice that they are making errors or to "learn from their mistakes". In short, people who have executive function impairments cannot readily put their energy and intelligence to work without assistance.

Causes of Injury

Injury to the frontal lobes may result from disease or from trauma. Strokes, meningitis, and any event which temporarily results in a lack of oxygen—such as drowning or cardiac arrest—may result in damage to frontal lobe mechanisms which underlie the executive functions. The frontal lobes are very susceptible to traumatic injury due to their position in the brain. Uneven bony surfaces overlay the frontal lobes and are adjacent to the frontal pole. Blows from the front, back or side of the head can all result in frontal lobe injury. Even a whiplash-type injury without an actual blow to the head, may result in bruising of the forebrain.

Consequences of Frontal Lobe Injury

The major role of the frontal lobes is the regulation of behavior. They coordinate attention, memory, language, perception, motor functions and social behavior as we go about

our daily living and vocational activities. In short, they put the human machine to work. When their function is impaired, all of the other cognitive systems are affected, even though they may remain individually intact. The frontal lobes have been likened to the pilot of a Boeing 747, without whom millions of dollars worth of highly complex technology would sit idle at the airport. Recognition and appreciation of these deficits is critical to rehabilitation efforts with the closed head injured population. These deficits can be classed generally and include:

- *Problems of Starting* - This may manifest as decreased spontaneity and initiation. Such individuals seem to lack motivation and may sit silently without apparent interest in or curiosity about surroundings until they are directed to do something.

- *Difficulties in Making Mental or Behavioral Shifts* - This includes rigidity or perseveration on a single idea or a single action. Individuals with these problems may be able to successfully verbalize solutions to problems, including plans necessary to meet goals successfully, yet be unable to put any plan into effective action.

- *Difficulties with Attention* - Individuals with frontal lobe deficits are often "captured" by extraneous aspects of a task. As a result, they may demonstrate behaviors which seem irrelevant, even bizarre, to the observer. Because they may be highly distractible, they often seem to shift focus continually, never arriving at a point which seems purposeful.

- *Problems in Stopping* - This may manifest as a more general deficit in self-monitoring. It may present as impulsivity or a quickness to anger, speaking too loudly, or carrying a joke or sexual innuendo too far.

- *Problems with Social Awareness* - This category would include deficits in the ability to appreciate the impact one makes on others, sometime resulting in rude or insensitive behavior or with a general lack of apparent concern about social conventions.

- *Deficient Self-Awareness* - Defective self-criticism may be associated with a tendency to be self-satisfied, to experience little

or no anxiety, and to fail to appreciate the existence and practical implications of deficits (limited insight).

- *A Concrete Attitude* - Some patients with frontal lobe lesions retain high-level conceptual abilities, but demonstrate a day to day literal-mindedness and loss of perspective.

Assessment and Treatment of Frontal Lobe Deficits

The assessment of frontal lobe functions poses a challenge. Stuss and Benson (1987) have stated correctly that "The commonly used neuropsychological test batteries are useful as screening tests but are not yet competent tools for detecting independent frontal lobe functions...". In addition, the very action of structuring a performance situation and defining expectations may effectively "bypass" the individual's need for frontal lobe involvement and thus mask problems in this area. Nevertheless, there are a variety of neuropsychological measures which are

known to be sensitive to frontal lobe deficits and a variety of qualitative aspects of performance which can suggest problems with this area. In all such cases careful observation and structured interview of both the individual and those around them is essential to the accurate diagnosis of frontal lobe deficits.

Effective rehabilitation of the brain injured adult demands recognition and development of approaches to work with frontal lobe dysfunction. Although clinicians are just now laying the groundwork in this area, most of the literature stresses the importance of providing structure, making expectations clear, providing immediate feedback about performance, and providing appropriate cueing to prompt either direct action or self-monitoring. Information and education about the consequences of frontal lobe dysfunction may be the most important tool in increasing family members' awareness and understanding of these disorders.

References

Lezak, M. (1983) *Neuropsychological Assessment*, Oxford University Press, New York.

Mesulum, M. (1985)*Principles of Behavioral Neurology*, F.A. Davis, Philadelphia.

Prigatano, G. et.al. (1986) *Neuropsychological Rehabilitation After Brain Injury*, John Hopkins University Press, Baltimore.

Sohlberg, M. M. & Mateer, C A. (1989) *Introduction to Cognitive Rehabilitation (Chapter 10; Remediation of Executive Function Impairments)*, *Guilford Press, New York.*

Strub, R. and Black, F.W. (1981) *Organic Brain Syndromes*, F.A. Davis, Philadelphia

Stuss, D.T. and Benson, F.D. (1986) *The Frontal Lobes*, Raven Press, New York.

© *Center for Cognitive Rehabilitation, July, 1987, Updated: August, 1990*

APPENDIX B

An example of one scale from the Profile of Executive Control System. This is a clinical evaluation of executive functions developed at the Good Samaritan Hospital in Puyallup, Washington.

Good Samaritan Hospital

Center for Continuing Rehabilitation

Profile of Executive Control System

PRO-EX

Patient Name: _____

Date of evaluation_____ Date of Birth

_____ Date of Injury _____

Context of Evaluation

Interview:

Name/Relationship of Person

Interviewed_____

Amount/Nature of Contact with

Patient_____

Observation:

Setting of

Observation(s)_____

Evaluator/Relationship to

Patient_____

Amount of Prior Contact with

Patient_____

Circle highest letter that best describes level of
functioning.

I.   <u>Goal Selection:</u>   Refers only to ability to
                          select a goal, not the ability
                          to actually achieve a goal.

   A.   Unable to indicate any goal

   B.   Only expresses goals to increase
        physiological comfort (e.g., verbalizes need
        to eat when hungry or cool off when hot)

   C.   Expresses feasible, short-term goals for
        highly desired actions (e.g., talks about
        needing to use phone to call family)

D.   Often expresses unfeasible goals (e.g., although unable to transfer independently, predicts s/he will walk by end of the week)

E.   Expresses feasible short-term goals for less desired activities; occasionally expresses intentions that are unrealistic (e.g., announces intentions to call mom to bring splint; occasionally expresses vocational goals that are not reasonable given limitations)

F.   Expresses feasible, short-term and long-term goals for moderately complex activities (e.g., talks about need to open a checking account in the area)

G.   Expresses feasible, complex, long-term goals (e.g., describes need to save money to make adaptation on car to accommodate physical disability when driving privileges restored)

Comments: _____

_____

_____

_____

Treatment Plan: _____

_____

APPENDIX C

An example from one patient of a hierarchy of training used to train generalization.

Hierarchy of Generalization Training

Level 1: Simple abstracting tasks, such as presenting three geometric shapes and determining which two are most alike.

Level 2: Abstracting tasks using semantic material, such as which two of three animals are most alike (where two are pets and one is a jungle animal).

Level 3: Learning to recognize similarities and differences between activities (for example, learning to recognize which two of the following three activities requires money; which two of the following three activities take more than an hour; etc.)

Level 4: Everyday difficulties—which of the following problems could use a particular solution.

Level 5: Problems are presented in session and possible solutions must be generated.

Level 6: A daily log of problems encountered in daily life is taken and spontaneous ability to solve problems is scored.

III

TREATMENT OF EMOTIONAL SEQUELAE

7

Psychotherapy Approaches

MCKAY MOORE SOHLBERG

It is now well recognized that the behavioral and psychological effects of mild traumatic brain injury (MTBI) can be the most enduring and debilitating (e.g., Andrasik and Wincze, 1994; Lezak, 1987; Rosenthal and Bond, 1990). This is particularly well illustrated by some MTBI patients who experience significant functional disability in spite of relatively minor physical and neuropsychological symptoms (Fann et al., 1993). Such persons may present years after injury with pronounced emotional distress and a lesser capacity for self-motivated work, but with minimal, if any, "objective" organic bases for their problems (Mateer, 1992). The complex interaction between biologic, psychological, and environmental variables poses a significant challenge to the assessment and management of these difficulties (Blanchard et al., 1995; Kay, 1993; Mateer, 1992).

The types of psychosocial, emotional, and self-regulatory complaints often vary according to the stage of postrecovery (Fann et al., 1995). This chapter focuses primarily on psychosocial and emotional issues that are common at later phases. Mateer (1992) describes the characteristic psychological problems in MTBI as emerging after patients' and/or caregivers experience prolonged inefficiencies in cognitive function and when self-confidence and preinjury productivity diminish. There may be changes such as irritability, frustration, depression, and anxiety with concomitant damage to relationships with family, friends, and colleagues.

Kay (1993) defines the primary psychological factors stemming from MTBI as those internal responses (which may have existed premorbidly or occurred as a reaction to or direct result from the injury) that affect a person's ability to function after a seemingly mild injury. These can include personality style, affective status, sense of self, social/environmental support and response to being in litigation.

"The lack of systematic medical explanation and management of their symptoms appeared to be contributing to increasingly dysfunctional scenarios. Discharged patients attempted to resume functional activities, failed, sought additional medical guidance (which did not constructively address their symptoms), and then became embroiled in cycles of failure, frustration, loss of confidence, anxiety, avoidance, depression, and eventual isolation, social alienation, and unemployment." (Kay, 1993, p. 375)

The Best Approaches to Managing Behavioral, Emotional, and Psychosocial Issues

Several approaches to the brain injury population have been taken, including behavioral interventions (Burke and Wesolowski, 1988; Wood, 1987), cognitive–behavioral therapy (Davis and Goldstein, 1994), and a variety of other forms of individual psychotherapy (Bock, 1987; Christensen and Rosenberg, 1991; Crossen, 1987; Prigatano, 1991). Behavior therapy is most useful when the goal is to decrease specific target behaviors such as aggression, or in systematic desensitization to anxiety provoking stimuli. Some examples of application are provided in Chapters 9 and 10.

Cognitive Therapy

Cognitive therapy is an active, directive, and time-limited approach, that assumes problems are caused, at least in part, by dysfunctional thoughts. Cognitive therapy focuses on identifying the aspects of these thoughts that are irrational and challenging the cognitive distortions with more rational thinking. Techniques include monitoring the negative thoughts, learning to recognize the connections between these thoughts, their feelings and behavior, examining evidence for and against the distorted thoughts, substituting more realistic interpretations, and learning to identify and alter the dysfunctional beliefs that distort a person's experiences (Beck, 1976). See Chapter 8 for a more detailed discussion of this approach.

Multimodal Approaches

Determining the source of functional disability after MTBI can be the most challenging part of developing a treatment plan. Problems might result from changes in brain functioning, from a reaction to real or perceived changes in ability across different domains, or from an interaction of these with premorbid personality style, methods of coping, and psychosocial history. Problems may respond best to different treatment strategies, depending on their origin. If, for example, an individual is experiencing anger-management problems due to damage to those brain mechanisms involved in impulse control, a therapist might implement behavioral interventions such as those described in Chapter 10. Alternatively, if the anger problems primarily stem from identity issues or discrepancies between perceptions of one's premorbid and postinjury self, a combination of education and counseling to increase adjustment may be most appropriate. If, before injury, the person was an overachiever with perfectionistic tendencies, there may also be a role for stress reduction and a more realistic framing of the problem. To develop an appropriate plan, the therapist needs to be grounded in both brain-behavior relationships, the nature of traumatic brain injury, and in traditional counseling methods.

Ruff et al. (1996) describe management of behavioral and emotional factors in four individuals with MTBI who demonstrated preexisting personality traits that compounded their symptom presentations. Whether psychosocial problems represent primary symptoms of the brain injury, secondary reactions, or preexisting traits, the clinician will need a variety of "tools" from which to choose in order to treat this population effectively.

Andrasik and Wincze (1994) describe a biopsychosocial approach that includes behavioral methods such as coping skills, training, and biofeedback, cognitive intervention, and family and individual counseling. It is well recognized that intervention intended to remediate *physical* problems (e.g., biofeedback, relaxation training targeting headaches) may also have emotional benefits (e.g., perceived increase in personal control). The current author has also frequently observed the emotional benefits of *cognitive* intervention. For example, if patients perceive their attention abilities are improving via attention training, many emotional symptoms (e.g., irritability, anxiety, feeling out of control or overwhelmed) appear to lessen.

Groups

Many survivors with MTBI report the desire for validation and knowledge that their symptoms are not unique. A group can provide such functions that may not occur in one-to-one rehabilitation settings. Functions served include (1) education and information, (2) regular opportunities for group discussions to share issues of mutual interest and concern, and (3) a vehicle to develop communication, share resources, and form a social network. Groups allow for frank sharing of feelings, mutuality of support, and friendship bonds. The small-group format has been shown to provide a temporary community in which individuals can be understood by peers (Yalom and Vinogradov, 1988). Recent literature in the use of group therapy and peer groups indicates their value in many populations. Group therapy has been described as beneficial in the TBI community both for group education and generalized problem-solving, and for group counseling to solve individual problems of group members. Members often reported receiving a reduction in social isolation, validation of their own experiences, and support as they began to understand the changes that had occurred in their life and to face the options available for their future.

Groups can take several forms. We have used two different types of groups with survivors of MTBI. The first type of group is a more traditional support group. In this group survivors came to monthly meetings whenever they felt a desire to do so. Typically there would be 15 to 20 members present, but no requirements were placed on attendance. A topic was picked for discussion each week. (A list of sample topics is provided in Appendix A). This was done for several reasons. The first was to allow group members to think about the topic in the preceding month, gather their thoughts, and write down important ideas. The other was to provide some focus to the group so that it did not become too difficult for members to follow the discussion. Each group initiated with introductions. We generally found it helpful to allow 10 minutes for new members to introduce themselves and 5 minutes for returning members. This kept members on track rather than feeling they needed to go into lengthy descriptions of their life history. This type of group has also spontaneously decided to work on legislative issues or to regularly distribute TBI literature in emergency room and neurology department waiting areas. At the end of approximately 2 years, the group was asked to rate their experience on the form presented in Appendix B. As can be seen in Table 7.1, this group felt that the group experience was helpful for short-term gains, but did not promote long-term change.

The second type of group was more insight oriented. This group had only approximately five to seven members. The group was closed so that new members were not permitted, in order to allow members to begin to

Table 7-1 The two groups on the self-report questionnaire in Appendix A.

	Mean (Standard Deviation)	
	Small, Insight-oriented	Large, Support
Insight	4.00	3.51
	(0.13)	(2.72)
Give feedback	4.33	3.62
	(0.52)	(2.12)
Receive feedback	4.67	3.62
	(0.12)	(1.79)
Self-esteem	4.67	2.38
	(0.54)	(2.57)
Socialize	4.33	2.75
	(0.36)	(2.79)
Depression	4.00	2.87
	(0.11)	(2.91)
Anxiety	4.00	3.38
	(1.00)	(2.01)

feel comfortable with each other. Each member was also asked to make a commitment to attend each month. Each session typically began with a check-in so that members could bring each other up to date and discuss pressing issues. Each member also provided the group with an issue that was of importance to them (e.g., being a better listener, being less impulsive, being more independent). The other group members were then asked to help the person examine the events of their life in the past month in terms of this issue. Table 7.1 presents the data from this group as well. Compared to the less structured group, these members reported more lasting changes, particularly in self-esteem and the ability to receive feedback.

Assessment Models for Guiding the Development of Psychological Interventions

The development of an individualized psychotherapeutic treatment plan begins with conducting a thorough assessment. Three assessment models are reviewed in this section.

P-I-E-O Concept

One conceptual model that continues to be useful in organizing an assessment of psychosocial functioning is proposed by Sbordone (1990). He suggests that it is important for clinicians to understand the person-injury-environment-outcome (P-I-E-O) interaction. The components of the model are described below:

- *Person*: The background of the individual who sustained the injury, including his/her history of achievements, specific intellectual skills or deficits, academic skills, social and behavioral skills, support system, personality style, stress management skills, and unique biological factors such as age, sex, and previous medical history.
- *Injury*: The injury variables such as severity, any loss of consciousness, or posttraumatic amnesia.
- *Environment*: The demands that the family and environment place on the patient after the injury. This component includes such factors as the degree of structure in the environment, financial–insurance resources, vocational, academic, and household responsibilities, previous commitments, financial burdens and responsibilities, etc.
- *Outcomes*: The specific successes or failures that a person experiences following the injury including such events as loss of relationships or job, inability to manage household affairs, etc.

Consideration of these four components may guide a clinician's assessment and subsequent planning of psychosocial intervention. Very similar interactive models have been put forward by Cicerone (1991), Lewis (1991), and Kay (1993).

The following profile of a patient who has sustained an MTBI illustrates application of the model. Before sustaining a brain injury in a motor vehicle accident, the patient was a high-achieving, driven individual whose identity was very much tied to her accomplishments (significant *person* variables). This information was gleaned through interview, review of academic/vocational/social history, and administration of a personality inventory. Interview and review of medical records suggested that relevant *injury* variables included the fact that there was no documented loss of consciousness, although the patient was disoriented to time and place when seen at the emergency room after the accident. When pursuing medical evaluation in follow-up, there were no neurologic findings supporting brain injury. A patient interview further suggested that important *environmental* variables were that the person attempted to return immediately to full-time employment and normal management of home responsibilities. Finally, review of medical records, phone interviews with the employer and significant other suggested that relevant *outcome* variables included the fact that the individual experienced headaches, decreased concentration, and problems with irritability following the injury. The patient had experienced several anger outbursts at work. She sought medical attention and was told that neurologically she appeared to have no residuals from the accident and was probably experiencing difficulties with stress management. Interview and a depression inventory further substantiated that the patient was feeling depressed and despondent.

Systematically considering each of the four components in Sbordone's (1990) model as a framework to organize assessment results thus revealed important information about the client: (1) She had a vulnerable personality preinjury (the "overachiever"). She may also have had perfectionstic tendencies and strong reactions to any imperfections she perceived in her work. These factors would put her at a higher risk for a dysfunctional response to a mild brain injury (Kay et al., 1992). (2) There was no hard evidence for an organic basis for her subjective complaints although emergency room records substantiated a significant blow to the head causing temporary disorientation. (3) She did not take any time to recover or gradually return to responsibilities. Thus, she may have experienced initial subtle but "real" impairments resulting in the development of negative emotional reactions. (4) She experienced significant "failure" since the accident without supportive education or intervention, resulting in loss of confidence, shaken identity, and depression. She may also have had a high stress level before the accident, and the additional stressors of the MTBI may have resulted in an overload, anxiety, and nonproductivity. Based on these findings the psychosocial plan might have included a plan to educate and support the individual and address the identity issues, while simultaneously recommending strategies to manage stress and real or perceived changes in attention/concentration (e.g., pacing, notetaking, etc.).

A combination of models is useful in guiding the psychosocial and emotional assessment and treatment planning for individuals with MTBI. The four components presented by Sbordone (1990) offer a clear taxonomy for categorizing information gleaned through interview, records review, formal psychosocial testing (e.g., personality or depression inventory), and neuropsychological or cognitive assessment. A complete assessment needs to evaluate each of the four components: person, injury, environment, and outcome. Kay's model (1993) stresses the influence and relative weight each neurologic, physical, and psychological factors have on functional outcome. It facilitates discernment between subjective and objective cognitive complaints. Superimposing Kay's (1992) dynamic view of assessment onto Sbordone's (1990) P-I-E-O taxonomy (i.e., evaluating the relationship between the four factors) can be profitable when developing psychosocial treatment plans after mild traumatic brain injury.

Intervention Strategies

Using the above assessment model may assist the clinician in organizing the results of an evaluation. When an assessment reveals that emotional and psychosocial and cognitive symptoms appear primarily neuropsychological in nature (i.e., a direct result of the brain injury), cognitive interventions such as those described in Chapters 4–6 may be the most effective. The interventions reviewed in the remainder of this chapter are designed for those patients whose psychosocial problems are *persistent* or do not appear to have a direct relationship to the patient's neurological status. This would include patients who do not receive initial intervention and develop negative emotional reactions in response to early symptoms that are not recognized, patients who exhibit a "shaken sense of self" (Kay, 1993), and/or patients whose *beliefs about their disability* may be discrepant with performance-based measures (Cicerone, 1991). All of these are consistent psychosocial profiles with a MTBI.

General clinical guidelines

Research carried out at the Research and Training Center on Head Trauma and Stroke at New York University Medical Center investigated the nature and treatment of functional disability after mild traumatic brain injury (Kay et al., 1992; Kay, 1992, 1993). Part of this work resulted in the development of clinical guidelines for treating the late management of persons with MTBI. These include the following:

1. Validate the experience of the person.
2. Do not prematurely confront emotional factors as primary.
3. Reestablish the shaken sense of self.
4. Involve the family.
5. Treat the emotional problems along with the cognitive problems.
6. Sort out primary from secondary deficits.

Cicerone (1991, 1992) discusses important components specific to the management of psychosocial issues after MTBI. Among his recommendations for patients whose cognitive symptoms are not primarily neuropsychologically based are the following:

1. Validate the *experience* that patients' report and encourage alternative *interpretations* of symptoms as appropriate.
2. Psychosocial treatment needs to reconcile any significant discrepancy between patients' own assessment of functioning and their performance-based competency.

Cicerone (1992) summarizes the goal of psychosocial therapy with persons who are challenged by MTBI by noting, "A common theme and 'final denominator' in psychotherapy after mild TBI will be the reconciliation of discrepancies among patients' own assessment of functioning and their performance-based competencies, sense of preinjury identity and ability, and their subjective expectations for future successful functioning."(p.139)

The remainder of this chapter offers some exercises and approaches to help structure and implement some of the therapy guidelines described above. They were developed in the mild brain injury program at Good Samaritan Hospital's Center for Continuing Rehabilitation and utilize an eclectic approach to psychosocial intervention as discussed previously.

Validating patients' experience

Clinical guidelines for working with individuals challenged by MTBI stress the importance of validating patients' experiences or reports of their symptoms. This is critical both for building a therapeutic alliance and for helping patients with some of the core identity issues resulting in a "shaken sense of self" or loss of confidence (e.g., Cicerone, 1992; Kay, 1993; Mateer, 1992). How does the therapist validate the patient's experience in a constructive manner (i.e., does not further focus on their deficits) that feels empathic yet not patronizing?

The current author has utilized the following three-step sequence with select MTBI patients when the goal is to ensure the patient feels validated. This is almost always an initial therapy objective for patients who have developed symptom maintenance or symptom magnification when they did not receive adequate explanation for their symptoms early after injury or who have experienced medical and/or social systems that minimized their problems.

1. *Interview Patient and Construct Most Troublesome Symptom List*: Taking time to foster an initial therapeutic relationship and establish a rapport characterized by trust and respect can be particularly important when treating persons with MTBI. Some patients may not perceive professionals as having recognized their symptoms, which heightens their vigilance toward their own symptoms and escalates their need for help (Cicerone, 1991). Beginning a therapeutic alliance by conducting an interview that allows patients to describe symptoms in an atmosphere where they do not feel they have to "convince" the therapist of the validity of their complaints can be extremely beneficial to being able to address emotional issues.

Such an atmosphere can be fostered when: (1) the therapist does not confront the patient early on about possible emotional underpinnings for reported physical and cognitive complaints; (2) the therapist offers options for explaining symptoms that include the possibility for an organic basis for symptoms; and (3) the therapist leaves the door open for improvement, but in a conservative manner that does not make the patient feel he or she will be "cured."

If the patient is being seen relatively soon after an injury, a number of preventative steps need to be taken including counseling the patient on a gradual return to work/school/home activities, and setting realistic time frames for symptom recovery. (See Kay, 1992.)

The following is an example of a therapist's summary statement during an interview designed to communicate validation and support:

> "You have mentioned a number of annoying symptoms with which you have had to cope since you fell. Although we don't fully understand why these problems occur, they are frequently reported by people who have had a fall such as yours. The good news is that most people can learn to manage the symptoms that persist so they do not get in the way of what they want to do. Once we identify those problems that are most troubling to you in your life, we will talk about options for addressing them. Right now I just want to make sure I have a good idea of what symptoms are bothering you the most."

Constructing a *Most Troubling Symptom List* (See Appendix C) may be a useful activity to assist with the interview process. The notion is to encourage the patient to prioritize those issues that interfere most with day-to-day functioning and to reflect on how she or he responds to them. The use of an established protocol may also assist in structuring the patient report to avoid "a stream of consciousness," where it is hard to discern needed information. In most cases, the recommendation would be to obtain the information via an interview format (vs. having the patient fill out the form independently). Hearing *how* the information is presented can be very important as to what is presented.

2. *Select Educational Materials.* An effective method for helping a patient feel validated while simultaneously increasing their knowledge about MTBI is to provide structured opportunities to review educational materials. The goal is to demonstrate to the patient that "experts" have written about issues with which they are personally confronted. The clinician can select written or visual materials containing helpful information for the patient. Example of materials might be a general article on MTBI written for survivors, families, or professionals, videotapes on different aspects of brain injury available from the Brain Injury Association (including one on MTBI called "The Unseen Injury"), or copies of pages from a book chapter that discusses topics germane to the patient. For example, the initial segment of Chapter 1 in this volume gives a general description of MTBI. The introductory paragraphs to articles or chapters often provide useful summaries of the nature of a specific problem. Alternatively, the clinician can construct a handout discussing different facets of MTBI. The therapist can then review the materials with the patient using some of the formats offered below.

3. *Structure Exercises to Personalize Educational Information.* After having selected the educational materials, the clinician will want to structure activities to enhance the validation experience. Examples of activities are listed below:

1. Giving assignments where the patient (*a*) summarizes the information, (*b*) writes down questions that the reading evokes, and/or (*c*) writes more paragraphs to go with the readings that specifically describe his or her situation;
2. Having the patient "present" the information to other patients in a group therapy situation, or to significant others.

The type of exercise that is selected will depend upon the needs of the particular patient. The psychosocial profile of the patient and stage in the treatment process will affect how the educational process might be carried out. Examples of assignments for individual patients are shown in Table 7.2.

Assisting patients with reconciling perceptions of past/present/future selves and abilities
As reviewed, some patients demonstrate discrepancies between their own assessment of their abilities and what their performance suggests about their capabilities. Similarly, patients may develop a distorted vision of their preinjury self and abilities. Such identity issues can interfere with the patient's expectations for the future. For example, displaying an inflated perception of their capabilities before injury is common for some patients, resulting in a catastrophic reaction to current problems. Symptom focus and symptom magnification are characteristic of patients with MTBI who exhibit difficulty reconciling perceptions of their self pre and post injury. Described below are two sample therapy activities to work on developing a more realistic and balanced sense of self.

Describing performance on activities at different phases
One activity that can be useful is to encourage patients to describe and/or predict how they would perform on a specific activity at different stages

Table 7-2 Exercise examples for different patient needs

Patient Displays	Therapy Exercise	Rationale
Loss of confidence; wonders if cognitive and physical symptoms indicate she is going crazy.	Patient reads general description of MTBI and underlines those symptoms that match the patient's personal experience.	Validate patient's symptoms as recognized problems after MTBI to help decrease secondary anxiety.
Unproductive focus on previous inadequate treatment by caregivers (i.e. displays excessive anger toward professionals that ignored problems).	Patient reads materials and develops handout for professionals to give future patients on signs and symptoms of MTBI.	Help patient begin to shift from a blaming mode to a management mode; provide constructive outlet for focus on problems.

pre and post injury. The therapist and the client begin by developing a list of specific activities that would be helpful in "exploring changes." Choosing discrete activities for which performance is measurable is important. Examples of activities might be performance on specific (1) cognitive activities such as academic or neuropsychological tests; (2) hobbies/recreational activities such as golf, woodworking, chess, knitting, etc.; (3) home management tasks such as balancing one's checkbook, cooking etc., and (4) work related tasks such as data entry, filing etc. Together the therapist and client fill out a protocol such as the one found in Appendix D. The patient describes the activity(ies) and offers an opinion for how she or he is currently performing on the task(s). The patient is also asked to look retrospectively and describe how she/he would have performed on the activity prior to the accident and 1 month after the accident. Finally, the patient is asked to anticipate performance in 1 year.

The therapist uses the above discussions to structure counseling by reviewing trends and encouraging a more balanced perspective between the different preinjury/postinjury "selves." For example, the therapist might note that the patient consistently describes a significant difference between perceptions of performance before the accident and current performance, with very high levels of achievement reported before the injury and consistently low levels reported for current performance. Having the patient focus on the interval of time right after the accident to the present time might be useful in helping such a patient appreciate improvement. Choosing a variety of activities to illustrate trends in the patient's perceptions is important. The goal is to increase the patient's awareness of how he or she is viewing changes and how these are affecting expectations by externalizing the perceptions. Implementing the activity at different phases in the rehabilitation process may also be useful.

Identifying residual strengths

Another activity that has been useful for patients is to construct a list of positive personal traits that have *not* changed because of the accident. Together the therapist and client fill out a list titled "Core Traits that Have Not Changed." These traits may include specific abilities such as math or writing skills as well as personality characteristics such as "being a caring person." The notion behind this task is to encourage the patient to build upon existing strengths and to decrease focus on symptoms. For some patients, it can be counterproductive to attempt to "cure" or even address "managing" persistent symptoms. For these patients, it may be most effective to validate their frustration with reported problems and to acknowledge the difficulty the symptoms present. Directing therapy at discussing how to exploit residual talents to achieve future goals (instead of addressing ongoing problems) can be a helpful way in which to approach treatment.

This type of exercise is most useful for those patients who are very invested in their symptoms and for whom validation, education, and counseling seem to result only in an increased symptom focus. The idea is for the therapist to "agree" with the patient about the gravity of the reported problems and to communicate that therapy will not reverse reported problems; instead it will be directed at maximizing preserved abilities as a vehicle to improve functioning. Sometimes this results in a reversed response by the patient and she/he actually begins to attempt to convince the therapist that the symptoms are manageable.

Behavior Modification

Another avenue for managing behavioral and emotional problems is to identify specific problem behaviors and feelings and to develop an individualized treatment plan. Examples of the types of areas that might be addressed include problems with stress, irritability, anger, and lability. This approach combines behavioral charting and monitoring techniques with counseling. The basic sequence of treatment is listed below:

Step 1. *Identify the Target Problem Behavior or Feeling.* This step will necessarily involve interviewing the patient and significant others and monitoring to determine the nature, frequency, and antecedents/consequences associated with the problem.

Step 2. *Generate a List of Options for Addressing the Problem.* During this phase the therapist describes and enumerates for the patient a variety of intervention options that might be helpful for coping with the identified problem. These might include both techniques to manage the response to a problem (e.g., stress management techniques for when a patient becomes confused) as well as specific compensatory techniques (e.g., a verbal mediation technique to decrease the onset of confusion).

Step 3. *Patient Selects Most Appropriate Option.* The idea in this step is that *the patient* reviews the list of options and selects the treatment approach she/he feels is most suited to her/his individual situation. The important factor is that the patient is given control over the selection to increase his or her investment in and comfort with the strategy's success. This process may involve modifying some treatment options.

Step 4. *Therapist Provides Training and Support for Implementing Treatment Strategy.* The patient receives information specific to how, when, and where to implement the selected treatment option. This phase of treatment may involve the patient and/or significant others completing incident logs and reports. The therapist may also develop some type of structured cuing system to remind the patient to implement the strategy (e.g., note in appointment book, reminder phone calls, reminder notes for refrigerator, etc.).

Step 5. *Encourage Independence and Self-Management of Symptom Behaviors.* The goal of this step is to make sure there are maintenance and generalization of the use of the strategy beyond the therapy environment. The therapist may gradually decrease the amount and type of cuing and decrease the frequency of visits, eventually placing the patient on a "follow-up" schedule.

Obviously, this approach to therapy is grounded in the principles of applied behavioral analysis, which have been described in depth in other sources (e.g., Wood, 1987). An important distinction, however, is the involvement of the patient in generating and selecting the specific treatment strategy. This helps the patient take responsibility for the success of the intervention. Involving the patient in the monitoring and reporting of the problem behavior or feeling is also important. Incorporating a self-evaluative approach for treatment strategies that the patient has endorsed as having potential to fit with his or her lifestyle/personality/abilities can be very affective for addressing some of the psychoemotional problems that tend to maintain emotional symptoms late after an injury.

The following case synopsis illustrates implementation of the above treatment sequence:

Case Study

A 33-year-old man sustained an MTBI in a work-related fall. After the fall he experienced a brief loss of consciousness but was not hospitalized. Before the accident the patient was a foreman for a construction crew. Neuropsychological testing completed several weeks after the fall suggested some reduced speed of information processing and difficulty with complex attention. The patient was seen 14 months after the injury for persistent complaints of irritability and anger management that were interfering with his performance at work.

Together the patient and therapist identified "anger outbursts" as the target behavior. The therapist spoke with the patient's employer and girlfriend who corroborated the patient's account of the problem. This information was carefully used to describe the nature and frequency of the outbursts. The therapist, with the patient, then generated a variety of options for managing the anger outbursts. This included the following: taking "time-outs" when the patient felt the onset of irritability; muscle relaxation techniques; use of relaxation tapes; self-talk strategies; deep breathing; visual imagery, etc. The different types of strategies were explained and listed for the patient. The patient felt that taking time-outs would work the best and would be possible at his particular job site. A more complete plan for taking time-outs was developed that included identifying the signals that precipitated the anger, and developing what the patient would say to his co-workers/peers when he implemented the time-out.

Therapy included actual practice carrying out the time-out strategy. The patient (and later his girlfriend) kept an "Anger Incident Log" on which anger incidents and time-out usage was documented. The therapist helped the patient write some reminder cue cards for his wallet, desk, and bathroom mirror. Therapy involved reviewing the incident logs, adjusting the technique as necessary, and gradually decreasing the therapist's involvement. The girlfriend and employer filled out "Anger Log Sheets" developed during therapy as requested by the patient. Eventually, the patient just received phone support for implementing the strategy. Other anger management strategies are provided in Chapter 10.

Summary

Persons with persistent behavioral, psychosocial, and emotional problems after MTBI can benefit from intervention that takes into account some of the idiosyncrasies specific to this population. Effective psychosocial therapy emanates from careful assessment of the variety of emotional, neuropsychological, environmental, and physical factors as well as the interplay between the relevant components. An eclectic repertoire of intervention approaches including behavioral and psychotherapy techniques as well as an understanding of the nature of MTBI is also important to delivering effective psychosocial therapy.

References

Andrasik, F., and Wincze, J. (1994). Emotional and psychosocial aspects of mild head injury. *Seminars in Neurology, 14*(1), 60–66.

Beck, A.T. (1976). *Cognitive Therapy and the Emotional Disorders.* New York, NY: International Universities Press.

Blanchard, E., Hickling, E., Taylor, A., and Loos, W. (1995). Psychiatric morbidity associated with motor vehicle accidents. *Journal of Nervous and Mental Disease, 183*(8), 495–504.

Bock, S.H. (1987). Psychotherapy of the individual with brain injury. *Brain Injury, 2,* 203–206.

Burke, W.H., and Wesolowski, M.D. (1988). Applied behavior analysis in head injury rehabilitation. *Rehabilitation Nursing, 13*(4), 186–188.

Christensen, A., and Rosenberg, N.K. (1991). A critique of the role of psychotherapy in brain injury rehabilitation. *Journal of Head Trauma Rehabilitation, 6*(4), 56–61.

Cicerone, K.D. (1991). Psychotherapy after mild traumatic brain injury: Relation to the nature and severity of subjective complaints. *Journal of Head Trauma Rehabilitation, 6*(4), 30–43.

Cicerone, K.D. (1992). Psychological management of post-concussive disorders. *Physical Medicine and Rehabilitation: State of the Art Reviews.* Philadelphia, PA: Hanley and Belfus, Inc., pp. 128–142.

Crossen, B. (1987). Treatment of interpersonal deficits for head-trauma patients in inpatient rehabilitation settings. *The Clinical Neuropsychologist, 1,* 335–352.

Davis, J.R., and Goldstein, G. (1994). Behavior therapy in brain injury rehabilitation. In A. Finlayson and S. Garner (Eds.), *Brain Injury Rehabilitation: Clinical Considerations.* Baltimore, MD: Williams and Wilkins.

Fann, J., Kayton, W., Uomoto, J., and Esselman, P. (1995). Psychiatric disorders and functional disability in outpatients with traumatic brain injury. *American Journal of Psychiatry, 152*(10), 1493–1499.

Kay, T. (1992). Neuropsychological diagnosis: Disentangling the multiple determinants of functional disability after mild traumatic brain injury. *Physical Medicine and Rehabilitation: State of the Art Reviews.* Philadelphia, PA: Hanley and Belfus, Inc., pp. 109–127.

Kay, T. (1993). Neuropsychological treatment of mild traumatic brain injury. *Journal of Head Trauma Rehabilitation, 8*(3), 74–85.

Kay, T., Newman, B., Cavallo, M., Ezrachi, O., and Resnick, M. (1992). Toward a neuropsychological model of functional disability after mild traumatic brain injury. *Neuropsychology, 6*(4), 371–384.

Lewis, L. (1991). A framework for developing a psychotherapy treatment plan with brain-injured patients. *Journal of Head Trauma Rehabilitation, 6*(4), 22–29.

Lezak, M.D. (1987). Relationships between personality disorders, social disturbances and physical disability following traumatic brain injury. *Journal of Head Trauma Rehabilitation, 2*(1), 57–69.

Mateer, C.A. (1992). Systems of care for post-concussive syndrome. *Physical Medicine and Rehabilitation: State of the Art Reviews.* Philadelphia, PA: Hanley and Belfus, Inc., pp. 143–160.

Prigatano, G.P. (1991). Disordered mind wounded soul: The emerging role of psychotherapy in rehabilitation after brain injury. *Journal of Head Trauma Rehabilitation, 6*(4), 1–10.

Rosenthal, M., and Bond, M.R. (1990). Behavioral and psychiatric sequelae. In M. Rosenthal, M. Griffith, M.R. Bond, and J.D. Miller (Eds.), *Rehabilitation of the Adult and Child with Traumatic Brain Injury* (2nd ed.) Philadelphia, PA: F.A. Davis, pp. 179–192.

Ruff, R.M., Camenzuli, L., and Mueller, J. (1996). Miserable minority: Emotional risk factors that influence the outcome of mild traumatic brain injury. *Brain Injury, 10*(8), 551–565.

Sbordone, R.J. (1990). Psychotherapeutic treatment of the client with traumatic brain injury: A conceptual model. In J.S. Kreutzer and P. Wehman (Eds.), *Community Integration Following Traumatic Brain Injury*. Baltimore, MD: Paul H Brooks.

Wood, R.L. (1987). *Brain Injury Rehabilitation: A Neurobehavioural Approach*. Rockville, MD: Aspen Press.

Yalom, I.D., and Vinogradov, S. (1988). Bereavement groups: Techniques and themes. *International Journal of Group Psychotherapy, 38*(4), 419–446.

APPENDIX A

Example topics to be discussed at a support group of individuals with mild traumatic brain injury.

Topics Generated By Members of Support Group

Do you tell friends or employers about the injury?
Alternatives to social isolation
Employment issues
Trouble thinking, remembering, concentrating
Stress and anger
Dealing with family (parents, spouse, children)
Giving up who you were before
Sexuality, love, relationships
Resources in the area
Dealing with physicians and other professionals
Changes in emotions
Insurance and financial issues
Sadness and depression
Individuation/Self-esteem
Loss of interest in activities, lack of motivation
Medications
Sleep and fatigue
Physical pain management
Unpredictability of symptoms

APPENDIX B

Rating form used by the mild traumatic brain injury support group in Seattle, Washington, to measure usefulness of the group.

Support Group Rating Form

Please rate each item on a scale of 0 to 5:

0 = has had no effect or has had a negative effect
1 = has had a minor effect while in the group
2 = has had a minor effect in my daily life
3 = has had a definite effect that is short-lived
4 = has had a definite effect in all aspects of my daily life
5 = has had a major effect in changing this aspect of my life

I feel that the group has had a direct impact on my:
_____ Insight
_____ Ability to give feedback to others
_____ Ability to receive feedback and understand it
_____ Self-esteem
_____ Ability to socialize with others comfortably
_____ Depression, and reducing feelings of despair
_____ Anxiety and learning to relax

APPENDIX C

A worksheet used to help persons with mild traumatic brain injury identify their most troubling symptoms and begin to gain insight about what causes them and their effects.

Most Troubling Symptom List

Describe Symptom	When Does It Occur?	What Do I Do When It Occurs?

APPENDIX D

A worksheet developed at the Good Samaritan Center for Continuing Rehabilitation in Puyallup, Washington, used to help individuals with mild traumatic brain injury begin to reconcile perceptions of their abilities before and after the injury.

Reconciling Perception of Past/Present/Future Self and Abilities

Activity	Current Performance	Performance Prior to Injury	Performance Immediately Following Injury	Anticipated Performance in ____ months	Notes/ Trend

8

Depression

SARAH A. RASKIN AND PAULA N. STEIN

Emotional processing occurs in the brain as a result of a widespread but integrated system, including interhemispheric and intrahemispheric networks (Borod, 1993), and injury to the brain can result in alterations of mood states. Depression is common following MTBI, though the nature, course, and causes of depression may be atypical compared with the depression seen in the nonbrain injured population (Cicerone, 1991; Saran, 1985; Schoenhuber and Gentilini, 1988).

When diagnosing depression following MTBI, being aware of potential complicating factors is important. Both overdiagnosis, due to reliance on overt affect, and underdiagnosis, due to reliance on the survivor's insight and awareness, are possible (Hibbard et al., 1992; Ross and Rush, 1981).

Within the context of a neuropsychological assessment, one might be concerned that cognitive deficits are due to the depression rather than to organic impairment from the TBI. This should be carefully evaluated in individual cases, but as a group evidence exists that refutes this concern. The presence of major depression does correlate with severity of reported symptoms and with functional disability, but not with objective cognitive impairments (Cicerone, 1991; Fann et al., 1995). In fact, symptoms of depression do not correlate with cognitive deficits (Raskin et al., 1998), nor does preinjury psychological treatment history (Karzmark et al., 1995). In addition, cognitive symptoms have been demonstrated early in MTBI, which would not be expected if they were due solely to the late development of a reactive depression (Cicerone, 1991). Thus, the presence of symptoms of depression should not be used as the sole explanation of cognitive deficits observed in individuals with MTBI.

Prevalence of Depression in Mild Traumatic Brain Injury

Subjective complaints of depression are reported in approximately one-third of the cases both immediately after the injury and 1 year later (Cicerone, 1991). This is essentially equivalent to findings of 39% on self-report rating scales (Schoenhuber and Gentilini, 1988).

Theories of Depression

Biological Theories

Jorge et al. (1993c) and Federoff et al. (1992) speculate that anterior brain injury, common in MTBI, interrupts biogenic amine- containing neurons as they pass through the basal ganglia or frontal subcortical white matter. These researchers suggest that the actual lesion to the anterior portion of the brain causes the depression. This is often difficult to validate in persons with MTBI due to the lack of objective findings on imaging techniques. However, in a single case study it was reported that an individual who developed rapid cycling bipolar disorder following MTBI demonstrated left frontal dysfunction on EEG and SPECT (Zwil et al., 1993).

Mobayed and Dinan (1990) separated individuals with MTBI into two groups. One reported evidence of depression on a self-report measure and the other did not. No subject in either group had a history of affective disorder, family history of affective disorder, epilepsy or cognitive impairment, alcohol abuse, or significant social stresses premorbidly. These two groups were then compared with a matched control group. The patients who developed depression showed a blunted prolactin response to buspirone challenge. The authors took this as support for their hypothesis that the serotonin system is affected by MTBI. They further hypothesize that the disruption of the serotonergic system occurs from damage to brain stem structures, including the raphe nuclei.

Thus, it remains unclear whether specific brain regions or, more likely, systems involving both cortical and subcortical structures are responsible for depression following MTBI.

Psychological Theories

Live events and challenges can also contribute to depression. Patients with MTBI often experience a variety of losses (e.g., physical, financial, future goals) and life changes (occupational, social, personal). These can affect a person's sense of well-being, confidence, and security. Emotional reactions and adjustment problems clearly contribute to the prolonged disability in some patients with MTBI (Willer et al., 1991).

Assessment

An important part of the assessment should include questions of premorbid tendency toward depression, coping styles, and history of substance abuse, because there may be multiple neurological, medical, and environmental factors that are causing or affecting the depression

(Alexander, 1994). To this end, Ross and Rush (1981) present a series of signs to aid in the diagnosis of depression in neurologically impaired patients. These include being aware of subtle symptoms, such as erratic recovery or deterioration after the neurological deficit has stabilized, and the content of statements in the presence of aprosodia.

Standard Measures of Depression Applied to Mild Traumatic Brain Injury

Due to difficulty sustaining attention or reduced awareness, when a self-report instrument is used (e.g., Beck Depression Inventory; Zung Self-Rating Scale of Depression), each item should be analyzed before making a diagnosis based on a total summed score.

Studies of MTBI using the Minnesota Multiphasic Personality Inventory (MMPI) have consistently demonstrated elevations of depression in this population. One study reported that the MMPI profiles of individuals with MTBI were similar to those with other neurological disorders (Diamond et al., 1988). Even with brain injury correction factors (Gass and Russell, 1991; Gass, 1991), the literature is mixed on whether depression measured by the MMPI in cases of MTBI is psychological or neurological (Karzmark et al., 1995). Several problems exist when relying on the MMPI to diagnose depression after MTBI. First, the MMPI is long and time-consuming and can be particularly difficult for individuals with poor sustained attention and concentration or fatigue. Those who experience fluctuation in attention may have difficulty comprehending the wording of questions. In addition, this scale also relies on self-report, the limitations of which are discussed above. As with the other scales, individual item analysis is essential, especially given the number of items relating to fatigue and to difficulty concentrating.

Alternative Measures of Depression Designed for Persons with Brain Impairment

Gordon and his colleagues have published a series of articles about the diagnosis of depression following stroke (Gordon et al., 1989, 1991; Hibbard et al., 1990b, 1993). Given that problems diagnosing poststroke depression are similar to problems following MTBI, this research will be applied to the diagnosis of depression in MTBI.

The above investigators created The Structured Assessment of Depression in Brain-Damaged Individuals (SADBD) (Hibbard et al., 1993). Two traditional measures of depression, the Beck Depression Inventory and the Hamilton Rating Scale for Depression, are embedded within the SADBD. Intrapsychic items are clearly delineated from somatic items to allow for subtotals of each domain. Reliability and validity of diagnosis were shown to be high.

These authors have further suggested that a Multimodal Approach to the Diagnosis of Depression (MMADD) be used with neurologically impaired persons (Hibbard et al., 1993). This involves not only the administration of the SADBD, but at least one outside observer's rating of the person's mood. Involving a family member or close friend is usually involved with MTBI. Further, a structured awareness questionnaire and a neuropsychological evaluation are included in the MMADD. Specific criteria for diagnosing depression are provided dependent on the outcome of these measures.

Treatment

Medications

Many antidepressant medications are often prescribed to survivors of MTBI with benefit (for a review see Glenn and Wroblewski, 1989), although some researchers have reported poor response in this population (Saran, 1985). While a comprehensive discussion of medications used to treat depression following brain injury is beyond the scope of this chapter, several considerations are addressed. First, for many individuals pharmacological treatment may be contraindicated due to coexisting medical problems related to the injury. Additionally, side effects of antidepressant agents may interfere with cognitive functioning. In particular, anticholinergic use (such as the tertiary amine tricyclics) should be closely monitored for increased confusional state, fatigue, and blurred vision. Fluoxetine can cause sleep changes and headache, and increase the risk of seizures. All non-MAO-I antidepressants can cause sedation. MAO-I antidepressants can be problematic in individuals with cognitive losses, due to the need to follow dietary restrictions. In addition, many individuals with MTBI prefer not to use medication to treat depression. Many people are already heavily medicated for coexisting conditions and may choose not to take more. Finally, as with any form of therapy, not everyone responds well to medication.

Psychotherapy

In discussing treatment of poststroke depression, Hibbard and her colleagues (Grober et al., 1993; Hibbard et al., 1990a) suggest that psychotherapy, as opposed to medication, may emerge as the treatment of choice for persons who have sustained stroke. Psychotherapy allows persons with neurologic dysfunction to learn new styles of coping, to improve impaired social skills, and to increase their sense of mastery and control, which can help prevent the recurrence of depression in the future.

Using the cognitive therapy model described below (Beck et al., 1979), Hibbard et al. (1990) outline a series of principles specific to treatment of poststroke depression that can be adapted for persons with MTBI. The principles identified are: (1) the level of cognitive functioning moderates the treatment strategies used; (2) cognitive remediation enhances the patient's ability to profit from therapy; (3) new learning and generalization may be difficult; (4) the patient's awareness of depressive symptomatology moderates the therapeutic strategy; (5) mourning is an important component of treatment; (6) premorbid personality, life style, and interests provide a context for understanding current behavior; (7) understanding the discrepancy between actual and perceived losses is essential to treatment; (8) reinforcing even small therapeutic gains improves mood; (9) emphasis on the collaborative therapeutic relationship facilitates a working alliance; (10) session flexibility is essential to ensure continuity of treatment; (11) fluctuations in medical status affect the course of treatment; (12) the distortions of family members must be addressed in therapy; (13) family members' mourning must be addressed; and (14) family members are important therapeutic helpers. When applied to traditional cognitive therapy, these principles offer the clinician specific tools to address the depression following neurologic injury.

Cognitive and behavioral approaches appear to be excellent intervention sources when working with the MTBI population. Persons with MTBI respond to an approach that targets these areas and teaches new skills appropriate to their cognitive abilities. It is, of course, axiomatic that despite the choice of therapeutic technique, the therapist must be a skilled clinician. In addition, since each person seeking treatment is affected differently by the MTBI an eclectic and individualized approach is necessary.

Cognitive therapy

Cognitive therapy is an active, directive, and time-limited approach. This approach assumes that depression is caused by dysfunctional thoughts (Beck et al., 1979). The cognitive triad of dysfunctional thoughts includes negative thoughts about oneself, the world, and the future. Cognitive therapy focuses on identifying the aspects of these thoughts that are irrational, and on challenging the cognitive distortions with more rational thinking.

In cognitive therapy, a series of strategies is used to determine and then test the individual's maladaptive assumptions developed from experience (e.g., "Because I have a brain injury, I can't do anything."). These techniques include monitoring the negative thoughts; learning to recognize the connections between these thoughts, feelings, and behavior; examining evidence for and against the distorted thoughts; substituting more realistic interpretations; and learning to identify and alter the dysfunctional beliefs that distort a person's experiences. The approach is one of collaborative empiricism. While the therapist initially structures the therapy sessions, she or he actively engages the survivor's participation and interpretations.

Persons are generally asked to keep a log of experiences that lead to feelings of sadness. As they are able to track these events, they learn to become aware of thoughts that lead them to feel sad at that moment. The person is then taught to recognize systematic errors in thinking. These include, for example, (Beck et al., 1979):

1. *Arbitrary inference.* Drawing a specific conclusion without evidence to support the conclusion (e.g., "Because I have a brain injury, I will never return to work.")
2. *Selective abstraction.* Focusing on a detail taken out of context, or ignoring more important details (e.g., "The doctor talked to me about my medication like I was stupid.")
3. *Overgeneralization.* Drawing a general rule or conclusion based on one or more isolated incidents (e.g., "I will always forget everything, just like I forgot my keys today.")
4. *Magnification or minimization.* Errors in evaluating the significance or magnitude of an event (e.g., "Forgetting to return that phone call is disgraceful and humiliating.").
5. *Personalization.* Relating external events to her/himself when there is no basis for the connection (e.g., "My friend canceled lunch because I have been so depressed.")
6. *Black-and-white thinking.* The tendency to place all experiences in one of two opposite categories (if not all good then all bad); (e.g.,"If I can't be a school principal I won't work at all.")

Behavioral interventions

As with traditional cognitive therapy, behavioral strategies are also an important component of treatment. A variety of behavioral interventions are easily incorporated into the psychotherapeutic process. Role playing can help a person with cognitive losses practice coping responses while enhancing generalization. Assertiveness training can help individuals with a "shaken sense of self" after MTBI regain a sense of competence. Relaxation training and anger control are also valuable tools and are discussed in Chapters 9 and 10. Often, behavioral homework assignments that are based upon work explored in session, are given as a way to challenge the dysfunctional thinking. For example, if a person's hypothesis is "because I have a brain injury I can't do anything well," then the therapist or treatment team may choose tasks that the individual can accomplish. These behavioral intervention assignments should also target the individual's symptoms of depression (e.g., loneliness) and schedule activities that were previously pleasurable.

Cognitive therapy is a particularly appropriate treatment for individuals with subtle cognitive losses, such as in MTBI, because it uses many principles already being learned in cognitive remediation sessions, and can be structured for retraining insight and awareness.

The cognitive and behavioral approaches work in a complementary fashion with cognitive remediation techniques. Most survivors are using some kind of memory compensation system, like a datebook, to help with memory and organization problems. An activity schedule can easily be included in their datebook. It is beneficial to discuss with survivors that while they may not initially "feel" like participating in the activity, finding out whether it will bring them pleasure is important. Therefore, one or two activities are scheduled in the memory log per week and then checked like any other homework. The activities should be relatively simple and free of postinjury difficulties including cognitive demands or a high financial cost. For instance, activities may include taking a walk with their partner or reading a newspaper. These homework activities not only challenge irrational statements, but treat the symptoms of depression (e.g., social withdrawal, worthlessness, helplessness). The number of pleasurable activities to be done each week is then slowly increased as appropriate until premorbid levels are approximated. Time is spent in session exploring the feelings surrounding the activity, before, during, and afterwards.

It may also be helpful to give handouts, notes, or summaries that reinforce the ideas discussed in session. Individuals with attention or memory deficits often appreciate the opportunity to review the information from sessions at home. Depending on the severity of the cognitive deficits, bibliotherapy can be a useful adjunct to treatment. One source of recommended reading is *Feeling Good* (Burns, 1980), which is designed to provide a lay description of cognitive therapy.

As the person progresses, a feelings log, and a log of dysfunctional thoughts, like that described by Beck et al. (1979), can also be added. An example is provided in Appendix A. Initially, individuals are asked to record feelings they have had over the past week only. When comfortable and proficient with recording their feelings, they are trained to recognize the thoughts that lead to the depressive feelings. Finally, they are trained to challenge their dysfunctional thoughts. All steps are individually tailored to meet the cognitive demands of the individual being treated.

The grieving process

Part of recovering from depression following a MTBI is analogous to the grieving process. Many losses may occur because of MTBI, not all of which may not be obvious to the survivor. These can include cognitive losses, loss of emotional control, loss of job or status at work, loss of self-esteem, loss of roles in the home, loss of autonomy, loss of a sense of self, loss of intimacy, loss of pain-free health, loss of control over how one spends one's time (going to appointments, fighting with insurance companies, etc.) and loss of future plans. Bowlby (1980) identified four phases of grieving that are applicable to the process of adjustment after MTBI. These are the phase of numbness (which includes some degree of denial), the phase of yearning and searching (trying to recapture the lost abilities with anger and irritability at the inability to do so), the phase of disorganization and despair (this includes depression with the realization that lost functions cannot or may not be recaptured), and finally the phase of reorganization (in which new attachments and a new definition of self are created).

The theoretical principles of Bowlby can be effectively used by practitioners who are treating persons with depression following MTBI. It is unclear whether denial, as originally formulated, occurs with persons with MTBI. However, denial may be observed as the person with MTBI begins to recognize that changes may be permanent. Many persons with MTBI believe initially that they will be "cured" and "the same as they were before." This may need to be discussed in therapy sessions, then tested as a hypothesis and replaced with less black-and-white thinking.

The anger stage is often complicated by the cause of the injury. Those who were victims are likely to focus their anger upon the perpetrator of the injury. Sometimes this can be a healthy outlet for the feelings. However, if litigation follows, and the decision is unfavorable, feelings of persecution and helplessness can be overwhelming. Conversely, those who were responsible for the injury themselves often develop self-blame and significant loss of self-esteem. This can be compounded by messages from significant others and society, especially if alcohol or drug use was involved.

Bargaining can often be seen within the therapy process itself. Some persons are willing to cooperate and do whatever is necessary for the course of recommended therapy because they believe they will be "back to normal" afterwards. The therapist has to be sensitive to the "good patient" and work on the distorted beliefs regarding treatment goals. The 1-year anniversary of the injury is often given great significance because many persons assume if they work hard on recovery for 1 year, by the end of that time it will all be over.

The stage of depression can be discussed as an important, perhaps inevitable, stage of recovery. This phase can occur at any point in the process, but usually accompanies the recognition that some losses will be permanent. This stage should not be rushed but worked through slowly in the processes described above. Acceptance or reorganization is, in part, achieved when the survivor learns to balance both his/her preserved premorbid abilities and actual deficit areas.

Groups, including peer support groups, can be very helpful in this process. Other group participants can serve as a mirror to changes that are taking place within one's self. These reflections can then be treated in individual therapy.

In sum, each of these treatment strategies can be employed, depending on the particular individual. Using a multidisciplinary approach at Good Samaritan Center for Continuing Rehabilitation, considerable improvement in self-reported depression was demonstrated in a group of individuals with MTBI who attended an outpatient program. These data are shown in Table 8.1.

Table 8-1 Scores on the Beck depression inventory
pre- and postmultidisciplinary MTBI treatment

	At Entry	At Discharge	(t)
Mean (sd)	20.1 (15)	9.3 (8.5)	4.21*

sd, standard deviation.
*$p < 0.05$

Partners of Persons with Mild Traumatic Brain Injury

Before concluding, it would be negligent to avoid exploring the adjustment and mood of significant others who also face the day to day difficulties of MTBI. Research has indicated that the prevalence of depression and anxiety in family members, especially spouses, of persons living with brain dysfunction is higher than 40% (Kinsella and Duffy, 1979; Stein et al., 1992). Given the prevalence of mood disorders, Stein et al. (1993) recommends that treatment be offered to the spouses of stroke patients as a natural outgrowth of the acute medical and rehabilitation process.

A thorough and detailed evaluation is necessary when working with family members of persons with MTBI. This evaluative process would serve to identify any unrealistic expectations about themselves or their partners, confusion or misinformation, and past and present coping strategies. This information would form the basis of an effective treatment plan. This is also particularly important, as the spouse's perception of their partner's functioning has been found to be a significant factor in determining the level of depression experienced (Stein et al., 1992).

The orientation and direction of partners' treatment would probably parallel that of the person who is living with MTBI. However, it is important not to assume treatment direction or view the partner as only a therapeutic agent for the person living with MTBI. Partners experience their own thoughts and feelings, based on their own losses and life challenges. Therefore, besides the necessity of mourning and education, a cognitive behavioral approach would be appropriate for working with partners and family members. Not only does this approach work on altering irrational expectations or self-statements, but also it offers a wide range of options to deal with actual stressors (Stein et al., 1993).

Conclusions

As with management aspects of MTBI, taking a flexible and multifaceted approach to the treatment of depression is important. Feelings of depression stem from an interaction of premorbid characteristics, a reaction to loss, and organic brain changes. Attempts to find a single source will not be fruitful. Similarly, the interaction of depression and cognitive functioning is complex. While it is possible that depression exacerbates cognitive loss, it is rarely useful to convey that all cognitive changes are due to emotional dysfunction. Such an approach can come across as discounting and trivializing a profoundly difficult change. This is likely to lead to an entrenchment of symptoms and a defensive posture by the survivor that disrupts any therapeutic relationship. Validation of perceived losses and emphasis on the interaction of emotion and cognition are more helpful. Simultaneous treatment of both, with feedback about improvement, can gradually lead to positive changes of all symptoms.

Case Study

AS is a 39-year-old right-handed man. He worked in construction for 11 years until the time of the accident. He never married and has no children. He has lived for the past 14 years with his girlfriend.

On the day of the accident AS was driving his pickup truck across an intersection and another truck struck his at the front left wheel. He reports that his left shoulder hit the side of the cab and the back of his head hit the back wall. He reports that he had bruises on the back and top of his head. He has no recall of the accident, nor of the preceding approximately 30 minutes. He does recall getting into his car at his home. His next memory is of being in the emergency room. He reports that he felt dizzy and disoriented.

His girlfriend currently reports that since the accident AS becomes angry and cries more easily than before. She reports that they had never fought before but immediately after the accident he became very critical of her. She reports that he would get days mixed up, wouldn't eat, and had difficulty getting along with anyone. She reports that at this time he is still more irritable than before, that his memory seems to "come and go" (i.e., some days he seems completely disoriented and others he seems much better). She reports that, in general, he forgets things she tells him. He forgets appointments even if she writes them on his calendar, and he has gone from being very independent to being fearful and dependent. She is also concerned because he seems to be paying less attention to his personal hygiene. She has noticed a gain in weight from 190 to 222 pounds, and reports that he has no interest in sex. She reports that he spends most of his time lying on the floor watching television.

AS was given a journal and asked to write down his feelings at each meal. This was then reviewed with him in weekly sessions. In this way, AS could see that he was, in fact, quite depressed. During this initial period, he was also provided with information on the effect of depression on things such as appetite, sexual interest, irritability, and memory.

AS was then asked to record his feelings more frequently. He was then trained to record his thoughts while having these feelings. AS tended toward errors of black-and-white thinking ("I will never be able to work again.") and personalization ("My girlfriend decided to work late so she can avoid seeing me.") Over time he learned to recognize these thoughts and substitute more rational thoughts.

At the same time, AS and his girlfriend were asked to slowly resume activities that had previously been pleasurable. Although their finances kept them from some activities, they could resume going to a movie one night per week and cooking a special dinner together one night per week.

Both AS and his girlfriend learned compensation strategies for AS's memory difficulties (see Chapter 5 for a discussion of these). In particular, AS was given one memory assignment each day to complete with the help of any memory strategy he chose. In this way he began to have memory "successes" each day.

After approximately 6 months of treatment, AS's mood was significantly improved. The combination of decreased depression and increased use of compensations also lead to a significant decrease in memory failures. This led to further increases in mood. AS then stopped labeling his dysfunctional thoughts but continued to use his journal to record feelings and maintain a level of insight into his mood.

References

Alexander, D. (1994). Depression and cognition as factors in recovery. In D. Good and J. Couch (Eds.), *Handbook of Neurorehabilitation*. New York, NY: Marcel Dekker, pp. 192–152.

Beck, A.T., Rush, A.J., Shaw, B.F., and Emery, G. (1979). *Cognitive Therapy of Depression*. New York, NY: Guilford Press.

Borod, J. (1993). Emotion and the brain-Anatomy and theory: An introduction to the special section. *Neuropsychology, 7,* 427–432.

Bowlby, J. (1980). *Attachment and Loss: Loss, Sadness and Depression* (Vol. III). New York, NY: Basic Books.

Burns, D. (1980). *Feeling Good*. New York, NY: Signet, New American Library.

Cicerone, K.D. (1991). Psychotherapy after mild traumatic brain injury: Relation to the nature and severity of subjective complaints. *Journal of Head Trauma Rehabilitation, 6*(4), 30–43.

Diamond, R., Barth, J., and Zillmer, E. (1988). Emotional correlates of mild closed head trauma: The role of the MMPI. *International Journal of Clinical Neuropsychology, 10,* 35–40.

Fann, J., Katon, W., Uomoto, J., and Esselman, P. (1995). Psychiatric disorders and functional disability in outpatients with traumatic brain injuries. *American Journal of Psychiatry, 152,* 1493–1499.

Federoff, J., Starkstein, S., Forrester, A., Geisler, F., Jorge, R., Arndt, S., and Robinson, R. (1992). Depression in patients with acute traumatic brain injury. *American Journal of Psychiatry, 149,* 918–923.

Gass, C. (1991). MMPI-2 interpretation and closed head injury: A correction factor. *Psychological Assessment: A Journal of Consulting and Clinical Psychology, 3*, 27–31.

Gass, C., and Russell, E. (1991). MMPI profiles of closed head trauma patients: impact of neurologic complaints. *Journal of Clinical Psychology, 47*, 253–260.

Glenn, M., and Wroblewski, B. (1989). The choice of antidepressants in depressed survivors of traumatic brain injury. *Journal of Head Trauma Rehabilitation, 4*, 85–88.

Gordon, W., Hibbard, M., Egelko, S., Riley, F., Simon, D., Diller, L., Ross, E., and Lieberman, A. (1991). Issues in the diagnosis of post-stroke depression. *Rehabilitation Psychology, 36*, 71–88.

Gordon, W., Hibbard, M., Grober, S., Aletta, E., Paddison, P., and Sliwinski, M.(1989). A multi-modal approach to the diagnosis of post-stroke depression. *Archives of Physical Medicine and Rehabilitation, 70*, A54.

Grober, S., Hibbard, M., Gordon, W., Stein, P., and Freeman, A. (1993). The Psychotherapeutic treatment of post-stroke depression with cognitive-behavioral therapy. In W. Gordon (Ed.), *Advances in Stroke Rehabilitation.* Boston, MA: Andover Medical Publishers, pp. 215–241.

Hibbard, M., Gordon, W., Stein, P., Grober, S., and Sliwinski, M. (1992). Awareness of disability in patients following stroke. *Rehabilitation Psychology, 37*, 103–120.

Hibbard, M., Gordon, W., Stein, P., Grober, S., and Sliwinski, M. (1993). A multimodal approach to the diagnosis of post-stroke depression. In W. Gordon (Ed.), *Advances in Stroke Rehabilitation.* Boston, MA.: Andover Medical Publishers, pp. 183–214.

Hibbard, M., Grober, S., Gordon, W., and Aletta, E. (1990a). Modification of cognitive psychotherapy for the treatment of post- stroke depression. *Behavior Therapist, 13*, 15–17.

Hibbard, M., Grober, S., Gordon, W., Aletta, E., and Freeman, A. (1990b). Cognitive therapy and the treatment of poststroke depression. *Topics in Geriatric Rehabilitation, 5*, 43–55.

Jorge, R., Robinson, R., and Arndt, S. (1993a). Are there symptoms that are specific for depressed mood in patients with traumatic brain injury? *The Journal of Nervous and Mental Disease, 181*, 91–99.

Jorge, R., Robinson, R., Arndt, S., Starkstein, S., Forrester, A., and Geisler, F. (1993c). Depression following traumatic brain injury: A 1 year longitudinal study. *Journal of Affective Disorders, 27*, 233–243.

Karzmark, P., Hall, K., and Englander, J. (1995). Late-onset post- concussion symptoms after mild brain injury: the role of premorbid, injury-related, environmental, and personality factors. *Brain Injury, 9*, 21–26.

Kinsella, G.J., and Duffy, F.D. (1979). Psychosocial readjustment in the spouses of aphasic patients. A comparative survey of 79 subjects. *Scandinavian Journal of Rehabilitative Medicine, 11*(3), 129–132.

Mobayed, M., and Dinan, T. (1990). Buspirone/prolactin response in post head injury depression. *Journal of Affective Disorders, 19*, 237–241.

Raskin, S., Mateer, C., and Tweeten, R. (1998). Neuropsychological assessment of individuals with mild traumatic brain injury. *The Clinical Neuropsychologist, 12*(1), 21–30.

Ross, E., and Rush, A. (1981). Diagnosis and neuroanatomical correlates of depression in brain-damaged patients. *Archives of General Psychiatry, 38,* 1344–1354.

Saran, A. (1985). Depression after minor closed head injury: Role of dexamethasone suppression test and antidepressants. *Journal of Clinical Psychiatry, 46,* 335–338.

Schoenhuber, R., and Gentilini, M. (1988). Anxiety and depression after mild head injury: A case control study. *Journal of Neurology, Neurosurgery, and Psychiatry, 51,* 722–724.

Stein, P., Berger, A., Hibbard, M., and Gordon, W. (1993). Treatment issues and interventions in the spouses of stroke patients. In W. A. Gordon (Ed.), *Advances in Stroke Rehabilitation.* Boston, MA: Andover Medical Publishers, pp. 242–257.

Stein, P., Gordon, W., Hibbard, M., and Sliwinski, M. (1992). An examination of depression in the spouses of stroke patients. *Rehabilitation Psychology, 37,* 121–130.

Willer, B., Allen, K., Liss, M., and Zicht, M. (1991). Problems and coping strategies of individuals with traumatic brain injury and their spouses. *Archives of Physical Medicine and Rehabilitation, 72,* 460–464.

Zwil, A., McAllister, T., Cohen, I., and Halpern, L. (1993). Ultra- rapid cycling bipolar affective disorder following closed head injury. *Brain Injury, 7,* 147–152.

APPENDIX A

Example of a worksheet to be used to record dysfunctional thoughts and to then provide a more rational response to these thoughts. Reprinted from Beck, Rush, Shaw, and Emery (1979).

Daily Record of Dysfunctional Thoughts

Date	Situation	Emotion(s)	Automatic Thought(s)	Rational Response	Outcome
	Describe: 1. Actual event leading to unpleasant emotion, or 2. Stream of thoughts, daydream or recollection leading to unpleasant	1. Specify sad, anxious, angry, etc. 2. Rate degree of emotion, 1–100.	1. Write automatic thought(s) that preceded emotion(s). 2. Rate belief in automatic thought(s), 0%–100%.	1. Write rational response to automatic thought(s). 2. Rate belief in rational response, 0%–100%.	1. Re-rate belief in automatic thought(s), 0%–100%. 2. Specify and rate subsequent emotions, 0–100.

Explanation: When you experience an unpleasant emotion, note the situation that seemed to stimulate the emotion. (If the emotion occurred while you were thinking, daydreaming, etc., please note this.) Then note the automatic thought associated with the emotion. Record the degree to which you believe this thought: 0% = not at all; 100% = completely. In rating degree of emotion: 1 = a trace; 100 = the most intense possible.

9

Anxiety and Posttraumatic Stress

DAVID HOVLAND AND SARAH A. RASKIN

Persons who have sustained a mild traumatic brain injury (MTBI) may experience anxiety when confronted with subtle, but functionally relevant, deficits. Some distress may also be associated with specific, challenging situations and/or with reminiscent aspects of the injury. In fact, while only a small percentage of this population will meet the DSM-IV criteria for posttraumatic stress disorder (PTSD), problems with anxiety may overlap substantially with issues of posttraumatic stress, whether the root trauma is the injury itself, the resulting deficits, or perceived functional difficulties. Therefore, an inquiry into the dynamics of anxiety and posttraumatic distress is an important aspect of rehabilitation for persons challenged by MTBI. Some evidence suggests neurologic changes in the brain following prolonged exposure to inescapable stress. Such exposure leads first to a massive over utilization of catecholamines, which is followed by depletion. This becomes conditioned to even mild stressors (Sherman and Petty, 1980). Evidence also exists of low levels of serotonin in the brain following this type of prolonged stress (Van der Kolk et al., 1985). Kolb (1987) suggesting that brain changes in the locus coeruleus may result in poorly modulated arousal and disturbances in memory (such as flashbacks and disassociation).

The relationship between posttraumatic stress and persistent physiological over-reactivity is also well documented. Hyperalertness or heightened arousal (measured by blood pressure, pulse rate, higher levels of urinary epinephrine and norepinephrine) is associated with experiences perceived as sudden, overwhelming, and in which the victim perceives him or herself powerless.

Not surprisingly, then, preliminary evidence has documented cognitive changes associated with prolonged posttraumatic stress. Impairments have been noted in executive functions (Gil et al., 1990) and memory (Bremner et al., 1995), and these deficits have been shown to persist many years after the trauma (Sutker et al., 1995).

These findings have two implications for survivors of MTBI. First, those individuals who develop PTSD secondary to brain injury may perform more poorly on cognitive measures because of the PTSD rather than the MTBI. Second, individuals who had experienced prolonged stress before the injury may experience greater cognitive impairment when compounded with an MTBI due to additive effects.

In fact, this second possibility appears to have received support by a recent preliminary study of childhood sexual abuse survivors who then experienced MTBI (Raskin, 1997). Four groups of subjects were administered measures of cognitive and emotional functioning. Groups included those with MTBI, those with a history of sexual abuse, those with both MTBI and sexual abuse, and normal control subjects. Individuals with MTBI demonstrated deficits in working memory, those with sexual abuse demonstrated deficits in executive functioning, and those with both MTBI and sexual abuse demonstrated the greatest number of deficits, which were in working memory, executive functioning, and verbal memory. Tests of anxiety, depression, and PTSD, while showing significant symptoms in all clinical groups, did not correlate with the neuropsychological tests that differentiated the groups. Results suggest some cumulative effects of stress and MTBI that are not explained solely by the current level of PTSD. They also suggest that some individuals may be more vulnerable to MTBI based on a variety of prior stressful life experiences.

Miller (1961) and others have suggested that MTBI has no organic basis; rather, anxiety was seen as the *cause* of functional difficulties. As research began to indicate the relationship between MTBI and neuropsychological impairment (Barth et al., 1983; Gronwall and Sampson 1974), the interaction with anxiety was further explored.

Rimel et al., (1981) wrote of an interaction between the original cognitive deficits and the accompanying emotional response. These authors suggested that any of three explanations for MTBI symptoms were possible. The first was organic central nervous system damage, the second was secondary gain, and the third was an interaction between the original cognitive deficits and the subsequent emotional responses.

The possibility of such an interaction has been conceptualized in several ways. Semfield (1985) suggested that chronic or delayed forms of untreated posttraumatic stress may result in maladaptive ingrained patterns that may not be entirely attributed to the original traumatic event. Levin (1985) hypothesized that residual cognitive deficits, thought to be fully recovered, might become manifest under stressful conditions. Kay (1986) noted that anxiety might become classically conditioned to performance-based tasks that had become challenging. In this model, cognitive difficulties first cause anxiety due to an inability to do tasks that previously could be done easily. Then, anxiety further reduces cognitive abilities. After a time this anxiety is elicited by cognitively challenging tasks, even if there has been improvement in cognitive functioning.

Assessment

A need exists for tools that can adequately assess anxiety and posttraumatic stress after MTBI. There are many available standard assessment measures of anxiety (Beck Anxiety Interview, Symptom Checklist-90) and PTSD (Blake et al., 1990). Questions or disclosures in an interview, however, can also reveal preliminary information regarding symptom etiology and history. The interview should include questions about specific eliciting situations, bodily sensations, thoughts at the time, and what the person did to relieve the anxiety. The following list of sample questions targets symptoms that may require further exploration:

Sample Questions Regarding Posttraumatic Stress/Anxiety Sequelae of Mild Traumatic Brain Injury:

1. Have you experienced any increase in nightmares or vivid dreams since the injury?
2. Have you experienced any increase in "flashbacks," sudden recollections, or mental images of the accident or situations associated with the injury?
3. Are there any situations that somehow remind you of the accident, or produce similar feelings?
4. How do you experience problems since your injury (what does it feel like if and when you notice yourself having problems)?
5. Have you experienced any increase in feelings of tension or alarm since the injury (when/how)?

It is important to experiment with alternate phrasing in the interview in order to attempt a common language of symptomology with the client, and to avoid pejorative terms within their psychosocial schema. For example, some clients treated for these issues have exhibited strong reactions to words such as "anxiety" or "panic." Emotional responses to problems experienced by many persons with MTBI may include an avoidance of psychosocial issues. At the root, this may represent a fear of "going crazy" or of having deficits dismissed as "all in your head." Thus, efforts toward rapport and openly addressing these issues are critical.

Some clients however, may have a premorbid history of anxiety or posttraumatic stress. Current symptoms, then, may represent either amplified premorbid traits or problems that may now be attributed *solely* to the injury. In assessing these issues, it may be helpful to frame premorbid traits as normal confluences within the profile of persons challenged by MTBI. For example, the therapist might ask/inform the client, "A lot of people find that brain injury makes certain tendencies simply *more* of a problem. Have you found this at all [regarding this issue]?" This approach is perhaps more likely to facilitate assessment of preexisting proclivities (e.g., test anxiety, sleep disturbances) because it emphasizes the common nature of multiple contributors to current symptoms. Nevertheless, interviews with significant family members and/or friends are an important additional source of information.

Finally, direct observations reveal a great deal about anxiety, and this is particularly true in neuropsychological testing. Observation or consultation with the tester provides information that can then be explored with the client in an interview. For a more detailed review of assessment issues, see Chapter 3.

Treatment

Like many of the issues outlined in this book, treatment for posttraumatic stress and anxiety related to MTBI encompasses a spectrum of approaches. Given the variable levels of cognitive capacity within the MTBI population, the necessity for all clients to maintain some sense of control, the diversity in backgrounds of those pursuing treatment, and the relatively abrupt onset of emotional difficulties (high functioning brain injury clients may be unaccustomed to therapeutic roles), flexibility in treatment planning is vital. Possible treatment options are reviewed below.

Ventilation and Validation

It is axiomatic that effective psychosocial treatment encourages and supports the client's exploration of issues. Posttraumatic stress may often require a safe environment for exploration. Some clients may not have fully described their symptoms or reactions to the trauma. Others may have received subtle disincentives for doing so. The importance, then, of ventilating and describing these issues in repeated sessions is critical. Some clients may become fixed or focused on experiences and be unable to move ahead. All clients will undoubtedly require information and assistance. Thus, a balance must be struck between ventilation and other therapeutic approaches.

To achieve a balance some structure may be necessary, which may take the form of a negotiated and specific time framework for the sessions. For example, it may be helpful to designate the first portion of each session as a time for describing frequency, intensity, and content of trauma-related dreams or flashbacks, symptoms of anxiety, and other pertinent issues. During this designated time, it is important to pursue, to the best of the client's ability and willingness, the emotional significance of these disclosures. This endeavor, however, often requires specific, limited parameters of time (with the degree of specificity depending upon the client's ability to switch focus). Setting a preagreed and specific time limit, such as "up to 20 minutes," functions as a dynamic metaphor for the client's effort to set aside the presenting issues for periods of time. Thus, the session models the goal of reducing perseveration while allowing for ventilation. The remainder of the session (clearly marked by the therapist noting the time for transition) then becomes available for other treatment approaches.

Establishment and Normalization of the Relationship between Arousal and Cognitive Functioning

Education and explanation can help to establish the link between arousal (i.e., tension, anxiety, stress, worry) and the ability to think clearly and work productively for the client. Research has shown that there is an optimal level of arousal that facilitates clarity of thought. When this level of arousal is exceeded, as it is when stress increases, cognitive efficiency diminishes. The therapist can help the client to understand this dynamic through educational approaches (see Figure 9.1 for structured, written exercises or articles). However, the therapist is usually most effective when the negative impact of stress on functioning is discussed in terms of the client's everyday activities, demands, and experiences.

For many clients, cognitively challenging endeavors or situations have become the posttraumatic stress trigger. It may be important, particularly in the early stages of treatment, to emphasize the notion of cognition-inhibiting arousal as a probable contributor to the difficulty in functioning.

Recognizing Changes in Personal Identity, Self-Concept, and Perception

Kay's model (1992) has been adapted by many of those who work with MTBI. Immediately following an injury or illness, daily functioning is often disrupted. Common tasks may become challenging or fatiguing. On some level, the injured individual's confidence and general sense of identity may then become eroded. This process, which may well occur on a subconscious level, facilitates profound self-doubt and changes in identity, such as: "What is wrong with me?"; "Am I going crazy?"; "I just can't function."; or "Am I ever going to feel better?" These changes may, in turn, affect the way the individual perceives or values his/her abilities. Cognitive difficulties may become perceptually salient, magnified, and more often remembered. This further erodes the individual's sense of identity and creates a self-fulfilling prophecy (see Figure 9.2). Thus, a cycle develops in which the cognitive inefficiency (or pain, etc.) increases stress, which increases cognitive inefficiency, etc.

The therapist can assist in helping the client to recognize this cycle and provide reassurance regarding its common and reversible nature. The client may also be asked to recall events or periods of time since the injury when he or she experienced changes in confidence. These may have begun to function as unconscious contributors to everyday difficulties in functioning. Most important, the therapist asks clients to attend to their own perception of their difficulties, and encourages reflective and bal-

Reduced cognition   Optimal cognitive performance   Reduced cognition

Sluggish   Alert, but at ease   Anxious, Tense

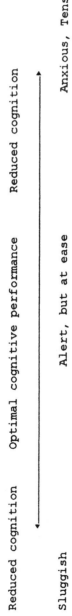

Figure 9-1 The relationship between arousal and cognition. (One might plot their own location upon this continuum for a given set of circumstances.)

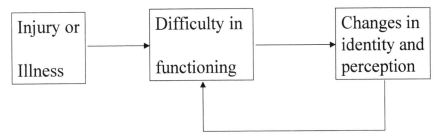

Figure 9-2 The cycle of changes in functioning and identity following mild head injury.

anced self-talk about these (e.g., "My difficulty with this task may be related to my injury, but everyone has difficulties at times and I may also be noticing my normal difficulties more.").

Training and Generalization of Brief Cognitive–Behavioral Strategies

While it is important to provide realistic information about the source of stress, it is also useful to provide strategies for managing symptoms of anxiety or posttraumatic stress. Many techniques for symptom management can be discussed with the client. Choosing those that appeal most to the individual is often helpful. Simple strategies are often the best, and creating a written list of these may be useful (particularly for clients experiencing problems with memory, topic maintenance, organizational skills, etc.). Knowing that these techniques are endorsed by the therapist and have been found helpful by others challenged by MTBI may also be critical aspects of accepting and adopting these new compensatory habits. Invariably, the client will have a number of spontaneous strategies already in place, such as, "I go outside for a breath of air." These may be reinforced and form the basis for a growing repertoire of stress reduction strategies.

Behavioral strategies might include techniques such as: taking a controlled, deep breath; attending to a behavior or sensation that signifies incipient symptoms (e.g., "Whenever I start to rub my forehead, I know I need to start using a technique."); progressive muscle relaxation (briefly tensing and then relaxing a specific part of the body); taking frequent, brief walks or stretching breaks before or at the first sign of symptom manifestation; improving sleep habits and increasing the overall amount of sleep; or giving self-suggestions regarding posttraumatic stress just before sleep (e.g., just prior to sleep, I tell myself, "I know why I am waking up and having these dreams, so there is no need for me to be alarmed. If I wake up or have a dream, I will simply use my techniques and try to go back to sleep.") Numerous resources for anxiety management reveal a comprehensive menu of techniques, but emphasis must be placed upon creatively personalizing various compensatory approaches for the individual (their preference, occupation, level of functioning, etc.).

Cognitive psychotherapeutic strategies for symptom management are described in Chapter 8 and might include specific coping statements or questions that the client frequently reads or recites to her or himself, such as the following: "I know more about why I am having these reactions now, so I can get through this"; "What is it I need to do here?"; or "One step at a time." It may also be helpful to relate these techniques to brain injury education, relating complex attention deficits to the need for consciously directing the mind back and forth from the situation at hand to the compensatory strategy. Finally, encouraging strategies for generalizing these techniques is important. For example, brief, written reminders might be placed on a page marker in the individual's daily organizer or a very small sticker might be placed in a highly visible location (such as on the individual's watch or telephone) to serve as a prompt to use techniques. An example of a divider from a client's daily organizer is presented in Figure 9.3.

```
                 Take a breath

              ↑ RELAXATION ↑

                 Pace myself

              It will get better.

                 How much is:

                    a) situation?

                    b) my reaction?

                 "Bear."
```

* Whenever he became stuck on a topic or an inappropriate solution to a problem, his wife and therapists were instructed to say "Bear to help him shift set. Eventually he was able to internalize this and cue himself.

Figure 9-3 Example of a reminder that can be placed in a date book.

Relaxation Training

Besides dealing with situational triggers for arousal or anxiety, individuals with posttraumatic stress often exhibit problems with cultivated (i.e., cumulative and ongoing) arousal. This cultivated and elevated arousal is often eclipsed by the clients' more intermittent symptoms, but should be addressed through more generic approaches such as relaxation training. Facilitating relaxation training by first explaining its need following MTBI from a neuropsychological perspective may be helpful. For example, the therapist might frame the need for relaxation training in terms of the fatigue/stress cost of the increased vigilance necessary to compensate for subtle but significant deficits in complex attention (whether these deficits result from organic deficits, psychosocial sequelae, or, as is more likely, both). The goal of this type of preparatory approach is to increase awareness of the need for relaxation training, even in clients who report that their symptoms appear unrelated to conscious anxiety (e.g., nightmares, panic attacks that occur "out of the blue," etc.). Also, the connection must be established between ability to enter a relaxed state under ideal circumstances, and generalizing this ability to other situations. Relaxation training, then, may take the form of therapist-guided exercises in sessions, or homework assignments, such as listening to similar exercises on a cassette. Many commercially produced cassettes are available (e.g., Jacobson and McGuigan, 1982) and, ideally, an effort should be made to find those that the client is most motivated to use. A guideline for relaxation training is also provided by Clark (1990). For individuals with poor prospective memory or follow-through, writing down or scheduling the relaxation training assignment may also be helpful.

Systematic Desensitization (and Generalization to the Environment)

In cases where the client's symptoms *are* related to specific trauma-related triggers, systematic desensitization entails relaxation and gradual exposure to the trauma-related triggers (or to descriptions of these triggers). In this way, the client improves control over his or her reactions to these triggers within treatment, and control can then be encouraged and generalized to daily living. Establishing the goal of improving control of (i.e., managing) symptoms at the onset of treatment is important. One approach to systematic desensitization is to ask for and write down descriptions of the images, activities, or situations that elicit stress-related symptoms, and organize these into a number of scenarios. Scenarios can then be ranked or rated by degree of associated distress. Given the instructions to signify increasing symptoms (e.g., "raise your hand") while maintaining a relaxed state, the client is asked to listen to relaxation instructions (or a relaxation tape). Following or during this, the therapist begins describing or otherwise facilitating gradual exposure to the triggers. If the client signals the experience of salient symptoms, the therapist ceases or decreases exposure to the trigger and facilitates relaxation alone. This process can then be experimented with as the therapist and client gradually attempt more challenging or graphic scenarios or prolonged exercises of systematic desensitization. Most important, however, the client learns to understand that this is an ongoing process which, ideally, would become his or her own undertaking in the community or at home. Essentially, the therapist conveys the message, "be careful, but deliberately elicit your own symptoms while using management strategies." Again, persons with MTBI may require a more structured approach toward this goal, including the use of written instructions, forms for data collection, or other forms of schedules/systems.

Case Study

Case 1

Ms. V sustained a mild brain injury when her automobile was struck from behind. Subsequently, she experienced subtle but significant problems with fatigue, sustained attention, and most importantly with posttraumatic stress/anxiety when faced with the following triggers (in rising order of severity): driving in traffic, sirens, emergency vehicle lights, and hospitals/emergency rooms. She participated in several structured sessions of relaxation, and descriptions of posttraumatic stress triggers were gradually introduced. Within these sessions, Ms. V required more frequent reminders to signify and compensate for the "butterflies in the stomach" she experienced with more intensive trigger descriptions. A total of six sessions was devoted primarily to systematic desensitization exercises, with two of these being tape recorded and later assigned as homework. Additionally, Ms. V was asked to envision and finally approach a nearby emergency room in stages. One week she was to drive by, the next week park nearby for 5 minutes, the next week get out of the car, etc. She was provided with written suggestions for use in the community, and, after 4 months, acknowledged cognitive benefits to her efforts.

Restructuring Difficult Adjustment Issues

Adjustment difficulties can be divided into several categories (e.g., posttraumatic stress, guilt, reactive anger), but perhaps two of the most basic distinctions might be termed awareness and acceptance. Problems with awareness include statements (or endorsement of statements) such as "this [difficulty] doesn't have *anything* to do with my injury," or "that [cognitive] testing doesn't tell you *anything* [or indicate problems related to my injury]." Problems with acceptance are inferred by statements/endorsements such as "I just *can't* accept what has happened to me," or "I *can't*

stop thinking about this [or about how things were before the injury]."
Like most adjustment difficulties, these issues inhibit the client's ability to
focus upon compensatory strategies and the ability to deal with the most
problematic sequelae of mild brain injury, including posttraumatic stress.

Mild brain injuries may, in some ways, entail more intractable adjustment issues for several reasons: The individual's relatively mild injury
may have elicited less medical follow-up or information regarding possible sequelae, thus allowing for more dysfunctional and cyclic response
patterns; the individual is often given less validation for having problems
or opportunities to explore them; or the individual may have no dis-
cernable causative factors to his/her symptoms and thus begin to seriously doubt themselves or their sanity (as discussed above).

Thus, addressing underlying adjustment issues may become a corner-
stone for treatment of psychosocial issues secondary to MTBI, and a necessary component of treating anxiety/posttraumatic stress. "Restructuring" refers to rethinking or restating adjustment issues in more balanced
or moderate ways. For example, the therapist might document extreme
statements (e.g., "This cannot be happening to me," "No one understands," etc.), provide models for restructured approaches (e.g., "It is hard
to believe this is happening to me," "It feels like no one understands, but
right now I am trying to focus on my own understanding and how I can
set this aside for periods of time," etc.), and then ask the client to restructure similar statements in their own words.

Case Study

Case 2

Mr. M suffered a toxic exposure resulting in minimal loss of consciousness, but sometimes has severe episodes of confusion, anxiety, and panic when in cognitively demanding situations (neuropsychological testing, crowds, etc.) or when exposed to chemically
based scents. For the first 2 months of treatment, he was provided
with daily therapy of education, support, and strategies for management of his symptoms, and found this helpful. He continued,
however, to exhibit difficult adjustment issues in the following ways:
Repeated statements indicative of rigid adjustment obstacles ("You
do not understand," "I cannot do anything," etc.); a tendency to insist upon repeated and prolonged periods of symptom description;
and a strong aversive response to the word "acceptance." He was
then provided with alternative phrasing for his adjustment ("Coming to terms with [problems related to the injury]"), supportive but
confrontive feedback regarding his adjustment issues/statements,
and assistance in generating goals for management of perseveration
and achieving longer periods of productivity. By the 4th month of

PACING

1. "Tomorrow is another day."

2. "I don't want to bother leader, but I'd still like

to be in the band."

3. "Do the best I can."

4. "Time out."   "Take a breath."

5. "Bear."

Figure 9-4 Examples of cognitive restructuring self-talk.

daily treatment, Mr. M appeared increasingly focused on his strategy for symptom management and was able to limit symptom descriptions or use them as material for discussion of compensatory approaches. Mr. M's self-talk reminder is presented in Figure 9.4.

References

Barth, J.T., Macciocchi, S.N., Giordani, G., et al. (1983). Neuropsychological sequelae of minor head injury. *Neurosurgery, 13,* 529–533.

Blake, D., Weathers, F., Nagy, L., Kaloupek, D., Klauminzer, G., Charney, D., and Keane, T. (1990). *Clinician-Administered PTSD Scale.* Boston, MA and New Haven, CT: National Center for Post- traumatic Stress Disorder.

Bremner, J., Randall, P., Scott, T., Bronen, R., Seibyl, J., Southwick, S., Delaney, R., McCarthy, G., Charney, D., and Innis, R. (1995). MRI-based measurement of hippocampal volume in patients with combat-related posttraumatic stress disorder. *American Journal of Psychiatry, 152,* 973–981.

Clark, D. (1990). Anxiety states: Panic and generalized anxiety. In K. Hawton, P. Salkovskis, J. Kirk, and D. Clark (Eds.), *Cognitive Behavior Therapy for Psychiatric Problems: A Practical Guide.* New York, NY: Oxford University Press, pp. 211–221.

Gil, T., Calev, A., Greenberg, D., Kugelmass, S., and Lerer, B. (1990). Cognitive functioning in post-traumatic stress disorder. *Journal of Traumatic Stress, 3,* 29–45.

Gronwwall, D.M.A., and Sampson, H. (1974). *The Psychological Effects of Concussion.* Auckland, New Zealand: University Press/Oxford University Press.

Jacobson, E., and McGuigan, F.J. (1982). Principles and Practice of Progressive Relaxation. New York, NY: BMA Audio Cassette Publications.

Kay, T. (1986). *The Unseen Injury: Minor Head Trauma.* Framingham, MA: National Head Injury Foundation.

Kolb, L. (1987). Neuropsychological hypothesis explaining posttraumatic stress disorder. *American Journal of Psychiatry, 144*, 989–995.

Levin, H.S. (1985). Outcome after head injury. Part II. Neurobehavioral recovery. In D.P. Becker and J.T. Povlishock (Eds.), *Central Nervous System Trauma. Status Report-1985.* Washington, DC: National Institutes of Health.

Miller, H. (1961). Accident neurosis. *British Medical Journal, ii*, 919–923; 992–998.

Raskin, S. (1997). The relationship between sexual abuse and mild traumatic brain injury. *Brain Injury, 11*(8), 587–603.

Rimel, R.W., Giordani, B., Barth, J.T., et al. (1981). Clinical and scientific communications: Disability caused by minor head injury. *Neurosurgery, 9*, 221–228.

Sherman, A., and Petty, F. (1980). Neurochemical basis of the action of antidepressants on learned helplessness. *Behavioral Neural Biology, 30*, 119–134.

Sutker, P., Vasterling, J., Brailey, K., and Allain, A. (1995). Memory, attention, and executive deficits in POW survivors: Contributing biological and psychological factors. *Neuropsychology, 9*, 118–125.

Van der Kolk, B., Greenberg, M., and Boyd, H. (1985). Inescapable shock, neurotransmitters, and addiction to trauma: Toward a psychobiology of posttraumatic stress. *Biological Psychiatry, 20*, 314–325.

APPENDIX A

An educational worksheet provided to individuals with brain injury to help them learn a series of techniques for thought-stopping when perseverative thoughts occur.

Good Samaritan Hospital Center for Cognitive Rehabilitation

Thought-stopping techniques. Preface: Many people find themselves dwelling on certain concerns. When it becomes difficult to stop thinking about a concern or the concern returns quite frequently, it is called "perseveration." Thought-stopping means specific techniques to *manage* (i.e., decrease, limit, etc.) perseveration.

1. *CASSETTE TAPE*
   Listen to a relaxation exercise on a cassette tape. Do this often. Every evening is a good time to listen, but you can practice the techniques throughout the day. Here are a few types:
   A. Physical tension reducers ("Tense your hand, then relax it.")
   B. Autogenic training (My left arm is heavy and warm.")
   C. Visualization (Picture yourself on a beach.")
   D. Psychoeducation ("One of the causes of insomnia is . . .")
   E. Mental relaxation ("You may find yourself feeling very relaxed.")

2. *SELF-TALK*
   When you find yourself tempted to perseverate, think to yourself or say something aloud to yourself. Try picking a few key *specific* phrases or reminders that work for you. For example:
   A. "Wait, there is nothing I can do about this right now. Part of me wants to keep thinking on this, but I *can't afford it.*"
   B. "Quiet thoughts."
   C. "I'm starting to perseverate. I know about that now, so I'll *redirect* myself."
   D. "Time for *mental control.* I'll think about that tomorrow."
   E. "*Easy does it:* What am I doing now?"

3. *WRITTEN PLAN*
   Construct a written thought-stopping plan and review it often. You may want to ask a therapist for help, or review examples of other written plans. Here are some things to consider:
   A. Put a copy by your bed or wherever you tend to perseverate.
   B. List the specific words/phrases that work for you.
   C. Consider making a place to keep track of how often thoughts occur. (Simply writing it down can actually decrease a recurrent thought.)
   D. Add to your plan as you go along.
   E. Write down *why* you want to work on thought-stopping (rationale).

4. *CHALLENGE DISTORTIONS*

   When you find yourself thinking in "distorted" ways, challenge yourself (in you mind or on paper) to think more clearly. There are many structured exercises and resources to help you with this. Examples:

   A. "I know things won't work out . . . Wait, this is a concern, but I can't tell the future for sure."

   B. "I can't handle anything . . . Wait, I'm having problems, but I'm handling quite a few things well."

5. *RECORD YOUR VOICE*

   What advice would you give yourself the next time you are perseverating? Make a tape recording of your own voice, encouraging yourself and reminding yourself of your techniques. Play this tape back for yourself when you need it most.

6. *DO SOMETHING PHYSICAL*

   This technique is not appropriate for late evening; but walking, stretching, or other exercises can be very helpful in managing perseveration.

7. *SELF-SUGGESTIONS BEFORE SLEEP*

   During the 5 to 10 minutes immediately before sleep, the brain enters a very relaxed state called "alpha." While the conscious mind still has a good deal of control in an alpha state, we are very open to suggestion (similar to deep relaxation or hypnotism). Many of us have had the experience of telling ourselves to awaken at a certain hour only to find ourselves waking up before the alarm clock. Likewise, we can make suggestions to ourselves not to wake up. For example, during the 5 minutes immediately before falling asleep, think to yourself:

   "There's no reason to wake up."

   "I know why I am waking up—I am concerned about things. But I don't need to wake up tonight. The more often I remind myself of this, the less I will wake up. If I do wake up, it will not concern me anymore. I will simply use my relaxation techniques and tell myself that this is not the time for concerns, etc."

8. *THINK OF SOMETHING ELSE*

   Consider making a list of things that are appropriate to wonder about. Try to make these things as interesting as possible (what gift to buy for someone, what menu items to plan for, etc.). Consult your list when tempted to perseverate.

9. *GRIEF MANAGEMENT*

   If the intrusive thoughts involve difficulty accepting certain losses, they may be a part of the grief process. In managing grief, it is important to explore and share your feelings, but it is also important to do much of this in set-aside time periods. Consider making an appointment with a therapist and/or setting aside some specific quiet times for yourself. Outside of these time periods, remind yourself that:

A. Grief is difficult, but it can be managed.

B. Perseveration, after a point, does not help the grief process.

C. You can make brief notes to yourself, to consider further in your set-aside time periods.

10. *USE AN OBJECT AS A SYMBOL*

Sometimes objects can be reminders for thought-stopping. When you see or feel a designated object, it can bring you back on track. For example:

A. A memento placed prominently in an area where perseveration tends to occur.

B. A rubber band worn on the wrist, which can be gently snapped to bring you "back on track."

C. A note with a written reminder/statement.

D. A photograph that symbolizes your thought-stopping work.

E. A written therapy appointment.

10

Irritability and Anger

DAVID HOVLAND AND CATHERINE A. MATEER

Increases in irritability and expressions of anger or frustration are frequently reported after not only moderate to severe, but also mild traumatic brain injury (MTBI). Anger and frustration may take the form of negative self-talk, verbal abusiveness to others (e.g., swearing or making denigrating comments), or of physical aggressiveness (e.g., throwing objects, hitting things, threatening postures, or actual assaults on others). Considerable stress and turmoil are created in the home and significant problems at work may occur when individuals exhibit such behaviors.

The effects of MTBI can be as subtle as they are disruptive. The fact that MTBI usually receives less intervention than more severe brain injuries contributes to the frustration of patients and their families. Multiple sources of frustration and anger experienced and exhibited by persons with MTBI may exist. It is often difficult to determine to what degree these individuals have underlying neurological bases for irritability or impulsivity and are more vulnerable to distraction and subsequent fatigue and agitation, or whether they are angry at their perceived losses, change of circumstances, or lack of support.

Considerable neural activity *inhibits* persons from overreacting or expending energy paying attention to too many things. Loss of such inhibition may result in problems with impulsivity, distractibility, fatigue, and irritability. However, premorbid personality and secondary emotional responses are also factors that contribute to emotional behavior. Anger can wear many disguises. Its truer sources may be more diffuse longer-standing issues that originated before or since the injury.

McKay et al. (1989), in discussing the psychological functions of anger, suggest that it can reduce stress by discharging or blocking awareness of painful levels of emotional or physical arousal. Anger may serve to dissipate painful affect, such as anxiety and fear, loss and depression, hurt, guilt, and shame, and feelings of failure, badness, and unworthiness. Anger also may reduce or eliminate painful sensations, such as those experienced from physical pain, overstimulation, muscle tension, tiredness, and overwork. Anger may release tension resulting from a frustrated drive, which arises out of blocked needs or desires, a sense that things are not as they should be, or the sense of being forced. Anger also may be a response to a threat, such as feelings of being attacked, engulfed, or abandoned. In our experience, many of these sensations and feelings are commonly endorsed by individuals who have experienced MTBI.

While much of the research on anxiety and depression (see Chapters 8 and 9) is relevant to other emotional responses/symptoms, little has been written regarding the issue of frustration and anger associated with MTBI. Such problems are, however, common among persons seeking support. Irritability has consistently been reported to be a symptom following MTBI. Rutherford et al. (1979) reported irritability in 5.3% of 131 patients with concussion at 1 year post injury. In the Middleboe et al. (1992) sample of 28 patients, 21% endorsed irritability at 1 year post injury. Edna (1987), reporting on a large sample of patients with concussion ($n = 485$), cited irritability in 18% of the group when they were followed up at 3–5 years post injury.

While the neural circuitry for irritability, anger, and aggression is not well understood, disruption of inhibitory influences of the prefrontal cortex over subcortical, and particularly limbic areas, has been hypothesized as a potential mechanism. Traumatic brain injury, including MTBI, has been shown to commonly involve disruption of prefrontal and frontal neocortex. Lesions of the frontal neocortex involving orbital regions are associated with impulsivity, difficulties in modulating behavior on the basis of social cues, and problems understanding and evaluating the way one is perceived by others (Damasio, 1985; Eslinger and Damasio, 1985; Luria, 1980).

From a clinical perspective, a conceptualization of orbital frontal dysfunction as an impairment in modulation of lower limbic activity, which can result in abrupt and violent responses to mild provocations, moves the behavior into a somewhat more reflexive arena. In this sense, aggressive or violent responses must not be seen solely as the result of impaired cognition (e.g., the absence of ability to be self-critical or the presence of altered social awareness). The ideational and contextual elements of orbital frontal aggression may not always be a key to the behavior, and a focus on the surface level context or content may not be useful.

Assessment

Before beginning a treatment program, evaluating the presence and nature of problems with negative emotions and behaviors is important. Persons experiencing problems with frustration and anger secondary to MTBI will often spontaneously reveal these issues. This is, however, somewhat dependent upon both their own insight into the problem and on their perception of the interviewer as being sensitive to MTBI issues, yet respectful of their identity and capacity to function (avoiding a view of them as "brain injured"). Initial assessment of emotional/behavioral functioning with this population requires that the therapist provide time, information, and support, without emphasizing limitations or a focus on brain injury per se. Approaches to assessment of irritability and anger may include interviews with the client and his/her family, checklists, use of personality inventories, and behavioral observations.

When interviewing a client, avoid leading the client toward endorsement of anger problems related to the injury, but make a point of assessing anger specifically. The client may not feel particularly distressed by problems with frustration or anger, although changes in these areas may be contributing to their functioning difficulties or relationship problems.

Sample interview questions regarding frustration/anger sequelae of MTBI include:

1. How have you been handling stress lately?
2. How have you handled stress in the past?
3. About how many times per week would you say you get frustrated or angry?
    . . . to the point where others would notice?
    . . . to the point of raising your voice?
    . . . to the point of physically showing your anger?
4. Do you think your ability to handle stress has changed?
5. What kinds of events or thoughts trigger feelings of anger or frustration?
6. Do angry feelings come and go suddenly, or do you feel angry for a long time?
7. How do you feel after you have been angry?
8. Are there times of day or situations that seem to result in more irritability?
9. What all do you suppose might be contributing to this [problem with anger/frustration]?

Interviews with family, friends, and significant others (with the client's permission) provide another important source of information. Often a brief telephone interview or written questionnaire reveals changes in the client's ability to manage frustration. Clients may have been unaware of the extent of these changes, or were embarrassed or reluctant to disclose them.

Reviewing a list of common triggers for anger may be helpful in identifying what, if anything, is precipitating or contributing to it. Table 10.1 contains a list of common triggers for irritability or anger. Identifying the common warning signs or behavioral correlates of irritability and anger

Table 10-1 Common irritability/anger triggers

Factors	
Stimulation	High noise or activity level
	Unexpected events
	Cognitive demands
Personal	Frustration
	Fear of anxiety
	Embarrassment, shame or guilt
	Discovery or confrontation of problems
Medical	Pain
	Fatigue
	Hypoglycemia (low blood sugar)
	Medications (levels low or high?)
	Alcohol or drugs

Warning Signs	
Verbal	Loud, high voice
	Cursing
	Name-calling
	Threats
Behavioral	Making fists
	Increased movement
	Angry face
	Moving towards the object of anger
	Breaking or throwing things
	Searching for or picking up weapons
	Hitting, kicking or other forms of violence
Physiological	Fast breathing
	Fast heart
	Sweating
	Over-aroused and alert
	Tense muscles
	Flushed face
	Bulging eyes
Mental	Fantasies of doing any of the speech or behavioral signs
	Confusion
	Feelings of frustration
	Feelings of fear or anxiety
	Feelings of embarrassment, shame or guilt
	Feelings of hurt

with the person or family also may be useful. These are listed in Table 10.1 as well. Using a standardized behavioral rating scale may be informative, such as the Overt Aggression Scale (Yudofsky et al., 1986). This scale is based on observable criterions and has been shown to have high interrater reliability. Aggressive behavior is broken down into four do-mains: verbal aggression, physical aggression against objects, physical ag-gression against self, and physical aggression against others.

Individuals with MTBI generally have better insight and awareness than individuals with more severe injuries. Cognitive abilities are also likely to be much better preserved. In many persons with MTBI, using one of the self-report anger scales may be helpful. An example is the No-vaco Anger Scale (Novaco, 1979), provided in Appendix A, which re-quires self-judgements about anticipated level of anger responses on a 5–point scale. (Little or no annoyance to very angry.) Having a family member complete the form to determine how aware the client is of his/her behavior may also be revealing.

Finally, it may be useful in the assessment process to query the per-son's perceptions, beliefs, and attitudes about anger and its management. The questionnaire in Appendix B can be given during the assessment phase (and again during or after treatment) and then discussed with clients to find out something about their levels of insight, potential for rigidity in thinking, and willingness to talk about or try strategies.

Approaches to Management of Frustration/Anger

The following list of treatment approaches and management strategies is hardly comprehensive, but is intended to increase awareness of multiple contributors to and approaches to dealing with anger problems follow-ing MTBI. There is a limited focus on approaches that would encourage therapeutic processing (e.g., open-ended questions to encourage ongoing exploration of issues that result in negative emotions). Many persons ex-periencing even a mild traumatic brain injury are challenged by issues of perseveration, topic maintenance, and lack of initiation or follow through, and these issues indicate a need for structured and strategy-focused treat-ment approaches. As with posttraumatic stress and other psychosocial is-sues, it has been found helpful to establish this therapeutic agenda in the initial sessions and to place limits upon time allotted for description of problems contributing to distressing or angry feelings. Finally, there is a very brief comment on pharmacological interventions.

Environmental Management

Early in treatment, if concerns arise regarding potential for escalating ag-gression or violence, steps should be taken to make the environment safe. This might include having potential weapons removed, removing alco-hol or drugs, or contacting adult persons at risk or appropriate agencies (e.g., Child Protective Services), according to state requirements. In a few cases, supervision of the person might be indicated. If response to envi-ronmental triggers is excessive, the person or family might be advised to reduce noise, turn down music, or prepare and leave available a safe, quiet place that the person might need to retreat to until the therapy is underway. The family or significant others might be advised of strategies such as leaving the person for a short period when warning signs of anger develop, or attempting to distract the person by changing the focus of conversation or activity.

Cognitive Behavioral Approaches

The cognitive–behavioral approach that we advocate for many individuals with TBI is similar to cognitive–behavioral approaches used for many affective and behavioral disorders. These approaches tend to be concrete, focused on measurable behaviors, data based, and hierarchical in nature. These factors are of benefit in working with individuals whose irritability and anger may have more of an organic than a situational base, and who have difficulty with abstraction, memory, attention, or self-awareness.

Luria's (1961) work on the normal development of children's self-control through internal speech was a precursor to subsequent approaches to anger control training. Anger control techniques were further developed by Meichenbaum (1977), whose research focused on impulsivity and poor verbal control of overt behavior. He viewed anger as an affective response to stress that occurs in the face of "demands that tax or exceed the resources of the system." Meichenbaum and Cameron (1983) identified three phases to coping skills training or stress inoculation: (1) education of the client, (2) skills training, and (3) practice under increasingly stressful circumstances. This third phase of "application and follow through" emphasized helping clients to analyze successes and failures and to enhance maintenance and transfer.

Novaco (1979) describe the stress inoculation approach to anger control as not attempting to suppress anger, but rather to minimize maladaptive effects and maximize adaptive function. Novaco identified several stages of such training: (1) preparing for provocation; (2) impact and confrontation; (3) coping with arousal; (4) subsequent reflection; (5) conflict unresolved; and (6) conflict resolved.

Wood (1984, 1987) has presented many cases describing use of strict behavior therapy in management of behavioral disorder in TBI patients (including aggressive behaviors). Only a limited number of studies have documented the effectiveness of behavior interventions for anger control in brain-injured individuals, and these have been in cases of moderate to severe injury (Lira, et al., 1983; McGlynn, 1990; Uomoto and Brockway, 1992).

Establish relationship between head injury and frustration/anger
When individuals with MTBI find themselves experiencing agitation, there are often issues of confusion, self-blame, and focus upon situational triggers. By providing information regarding the common occurrence of

anger and frustration problems following brain injury, the therapist assuages these concerns and paves the way for the work ahead. Give the client lists of common psychological responses or articles and videos regarding head injury sequelae. Often these can be obtained through The National or State Brain Injury Association. One video, "Mild Brain Injury: When Problems Remain," has been found particularly appropriate and inspirational for this population.

It may be helpful to highlight sections regarding anger and frustration, to review some of these in a session, or to assign structured exercises (e.g., written questions). In Appendices C and D are examples of an information sheet ("Ten Things You 'Should' Know about Your Anger") and corresponding questions about anger can be read and then discussed with the therapist. Providing information regarding anger problems following brain injury is another form of normalizing, and tends to reduce the secondary emotional sequelae (feelings about the problem itself). Other literature focusing on beliefs about anger, such as "The Advantages and Disadvantages of Anger" found in Appendix E, can also be used at this stage of developing awareness and providing information.

It is particularly helpful for the therapist to work in tandem with the neuropsychologist or speech–language pathologist/cognitive therapist in establishing the connection between subtle cognitive deficits and frustration, such that under conditions of greater cognitive demand, frustration is likely to escalate. For example, the cognitive therapist may be addressing problems with distractibility, and this issue can be fairly easily segued to issues of irritability, stress, and ultimately to frustration and anger. Subtle problems with divided and alternating attention can be viewed as adversely affecting tasks, but can also be viewed as adversely affecting emotional homeostasis. Thus, attention deficits also indicate probable difficulties alternating and simultaneously focusing upon tasks and upon the internal "self talk" with which we all keep our emotions in check.

Anger/frustration is explained to the clients to be a direct result of subtle cognitive deficits and changes in reactivity of their emotional response, as well as a common reaction to the functional difficulties themselves. In addition, cognitive remediation may be using similar techniques, such as self-talk for cognitive deficits.

Finally, it is of significant benefit to provide information to the client's significant other, family, friends, co-workers, and/or employer. As far as persons in the environment view the client's anger problem as related to his/her injury, they will more than likely exhibit less resentment and contribute unintentionally to stressful reactions.

As a cautionary note, some individuals with brain injury may be suggestible, dependent, or may become too invested in their identity as "brain injured" (vs. having *experienced* a brain injury that may well be contributing to current problems). Such individuals may tend to focus upon symptoms or internalize and subsequently claim new symptoms as they are presented in psychoeducation. If the therapist has any such concerns, editing or controlling the amount and/or type of information given is important.

Much of the focus in treatment itself is on identifying what has been termed the Angry Behavior Cycle (Goldstein et al., 1987) and its a–b–c's—antecedent, behavior, and consequences. Sessions focus on (*a*) recognizing anger cues, the cognitive and somatic precursors to anger; (*b*) using relaxation techniques and other anger reducers; (*c*) knowing and recognizing one's own "triggers," and (*d*) implementing self-coaching, self-evaluation, and self-rewarding. Anger provoking situations are role-played in the clinic and information is gathered about behavior outside sessions through completion of anger management charts or logs.

Identify methods to reduce situation stressors
It is a fundamental tenet of behavioral interventions that the antecedent of a behavior is often overshadowed by its consequence. Thus, the therapist not only directs attention to the clients' "warning signs" of anger, but to the types of situations where anger most frequently becomes a problem. The client is asked to analyze common time frames, events, or locations that may be more frequently associated with anger problems. These scenarios are then used in anticipating, describing, and rehearsing the use of compensatory approaches. An example of a simple anger management chart for listing anger episodes is given in Appendix F. This chart includes the time and date, a description of the situation, the event that resulted in an angry response, what the behavioral response was, and asks the person to suggest how they might have better handled the situation.

For many clients, two frequent themes may be associated with anger: situations with multiple distractions (noisy, active environments) and fatigue. Most clients experiencing MTBI continue to lead somewhat active lives and those around them tend to have difficulty understanding or maintaining awareness of their limitations. These issues, then, require special attention.

When in a distracting environment, the client is asked to take frequent, short breaks in a quieter room or space. The therapist provides a brain injury-based rationale for the cognitive and emotional cost of prolonged exposure to stimulation. The client might be encouraged to turn the radio off while driving, to read the paper after children have gone to bed, or to avoid or limit time in highly stimulating or crowded situations, such as malls or spectator sports events. Family education and participation are often used here. For example, it might be explained to children that, since the accident, the client sometimes hears too much noise at once. A particular room might be designated as their "quiet room," a space where it is quiet and the client can remain undisturbed for a period of time.

For problems with fatigue, again, family involvement and education are important, while clients are directed toward fatigue management or "pacing," strategies. Wearied by the unconscious effort of suppressing continual distraction, the client also often needs an explanation of the source of their fatigue in order to predict and manage the frustration it engenders. It is as if energy meant for maintaining homeostasis is spent on buffering distractions and processing what was once automatic, with the ultimate price being frustration and anger. To compensate, therapist and client again generate specific strategies, such as nutrition breaks just before anticipated periods of fatigue or an earlier bedtime. It may be helpful to plan high energy or cognitively demanding activities at the beginning of the day or after a rest, and to limit the activity in one day.

Identify somatic precursors to anger
Many individuals with MTBI describe their episodes of anger as occurring "out of the blue." This may be due in part to the nature of problems with impulsivity and also to the increased effort given to attending to environmental stimuli at the expense of attention to physiological cues. The notion that anger occurs without any warning must be dispelled, and the client must learn to conceptualize these responses as simply occurring much faster and perhaps with less attention given to warning cues. Once this has been established, therapeutic efforts can begin to focus on delineation of the somatic cues that signify escalating tension and anger. Checklists of common warning signs for anger and frustration in individuals with MTBI may be helpful, but clients can probably generate the most accurate sensations that precede episodes of anger. Case examples of anger warning signs are listed in Table 10.1. The client is asked to learn his/her own cues, and here again a written cue card, sticker, or note in his/her daily organizer or nototebook may be very helpful. The usefulness of these cues is presented to the client as a type of natural biofeedback that signals them to employ some sort of compensatory strategy (see below). A typical cue card for anger might look like this:

MY ANGER SIGNS:
   Loud voice
   Tense muscles
   Thoughts of hitting
   Confusion
BACK OFF:
   Say: "I am feeling angry. I need to back off."
   Leave the room.
   Sit, close my eyes, slow, deep breaths, Relax muscles.
WHEN I CAN SMILE:
   Explain? Apologize? Talk about it?

There will likely be a training phase in recognizing precursor signs and referring to the cue card. Initially the therapist may indicate the onset of anger signals in the client in both natural and contrived situations that are likely to trigger anger. Then having the client mentally visualize various scenarios in which the client notices these warning signs can be incorporated.

Case 1

Mr. T sustained a mild brain injury in an industrial accident that left him with subtle but significant cognitive deficits, debilitating fatigue, and increased irritability and anger. For his wife and son, it was his problems with anger (abruptly yelling) that were most upsetting. Mr. T, however, felt helpless to address these episodes, stating "they just happen." With training he could identify several somatic cues that briefly preceded his yelling behavior (face feeling "flushed" and clenched teeth) and ultimately improved his ability to notice these cues in vivo. Inside his notebook was a chart where he indicated the time of day each time he sensed the warning signs.

Teach coping techniques and anger reducers
Lacking a remedy for behavioral problems subsequent to brain injury, compensatory approaches are often the focus of training. Just as a client must learn to increase his/her use of other compensatory systems (daily organizer/note-taking, lists, etc.), there is a need to specify, personalize, and generalize strategies to compensate for frustration and anger. Establish this common goal with the client by way of analogy with more concrete examples of compensation. Anger management is often a volatile issue, and the goals of compensation and management help to reduce resistance to strategies that do not "work" (fix the problem), but rather "help" (manage the problem). For individuals with MTBI, the introduction of compensatory strategies can feel patronizing, embarrassing, or insulting. Framing simple anger management strategies as helpful for a sizable population of those in similar circumstances mollifies this resistance, as do recurrent acknowledgments that such strategies were previously unnecessary for them.

Compensatory strategies include relaxation techniques (e.g., sitting, closing eyes, deep controlled breathing); cognitive/self-talk techniques (e.g., silently telling oneself, "It is just not worth it to get so upset."); logistical approaches (e.g., taking a break from the situation, going outside and walking); and prearranged responses/cues from significant others (e.g., the spouse employs a specified signal to increase awareness of rising anger, briefly leaves the situation his/herself, etc.). Each of these strategies is discussed briefly below.

The effect of increased vigilance and effort in daily functioning is increased tension. With the chronicity of this tension following TBI and subtle cognitive deficits, the body "forgets" what the absence of tension feels like at all. Consequently, *relaxation training* is a vital component of anger management therapy for persons challenged by MTBI. Relaxation training is described in the previous chapter on anxiety and posttraumatic stress. It is important that clients spend some time relearning the sensations of reduced arousal, be it 5 minutes in session or 30 minutes of homework with a relaxation cassette.

Cognitive "self-talk" techniques derived from Luria's (1961) early work on self regulation. Some evidence exists that verbal self-regulation strategies can be trained and used effectively by individuals with MTBI (see Chapter 6 on executive function training). In theory, these self-regulation strategies reinstate a level of control that would normally be automatically triggered by prefrontal systems that are now dysfunctional. It is a top-down model that proposes that one substitute a more conscious regulation of what become more reflexive emotional and behavioral responses following brain injury. This approach also addresses issues of possible rigidity or black-and-white thinking, and in that sense shares commonalities with management of other dysfunctional thoughts (see Chapter 9 on management of anxiety disorders). Examples of self-statements for dealing with anger both in anticipation of and during stressful or arousing experiences is given in Appendix G. Another exercise involves having the client generate specific strategies or self-statements to deal with different stages of anger as shown in Appendix H.

Compensatory approaches, such as taking a break from the situation, are ones that serve to remove or decrease the situational stressors or triggers. This allows the person to both deescalate and to use techniques to control angry or upset feelings more effectively. It is sometimes easier done at home than in a work environment, although accommodations might even be made in more structured circumstances.

Prearranged responses or cues from significant others can be useful in the early stages of training before the person has learned to identify the warning signs him/herself. It provides for a potentially more adaptive response on the part of a significant other who might otherwise be confused, hurt, or upset by the client's responses and actually contribute to the escalation of angry behavior. Practice in therapy sessions and agreement to the plan by all parties is essential.

Each person may respond best to a different constellation of approaches. It is therefore important to encourage clients to try different things and ultimately to become specific about the techniques they will use. Under circumstances of both increased agitation and reduced cognitive functioning, vague strategies (e.g., "I will just try to calm down.") will be more difficult to recall and employ. The clients are encouraged to write down their specific techniques (or the therapist writes these for them), which are then frequently referred to in session. Generalization is supported by review and anticipation of strategy use in specific situations, although it may initially require use of environmental cues and the cooperation of significant others.

Case 2

Mr. G entered a rehabilitation program after he was unable to return to his previous work following a mild brain injury. His wife was considerably distressed that his "temper (was) much worse" and that Mr. G appeared to dismiss this problem. With Mr. G's permission, the therapist was able to videotape Mr. G's agitation when discussing a recent and frustrating event. Viewing this video was helpful in increasing his awareness of how quickly and dramatically his anger tended to escalate. He was then given several suggested strategies for compensation. When an approach was selected, key words from these strategies were placed on the front of his daily organizer (which was often within his sight). His key words were "Back off; Calm down; Try again." *"Back off"* involved leaving the situation when anger warning signals appeared. *"Calm down"* included deep breathing, listening to soft music, closing his eyes, and/or physical exercise. Once calm, he was encouraged to prepare to return. Possible preparation included reviewing a list of questions ("Do I need to apologize?" "Do I need to explain why I left?") or rethinking the situation. *"Try again"* involved returning to the situation and apologizing, talking through the issue, or resuming what he was doing. Approximately 6 weeks of training (twice per week sessions) was required. He agreed that his wife might help him in using these strategies by asking her to signal him (touching her finger alongside her nose) at the first signs of escalating anger. In this way, Mr. G could "save face" when others were present and to avoid engaging with his wife regarding her verbal responses. His problems with anger continued sometimes in community situations, though his wife reported substantial improvements in the home. A decrease in the number of anger outbursts per day was documented in an anger management chart.

Overall, the anger management approaches discussed here progress in a hierarchy, involving recognition of anger and anger precursors and then employment of compensatory strategies, first on cue from others, then gradually with self-cuing. Training moves from simple controlled settings (e.g., an office), to more complex, interactive, but still controlled settings (e.g., a clinic with other clients), to complex and demanding naturalistic settings at home, at work and in the community.

Reactive Anger

Besides the physiological, cognitive, and situational factors described above, problems with adjustment to and acceptance of losses and a component of "reactive" anger may also exist. For a subset of persons experiencing a mild brain injury, there may be a psychosocial and emotional underlay to anger that may exert itself in situations where the individual is not entirely aware of this process (and may be focused upon the immediate situation). For example, the individual may be deeply angry at his/her perceived losses in functioning, at his/her lack of validation and support from others, or at the person(s) responsible for the injury. He/she may be angry at the perceived cause of an injury such as a drunk driver or an assailant.

Anger can also be one aspect of a grief reaction. Poor memory or judgement, or a perception that others don't understand or believe them, can complicate grief reactions. For some individuals, grief therapy or the facilitation of symbolic or ritualistic anger at the perceived source of problems may be beneficial. For a discussion of the grieving process, see Chapter 8 on treatment of depression.

Persons with reactive anger frequently tend to bring up certain issues related to their injury and will often disclose their angry feelings if queried by a supportive therapist. Once such issues have been recognized, the therapist should attempt to increase awareness of how such feelings may be a confluence to situational anger. The therapist provides a direct and balanced message to the client: that reactive anger is "normal," even condign, but that it is also an ill-afforded distraction, an obstacle to improvement, and often an undeserved and unfair response to others.

Finally, people who have had brain injuries still have legitimate reasons to get angry. Angry behaviors can be appropriate or inappropriate, but legitimate concerns and complaints should certainly be addressed.

Pharmacological Approaches

A discussion of pharmacological management of irritability and anger is well beyond the scope of this chapter, but a few remarks are in order. Many neurochemicals, but particularly the neurotransmitter serotonin, appear to be involved in the regulation of aggressive and other impulsive behavior. Serotonergic drugs, such as Trazodone, Fluoxetine, and Busparone, have been reported to reduce aggression. Some of these have been used successfully in patients with MTBI. Carbamazepine (Tegretol) is also sometimes helpful in managing aggression, raising the question of whether an unrecognized epileptic disorder may be at the root of some aggressive behavior. In states of aggression related to high anxiety levels, antianxiety agents such as benzodiazepines (and perhaps Busparone) are potentially beneficial, although there is little in the literature that addresses its effect on individuals with MTBI.

Conclusions

Frustration, irritability, and anger are common problems following brain injury. Their presence and presentation usually involve complex interactions between premorbid personality and predispositions, the nature of neurological injury, situational demands, and environmental stressors and reinforcers. Many individuals with MTBI possess sufficient cognitive skills and capacities for development of self-monitoring and self-control that they can benefit from cognitive behavioral strategies to reduce the impact of negative emotions and behaviors.

References

Damasio, A.R. (1985). The frontal lobes. In K.M. Heilman and E. Valenstein (Eds.), *Clinical Neuropsychology*. New York, NY: Oxford University Press, pp. 339–376.

Edna, T.H. (1987). Disability 3–5 years after minor head injury. *Journal Oslo City Hospital, 37*, 41–48.

Eslinger, P.J. and Damasio, A.R. (1985). Severe disturbance of higher cognition after bilateral frontal lobe ablation: Patient EVR. *Neurology, 35*(12), 1731–1741.

Goldstein, A.P., Glick, B, Reiner, S., Zimmerman, D., and Coultry, T.M. (1987). *Aggression Replacement Training: A Comprehensive Intervention for Aggressive Youth*. Champaign, IL: Research Press.

Lira, F.T., Carne, W., and Masri, A.M. (1983). Treatment of anger and impulsivity in a brain damaged patient: A case study applying stress inoculation. *Clinical Neuropsychology, 3*(5) 159–160.

Luria, A.R. (1961). *The Role of Speech in Regulation of Normal and Abnormal Behaviour*. London: Pergamon Press.

Luria, A.R. (1980). *Higher Cortical Functions in Man 2*. Revised and expanded edition translated by Basil Haigh. New York, NY: Basic Books.

McGlynn, S.M. (1990). Behavioral approaches to neuropsychological rehabilitation. *Psychological Bulletin, 108*, 420–441.

McKay, M., Rogers, P.D., and McKay, J. (1989). *When Anger Hurts: Quieting the Storm Within*. Oakland, CA: New Harbinger Publications, Inc.

Meichenbaum, D. (1977). *Cognitive-Behavior Modification: An Integrative Approach*. New York, NY: Plenum Press.

Meichenbaum, D. and Cameron, R. (1983). Stress inoculation training. In D. Meichenbaum and M.E. Jaremko (Eds.), *Stress Reduction and Prevention*. New York, NY: Plenum Press, pp. 115–154.

Middleboe, T., Birket-Smith, M., Anderson, H.S., et al. (1992). Personality traits in patients with postconcussional sequelae. *Journal of Personality Disorders, 6*, 246–255.

Novaco, R.W. (1979). The cognitive regulation of anger and stress. In P.C. Kendall and S.D. Hollon (Eds.), *Cognitive Behavioral Interventions: Theory, Research and Procedures*. Orlando, FL: Academic Press, Inc., pp. 241–278.

Rutherford, W.H., Merrett, J.D., and McDonald, J.R. (1979). Symptoms at one year following concussion from minor head injuries. *Injury, 10*, 225–230.

Uomoto, J.M. and Brockway, J.A. (1992). Anger management training for brain injured patients and their family members. *Archives of Physical Medicine and Rehabilitation, 73*, 674–679.

Wood, R.L. (1984). Behavioral disorders following severe brain injury: Their presentation and psychological management. In N. Brooks (Ed.), *Closed Head Injury: Psychological, Social and Family Consequences*. Oxford: Oxford University Press, pp. 195–219.

Wood, R.L. (1987). *Brain Injury Rehabilitation: A Neurobehavioral Approach.* Rockville, MD: Aspen Press.

Yudofsky, S.C., Silver, J.M., Jackson, M., Endicott, J., and Williams, D. (1986). The Overt Aggression Scale: An operationalized rating scale for verbal and physical aggression. *American Journal of Psychiatry, 143*, 35–39.

APPENDIX A

A self-rating scale of anger developed by Novaco.

0   You would feel very little or no annoyance.

1   You would feel a little irritated.

2   You would feel moderately upset.

3   You would feel quite angry.

4   You would feel very angry.

Mark your answer after each question:

NOVACO ANGER SCALE

1. You unpack an appliance you have just bought, plug it in, and discover that it doesn't work. _____

2. Being overcharged by a repairman who has you over a barrel. _____

3. Being singled out for correction, when the actions of others go unnoticed. _____

4. Getting your car stuck in the mud or snow. _____

5. You are talking to someone and they don't answer you. _____

6. Someone pretends to be something they are not. _____

7. While you are struggling to carry four cups of coffee to your table at a cafeteria, someone bumps into you, spilling the coffee. _____

8. You have hung up your clothes, but someone knocks them to the floor and fails to pick them up. _____

9. You are hounded by a salesperson from the moment that you walk into a store. _____

10. You have made arrangements to go somewhere with a person who backs off at the last minute and leaves you hanging. _____

11. Being joked about or teased. _____

12. Your car is stalled at a traffic light, and the guy behind you keeps blowing his horn. _____

13. You accidentally make the wrong kind of turn in a parking lot. As you get out of your car someone yells at you, "Where did you learn to drive?" _____

14. Someone makes a mistake and blames it on you. _____

15. You are trying to concentrate, but a person near you is tapping their foot. _____

16. You lend someone an important book or tool, and they fail to return it. _____

17. You have had a busy day, and the person you live with starts to complain about how you forgot to do something that you agreed to do. _____

18. You are trying to discuss something important with your mate or partner who isn't giving you a chance to express your feelings. _____

19. You are in a discussion with someone who persists in arguing about a topic they know very little about. _____

20. Someone sticks his or her nose into an argument between you and someone else. _____

21. You need to get somewhere quickly, but the car in front of you is going 25 mph in a 40 mph zone, and

you can't pass. _____

22. Stepping on a gob of chewing gum. _____

23. Being mocked by a small group of people as you pass them. _____

24. In a hurry to get somewhere, you tear a good pair of slacks on a sharp object. _____

25. You use your last dime to make a phone call but you are disconnected before you finish dialing and the dime is lost. _____

Now that you have completed the Anger Inventory, you are in a position to calculate your IQ, your Irritability Quotient. Make sure that you have not skipped any items. Add up your score for each of the twenty-five incidents. The lowest possible total score on the test would be zero. This would mean you put down a zero on each item. This indicates you are either a liar or a guru! The highest score would be a hundred. This would mean you recorded a four on each of the twenty-five items, and you're constantly at or beyond the boiling point.

You can now interpret your total score according to the following scale:

0-45:   The amount of anger and annoyance you generally experience is remarkably low. Only a few percent of the population will score this low on the test. You are one of the select few!

46-55:   You are substantially more peaceful than the average person.

56-75:   You respond to life's annoyances with an average amount of anger.

76-85:   You frequently react in an angry way to life's many annoyances. You are substantially more irritable than the average person.

86-100: You are a true anger champion, and you are plagued by frequent intense furious reactions that do not quickly disappear.

APPENDIX B

Understanding and Managing Anger

DAVID HOVLAND, M.S.W.

A worksheet developed at the Good Samaritan Center for Continuing Rehabilitation in Puyallup, Washington, to help individuals learn more about anger and its antecedents.

UNDERSTANDING AND MANAGING ANGER

David Hovland, M.S.W.

1. Why would you want to work towards being less angry? (check below)

    a.   Anger is a type of unhappiness. I want to feel better.

    b.   Anger is stressful on the body. I want to be healthier.

    c.   Something/someone requires me to be less angry.

    d.   Anger doesn't always help the situation any.

2. Anger <u>seems</u> to be caused by situations/other people. For the most part, it is not. (Circle below for True or False)

    T or F   We are totally helpless to our emotions.

    T or F   What we think about someone determines our reaction much more than just what they say or do.

    T or F   A situation can have very different effects on us, depending on our mental state and thoughts at the time.

3. Anger comes from 3 main sources: Grief/Acceptance (loss)

                                          Physical causes (biology)

    Match the examples below: Distorted Thinking (thoughts)

    Loss   You drink a lot of coffee and become irritable.

    Biology   You <u>know</u> someone "shouldn't" do that.

    Thoughts   You lose something important to you.

                  You don't get any exercise and become edgy.

                  Someone treats you, in <u>your</u> opinion, unfairly.

4. Often, anger comes from problems in our thoughts. Part of us believes that people and things "should (ought to) go a certain way (false).

    T or F   Human beings are imperfect by nature.

    T or F   Irritating things are examples of human imperfections.

    T or F   Therefore, people should behave in irritating ways.

    This doesn't make sense, does it? Neither does it make sense that people "should" behave perfectly or as we want them to.

5. It isn't easy, but we can change the way we think about people and things. What might be wrong with the following statements?   I ought to be able to do this. →

    I can't stand it when things are unfair. →

    You "make" me mad. →

6. Check the coping skills below that you would be willing to try:

    a.   Go for walks and do some brief stretching

    b.   Listen to a relaxation tape regularly

    c.   Take short breaks and do some controlled breathing

    d.   Get in touch with your "shoulds" and rewrite them

    e.   Switch to decaf coffee

    f.   Your own idea _____

7. I have done the exercises above and I agree with most of these points. I commit to myself to work on my anger with these skills.

    Signed/Date _____

APPENDIX C

An educational flyer developed at the Good Samaritan Center for Continuing Rehabilitation in Puyallup, Washington, to provide information about anger.

Ten Things You "Should" Know About Your Anger

1. The events of this world don't make you angry. Your "hot thoughts" create your anger. Even when a genuinely negative event occurs, it is the meaning you attach to it that determines your emotional response.

The idea that you are responsible for your anger is ultimately to your advantage because it gives you the opportunity to achieve control and make a free choice about how you want to feel. If it weren't for this, you would be helpless to control your emotions; they would be irreversibly bound up with every external event of this world, most of which are ultimately out of your control.

2. Most of the time your anger will not help you. It will immobilize you, and you will become frozen in your hostility to no productive purpose. You will feel better if you place your emphasis on the active search for creative solutions. what can you do to correct the difficulty or at least reduce the chance that you'll get burned in the same way in the future? This attitude will eliminate to a certain extent the helplessness and frustration that eats you up when you feel you can't deal with a situation effectively.

If no solution is possible because the provocation is totally beyond your control, you will only make yourself miserable with your resentment, so why not get rid of it? It's difficult if not impossible to feel anger and joy simultaneously. If you think your angry feelings are especially precious and important, then think about one of the happiest moments of your life. Now ask yourself, how many minutes of that period of peace of jubilation would I be willing to trade in for feeling frustration and irritation instead?

3. The thoughts that generate anger more often than not will contain distortions. Correcting these distortions will reduce your anger.

4. Ultimately your anger is caused by your belief that someone is acting unfairly or some event is unjust. The intensity of the anger will increase in proportion to the severity of the maliciousness perceived and if the act is seen as intentional.

5. If you learn to see the world through other people's eyes, you will often be surprised to realize their actions are *not* unfair from their point of view. The unfairness in these cases turns out to be an illusion that exists *only in your mind.* If you are willing to let go of the unrealistic notion that your concepts of truth, justice, and fairness are shared by everyone. much of your resentment and frustration will vanish.

6. Other people usually do not feel they deserve your punishment.

Therefore, your retaliation is unlikely to help you achieve any positive goals in your interactions with them. Your rage will often just cause further deterioration and polarization, and will function as a self-fulfilling prophecy. Even if you temporarily get what you want, any short-term gains from such hostile manipulation will often be more than counterbalanced by a long-term resentment and retaliation from the people you are coercing. No one likes to be controlled or forced. This is why a positive reward system works better.

7. A great deal of your anger involves your defense against loss of self-esteem when people criticize you, disagree with you, or fail to behave a you want them to. Such anger is *always* inappropriate because only your own negative distorted thoughts can cause you to lose self-esteem. When you blame the other guy for your feelings of worthlessness, you are always fooling yourself.

8. Frustration results from unmet expectations. Since the event that disappointed you was a part of "reality," it was "realistic." Thus, your frustration always results from your *unrealistic* expectation. You have the right to try to influence reality to bring it more in line with your expectations, but this is not always practical, especially when these expectations represent ideals that don't correspond to everyone else's concept of human nature. The simplest solution would be to change your expectations. For example, some unrealistic expectations that lead to frustration include:

a. If I want something (love, happiness, a promotion, etc.), I deserve it.

b. If I work hard at something, I *should* be successful.

c. Other people *should* try to measure up to my standards and believe in my concept of "fairness."

d. I *should* be able to solve any problems quickly and easily.

e. If I'm a good wife, my husband is *bound* to love me.

f. People *should* think and act the way I do.

g. If I'm nice to someone, they *should* reciprocate.

9. It is just childish pouting to insist you have the *right* to be angry. Of course you do! Anger is legally permitted in the United States. The crucial issue is—is it to your advantage to feel angry? Will you or the world really benefit from your rage?

10. You rarely need your anger in order to be human. It is not true that you will be an unfeeling robot without it. In fact, when you rid yourself of that sour irritability, you will feel greater zest, joy, peace, and productivity.

APPENDIX D

A short quiz to accompany Appendix C in providing education about anger.

Good Samaritan Hospital Center for Cognitive Rehabilitation

ANGER QUIZ

From: Ten Things You "Should" Know About Your Anger

1.   Do events trigger your anger?

2.   Is anger caused by what happens?

3.   Are you free to make a choice about how you want to feel?

4.   Does anger provide you with a productive purpose?

5.   Does anger cause you to be stuck in a non-productive state?

6.   Should you let go of anger and search for a solution?

7.   Can you feel anger and joy at the same time?

8.   Are anger thoughts distorted?

9.   Will looking at the situation from the other person's point of view help you control your anger?

10.   Does punishing the person usually help the situation?

11.   Does punishment work better than positive rewards for changing others' behavior?

12.   Is it O.K. to blame the other guy for your feelings?

13.   Do realistic expectations result in anger?

14.   Do you have a "right" to be angry?

15.   Is it to your advantage to be angry?

16.   Could changing unrealistic expectations reduce your frustration?

17.   Is this statement realistic: "If I work hard at something, it should go well."

18.   Do most people feel they deserve your punishment?

19.   Is anger needed for being human?

20.   Are you responsible for your anger?

APPENDIX E

An informational flyer developed at the Good Samaritan Center for Continuing Rehabilitation in Puyallup, Washington, to provide education about anger.

The Advantages & Disadvantages of Anger
David Hovland, M.S.W.

DIRECTIONS: Although anger may be causing you some real problems, you may also be deriving a variety of secondary gains through this emotion. Rate each example below as to how much it applies to yourself.

        1 = not at all
        2 = somewhat
        3 = about half
        4 = quite a bit
        5 = definitely

After rating each example, write at lease one advantage of your own (be specific). Try to remember these disadvantages when you <u>start</u> to get frustrated.

ADVANTAGES

____ In a way, it feels good.

____ I feel strong.

____ I have the <u>right</u> to get mad.

____ They'll see that <u>I'm</u> right.

____ I'll show them I won't be taken advantage of.

____ They will suffer.

____ I get revenge.

My example(s):

DISADVANTAGES

____ It sabotages my relationships.

____ I feel rude.

____ It interferes with my desire to respect others.

____ Being so "right" interferes with my desire to learn from other perspectives.

____ My anger gets in the way of finding a solution.

        ____ I don't <u>really</u> want to cause suffering.

____ They might try to get back at me; they might just succeed.

____ They might not want to be around me any more.

____ They might see me as immature.

____ I hate it when my moods go up and down like this.

____ The unpleasant feelings make my life miserable.

____ Life becomes a bitter experience when you often give in to anger.

My examples:

APPENDIX F

A worksheet designed to help individuals identify triggers for anger and begin to consider alternative responses.

Good Samaritan Hospital Center for Cognitive Rehabilitation

ANGER MANAGEMENT CHART

Date/Time	What was I doing before I became angry?	What happened that I got angry about?	What did I do when I got angry?	what could I have done to handle the situation better (if anything)?

APPENDIX G

A list of self-statements to help individuals with brain injury restructure
thoughts that can lead to anger.

SELF STATEMENTS FOR ANGER MANAGEMENT RELATED TO HEAD INJURY

Check the statements below which would be most helpful to you:

____ I'm starting to get those warning signs . . . I need to check myself.

____ This is making me mad, but I also know my injury could be making me over-react.

____ I need to take a break from this so that I can think abut how it might be the situation AND my injury.

____ Getting angry here doesn't help the situation at all.

____ I can handle this . . . I know how my anger is partially related to my injury and how I can manage it.

____ I'm not going to let this situation get to me, and I'm not going to let my injury fuel my anger either.

____ This isn't right! . . I need to just take a deep breath and slow myself down a bit.

____ I need to stop for a minute and think . . How do I want to handle this?

____ This situation and my injury make me want to just REACT, but I am going to RESPOND with self-

control.

____ Now is the time I need to remind myself of my pattern of reacting, and how I usually feel afterwards.

____ I'm not going to put up with this, but I'm not going to give in to my anger either.

____ This might seem worse than it is right now . . . could I be making too much of this?

____ I need to ask myself what all could be contributing to my anger right now . . . am I fatigued, distracted,

etc.?

Your own statement:

APPENDIX H

A quiz designed to help individuals learn techniques of cognitive restructuring for events that lead to anger.

Good Samaritan Hospital
Center for Cognitive Rehabilitation

ANGER MANAGEMENT QUIZ
David Hovland, M.S.W.

List the four steps of anger:

    1.   *The event, what happens, the person, etc.*
    2.   *Your thoughts, your mental response, etc.*
    3.   *Your physiological response, adrenaline, etc.*
    4.   *The "feeling" of anger.*

Write one 'self statement" to help you with step No. 1 above:
What two steps do we tend to focus on?

Examples: *"I will be tempted to focus on #1, but I can't change that."*
           "It's hard not to get preoccupied with the event."
           "The incident tries to get all my attention."

List two techniques to help you with step No. 2 above:

Tell myself, "Wait, there is no should - I simply don't like this."
Tell myself, "Part of me thinks . . . but part of me also knows . . ."
Ask myself, "Who is really worse off if I react to this?"
Count to ten.

List two techniques to help you with step No. 3 above:

Take one deep breath. Or, exhale, then exhale twice again.
Tense/relax specific parts of your body (autogenic).
Stretch specific parts of your body (your fingers, your face, etc.)
Switch positions.
Take a break.

What is the difference between "assertive" and angry?

Assertive is direct, but respectful/polite. Anger is intimidating.
Assertiveness is a more thoughtful expression. Anger is reacting.

List one strategy for generalization:

        Practice during minor incidents.
        Put post-it notes up as reminders.
        Put up this test where you will see it.
        Study this.

IV

VOCATIONAL AND COMMUNITY INTEGRATION

11

Vocational Rehabilitation

GINGER D. HURT

Previous chapters have outlined a variety of physical, cognitive, and psychoscocial difficulties associated with mild traumatic brain injury (MTBI). Many of these difficulties are relatively subtle and their impact is often not appreciated until the injured individual resumes preinjury activities. In some cases, it is only following attempts to return to work that problems surface. Employment commonly places demands on endurance, sustained attention, the ability to deal with distractions, memory, and organization. Weaknesses in these areas are familiar features of the postconcussive syndrome. In combination with mental and physical fatigue, and perhaps with persistent pain or other physical limitations, such difficulties may alter the individual's ability to cope effectively in the workplace.

It is acknowledged that the great majority of individuals who sustain MTBI are able to return successfully to preinjury employment status within a relatively short time following injury. In some cases, however, the individual is not successful in maintaining employment after injury, or feels that their safety and/or productivity at work has been compromised. Indeed, some research has suggested that although most individuals with MTBI do return to employment, they are often at a level below their preinjury positions (Steambrook et al., 1990).

Despite evidence that mild brain injuries comprise a substantial percentage of all brain traumas (Kraus and Nourjah, 1989), little attention has been directed toward the vocational rehabilitation needs of this population. Veach and Taylor (1989) outlined the utility of job trials, physical reconditioning, and psychosocial counseling to the vocational success of this population. Hurt (1991) described critical factors in vocational rehabilitation and provided a structured systematic model for delivery of vocational services to individuals with MTBI. This chapter elaborates on that model and provides additional information needed for successful vocational programming with this population.

Vocational Implications of Mild Brain Injury

Successful return to employment can be affected by difficulties in a variety of physical, cognitive, affective, and psychosocial domains, each of which is discussed below.

Physical Deficits

The physical sequelae that most commonly affect return to work in individuals with MTBI include: (1) chronic fatigue due to general deconditioning and effortful cognitive processing; (2) chronic pain; (3) impaired balance and coordination; and (4) visual difficulties.

Chronic fatigue can have a dramatic effect on physical stamina and work tolerances (Veach and Taylor, 1989). Individuals may be unable to work a full 8–hour day or a 40–hour week. Lack of physical stamina and poor work tolerances may result in: cognitive breakdown as the person fatigues, physical complaints of exhaustion and headaches, general irritability, and interpersonal problems on the job. As a result, gradual return to work, with a gradation from simple to more complex job tasks as work endurance and cognitive skills improve, can often prevent failure and compromised self- esteem. Problems with endurance can be addressed through the individual's participation in a work hardening program or structured exercise program aimed at aerobic conditioning, overall strengthening, and pacing of physical activity. There also should be a focus on facilitating regular sleep patterns.

Chronic pain, secondary to persistent headache, or to disabling neck or back pain, is frequently co-morbid with persistent MTBI symptomatology. Indeed, there are many commonalities between the two disorders and it may be difficult to disentangle the influences of each on work behaviors. Neurological work-up and treatment and, in some cases, participation in a chronic pain program may be appropriate.

Persistent problems with balance and dizziness can impact the ability to work at jobs that involve climbing, working at heights, walking on uneven terrain, moving quickly in hazardous situations, and safely operating machinery and/or equipment. It is important during the initial phase of vocational planning to request a static/dynamic balance evaluation for those individuals whose reported balance difficulties may impact return to work. Such evaluations are typically available through specialized physical therapy services where the individual, once assessed, can learn compensatory strategies for balance deficits. If balance problems persist, it may be necessary to avoid any occupations that involve climbing or working at unprotected heights.

Individuals with persistent visual complaints may experience problems at work sites that place heavy demands on driving, reading, blueprint analysis, clerical work, and/or computer use. Optometric and/or opthalmologic examinations may identify correctable conditions. In addition, compensations can be made in the selection of computer monitors and print size. There may also be benefit from therapeutic visual exercises by a vision specialist.

Cognitive Deficits

Cognitive impairments may manifest in a variety of difficulties both on and off the job and are described in detail in Part II in this volume. Memory deficits may impact the ability to learn new information and remember job tasks. Attention/concentration problems may result in difficulties staying on task due to distractability, problems paying attention to more than one task or aspect of a task simultaneously, and difficulty returning to a task after an interruption. Many individuals may also experience slowed speed of task performance and as a result, reduced levels of work productivity.

Deficits in executive function may result in reduced ability to organize, plan, set goals, establish priorities, and monitor behavior. Individuals with such deficits may feel overwhelmed by complex or nonrepetitive tasks. Impaired reasoning skills may impact the individual's ability to grasp abstract concepts and apply these to specific work situations.

Psychosocial Problems

Many individuals with MTBI demonstrate changes in emotional regulation and interpersonal behavior that can have a negative impact in the work environment. Irritability, anger outbursts, and insensitivity to others are common contributors to social and work-related difficulties (Lezak, 1978; Zasler, 1989). The physical and cognitive changes experienced by an individual with a mild brain injury can also result in altered perceptions of self that can impact the potential for successful return to employment. Premature return to work can result in a failure to meet former work performance standards. The consequence of a failed work experience is often a severe decline in the individual's self-esteem and a marked reduction in their confidence in work skills (Fogel and Paul-Cohen, 1992; O'Hara, 1988; Zuger and Boehm, 1993). Return to a stressful job, when cognitive recovery is incomplete, can play a significant role in the persistence of cognitive problems and the development of emotional difficulties (Wood et al., 1984). Anxiety and depression, due to previous work failures, may result in the individual being afraid to try compensatory strategies, and thereby, risk another failure. Unresolved grief issues related to the loss of a vocational dream and feelings of work competence may also impact the individual's ability to return to work successfully (Lezak, 1978; Prigatano et al., 1987).

Cicerone (1991) noted however that neuropsychological impairments related to the ability to integrate cognitive and affective information can lead individuals with MTBI to overestimate their competency and make inappropriate vocational choices. Individuals may be strongly influenced by intact memories of previous vocational capacities and may subsequently be resistive to activities that seem unchallenging to this "premorbid" sense of self. This may result in "pacing" difficulties, unawareness of the time needed to complete tasks, the setting of unrealistic goals, over extending themselves, and disregarding fatigue and pain. The individual's readiness for vocational planning is highly dependent upon his/her capacity for becoming aware of both his/her vocational strengths and limitations.

Such factors highlight the importance of exploring and understanding the subjective experience and perceptions of the client regarding his/her competencies, difficulties and overall functioning.

The Process of Vocational Rehabilitation

The process of vocational intervention is usually divided into several distinct components—intake/records review, vocational assessment, treatment plan and counseling, job placement/development, and postemployment job maintenance/follow-up services.

Intake/Records Review

Prior to beginning vocational planning, the vocational rehabilitation counselor usually reviews all available records to determine the client's needs and specific goals for vocational services. Current medical reports can provide important detail regarding the severity of the brain injury and related symptoms, unrelated medical problems, current medications, and medical restrictions, if any. If available, a current functional physical capacities evaluation will provide the counselor with valuable information on physical abilities and the appropriate level of work.

Vocational training and experience prior to the injury should be carefully reviewed. This will provide crucial information as to what the individual's prior capabilities were. If jobs were held or attempted after the injury, they can provide valuable information about the client's current functional skills and problems experienced due to brain-injury related difficulties. Educational records may also provide information about the individual's premorbid abilities.

Recent and detailed neuropsychological evaluation information often provides the best foundation for identifying areas of difficulty and vocational needs (Hallauer et al., 1989). Appendix A contains a checklist for organizing information from a neuropsychological assessment in functional terms that are relevant to vocational rehabilitation (Young et al., 1993).

Other areas that should be explored during the intake interview with the individual and, if possible, a significant other include: (1) history of substance abuse and treatment; (2) history of psychiatric or psychological treatment; (3) current financial status and source of income, including any financial incentives and disincentives for return to work; (4) current use of strategies to compensate for brain injury-related deficits; (5) current vocational interests and goals; (6) family support for return-to-work efforts; (7) current emotional status (i.e., depression, anxiety, anger management problems); and (8) cultural or lifestyle issues that may affect employment options.

Vocational Assessment

The vocational assessment itself includes both formal vocational testing and experiential activities designed to clarify vocational strengths/limitations, work values, interests, and needs. Traditional vocational assessment tools are often of limited benefit in that they measure aptitudes, but not the ability to consistently apply them. Behavioral and cognitive abilities, self-awareness, the capacity for adapting to novel situations, and skills generalization are not measured. For this reason functional assessments are an important adjunct to other sources of information. Functional assessments should address the ability to perform tasks, consistency in carry over and follow through, interpersonal skills, impulsivity, distractability, flexibility, and temperment while engaged in work tasks.

Treatment Plan and Intervention

The treatment plan follows from the assessment. If the person is not currently working, a determination is made as to whether the goal is to return the individual to work with the prior employer or another employer, and in the same or an alternate job position. This is done in conjunction with the individual and the employer. The treatment plan may involve a current work site evaluation, work monitoring, development of compensations in the work site, as well as a physical conditioning component, cognitive interventions, and individual and/or group counseling.

In some cases it is helpful to utilize a Job Therapy Experience (JTE; Hurt and Raines, 1993). This is an evaluation/treatment tool that allows clients the opportunity to practice existing skills or to learn new skills in a real work setting. It provides an opportunity for staff to evaluate work behaviors and work readiness and assists in building physical tolerances, and an opportunity to determine cognitive, physical, and psychosocial areas that require further remediation. It can also assist in development of realistic vocational goals, and it can promote self-confidence and improve self-esteem.

Attempts are made to increase the level of task difficulty while decreasing the amount of structure over the course of the job therapy experience. Renewed self-confidence and work skills tend to flourish as the individual realizes that he or she can adequately perform work tasks utilizing newly learned compensatory strategies. Examples of JTE sites used in a hospital-based treatment program include collating and simple machine operation in a print shop; computer research and light data entry in a microfilm department; computer-aided drafting and blueprint reading in an engineering department; equipment trouble-shooting and repair in a hospital maintenance department; stocking, cashiering, and waiting on customers in a gift shop; and custodial tasks.

Group counseling can provide a valuable adjunct to the actual work experience. It provides a forum for discussion of such topics as: (1) injury-related vocational losses; (2) fears related to return to work; and (3) needs and values as they relate to work. As O'Hara (1988) points out, "The opportunity for processing emotional reactions with others who have sustained minor brain injury in a small group setting allows most patients to come face-to-face, for the first time, with others who have shared the confusion, frustration, and trauma of minor brain injury." Individuals in vocational groups find a venue for discussing issues such as loss of earning potential, status, seniority, benefits, and opportunities for promotion. Fears related to return to work are discussed openly and dealt with empathically by peers. Some of the common fears expressed include: fear of impaired work performance and poor performance evaluations; termination; fear of demotion to a lower skill level job; fear of being "found out" at the work place and treated differently due to the brain injury; lack of ability to work required overtime; and effects of fatigue on the quality of work.

Job Development/Placement

This phase of vocational intervention focuses on identification of alternatives for future employment when a prior job or position is no longer viable. Each individual completes a written analysis of transferable skills and makes an oral presentation to the vocational group. This exercise is designed to assist the individual in learning to verbalize his vocational assets and limitations. Group members then provide feedback regarding skill levels and also discover possible vocational goals given that person's unique work history. The dynamics of peer influence are especially effective here in assisting the individual in assessing the appropriateness of his or her goals. This process facilitates and encourages accurate self-appraisal of skills.

The feasibility of vocational alternatives are then further assessed by the individual and the vocational rehabilitation counselor through Job Therapy Experience (JTE) Program involvement, job/task analysis, and administration of specific work samples in the areas of interest. Individuals are encouraged to become involved in conducting labor market surveys and informational interviews to gain further information about a particular occupation of interest. Throughout this process, the cognitive and psychosocial therapists provide significant input regarding the feasibility of the proposed vocational goal from their particular treatment perspective.

Should the individual with a brain injury return to a previous employer at the same job or at a lower skill level job, a number of employer concerns may need to be addressed by the vocational counselor. Supervisors and co-workers may tend to view the individual with a brain injury as having the same skills as they had prior to the injury, leading to an over-estimation of work abilities and inaccurate feedback on task performance. However, the employer may view the individual as being more impaired or restricted than they actually are, thereby underestimating work skills. Fellow employees may attempt to "cover up" the individual's work mistakes or minimize work difficulties. These issues should be discussed with the employer and work supervisors, as well as the individual with the brain injury, prior to the transition back to work.

Job Maintenance/Follow-up Services

Follow-up is often critical to achieving long-term vocational adjustment. During this stage, the vocational rehabilitation counselor can provide crisis intervention services due to the individual's susceptibility to emotional or behavioral breakdown during times of personal and/or environmental stress. Frequent contact by the vocational counselor with the supervisor and/or co-workers on the job results in timely resolution of work-related difficulties and a greater likelihood of adjustment to employment and long-term job retention.

Case Study

Pertinent History

J is a 29–year-old married man who sustained an MTBI in an industrial accident when a truck tire exploded in his face. No loss of consciousness was reported, and he was hospitalized for only 6 hours, although reports suggested that posttraumatic amnesia lasted at least 24 hours. An MRI was unremarkable, but his EEG showed mild left temporal slowing. Physical sequelae included blurry/double vision, hearing loss, left-sided weakness, headaches, fatigue, and altered sleeping patterns. Cognitive deficits included decreased attention/concentration, memory problems, reduced speed of responding, difficulty initiating and completing activities, and word-finding problems. Psychosocial problems were characterized by anger, irritability, and depression.

Education/Work History

J had completed the 10th grade prior to withdrawing from high school to seek full-time employment. At the time of the injury, he had been employed as a truck mechanic and shop foreman by a local logging company for 8 years. Prior to employment as a mechanic, J had worked as a logging chokesetter, a laborer in an auto wrecking yard, and a gas station attendant.

Prior to treatment, John had attempted to return to his job on five separate occasions, but was unsuccessful due to fatigue, headaches, slowness in performing tasks, and low frustration tolerance with angry outbursts at other employees. Each of the work attempts lasted only 8 weeks. Upon entrance to an MTBI program, he had been unemployed for about 18 months.

Vocational Programming

The initial 2 weeks of the program included comprehensive testing of J's physical, cognitive, and psychosocial function and his vocational abilities. Results of a functionally based physical capacities evaluation indicated he could work at "medium" level work. A JTE was developed in the hospital's stores department. Duties in the JTE included: (1) stocking shelves; (2) making deliveries; and (3) filling orders. Goals of the JTE were to increase work tolerances, to assist J in recognizing mental fatigue and taking breaks as needed, to improve attention and speed of processing, and to increase his use of memory aids. Goals in the psychosocial area included improving frustration tolerance and anger management. J participated in the JTE for 2 hours per day, 3 days per week for 4 weeks. He then participated in a second JTE in the hospital's maintenance department, where he worked for 3 hours per day, 4 days per week for another 4-week period. Duties included welding, maintenance and repair of equipment, and general maintenance work.

During this phase, a detailed job analysis of J's job at the logging company outlined the following duties: (1) "hands- on" repair of log and dump trucks; (2) routine maintenance on trucks and large equipment; (3) dispatching 10 to 20 trucks daily to loading sites; (4) supervision of other employees; (5) shop maintainance; (6) purchase of replacement parts; and (7) logging of equipment repairs and maintenance.

The employer identified the following cognitive skills as most important to performance of the job: strong organizational skills; good problem solving skills and the ability to "think on your feet"; the ability to plan ahead and set priorities; and the ability to deal with multiple distractions in a stressful environment. During the last 60 days of rehabilitation, J returned on a part-time basis to his previous employer through the JTE program. He worked three 8-hour days per week during this period and was assisted and monitored by a job coach. The employer was provided with education and training on how to assist J in implementing compensatory strategies at the work site. J returned to paid employment with his previous employer as a truck mechanic, rather than as a foreman, at his previous wage. He was followed up by phone on a monthly basis for 4 months. Follow-up with J 1 year post discharge revealed that he was not only continuing to work successfully, but had been able to resume his previous duties as a foreman.

Vocational Outcomes

The previously described vocational rehabilitation model was utilized with program participants involved at the Mild Head Injury Program at the Center for Continuing Rehabilitation in Puyallup, Washington. Vocational outcomes were examined for 20 consecutive patients. Subjects in this analysis ranged in age from 21 to 51 years old (mean 34 years old). Sixty percent were men, 40% were women. Months postinjury ranged from 8 months to 8 years with an average length of time since injury of 29.5 months.

Of the 20 participants treated during this period, 18 were placed in competitive positions (90%) upon program discharge. Of these 18, 5 were employed at program entry, but experiencing significant work difficulties that threatened job retention. All five were able to remain with their employer post treatment, although three were in less demanding positions.

Six other individuals, who had remained unemployed for more than a year after injury, returned to jobs with their previous employer; four to their job at time of injury, and two to lower skill level positions. In all cases, return to work was negotiated with the employer by the vocational rehabilitation counselor. The remaining eight participants returned to different jobs with new employers.

Twelve of these individuals were followed for 1 year post discharge and were able to successfully maintain adequate work performance levels. One individual was unable to continue employment due to chronic pain related to a back injury; and one was reinjured sustaining a severe brain injury in a home accident.

Summary

Successful return to work can be challenging for individuals who have sustained MTBI. Vocational counselors can play an important role in functional evaluation, work related interventions, and job placement and maintenance. They also play an important role in facilitating adjustment to the changes in vocational role and self-image experienced by many individuals with MTBI.

References

Cicerone, K.D. (1991). Psychotherapy after mild traumatic brain injury: Relation to the nature and severity of subjective complaints. *Journal of Head Trauma Rehabilitation*, 6(4), 30–43.

Fogel, K., and Paul-Cohen, R. (1992), Vocational rehabilitation after concussion. In L. Horn and N. Zasler (Eds.), *Rehabilitation of Post-Concussive Disorders*. Philadephia, PA: Henley and Belfus.

Hallauer D., Prosser R., and Swift K. (1989). Neuropsychological evaluation and the vocational rehabilitation of brain injured clients. *Journal of Rehabilitation*, 20(2), 3–6.

Hurt G. (1991). Mild brain injury: Critical factors in vocational rehabilitation. *Journal of Rehabilitation*, 4, 36–40.

Hurt, G., and Raines, J. (1993). Job Therapy Experience: Developing and Implementing JTE Programs. (manual) Good Samaritan Rehabilitation Center, Puyallup, WA.

Kraus, J., and Nourjah, P. (1989). The Epidemiology of Mild Head Injury, in Mild Head Injury. New York, NY: Oxford University Press.

Lezak, M.D. (1978). Living with the characterologically altered brain injured patient. *Journal of Clinical Psychiatry*, 39, 592–598.

O'Hara, C. (1988). Emotional adjustment following minor head injury. Cognitive Rehabilitation, 6(2), 22–24.

Prigatano, G., Klonoff P., and Bailey I. (1987). Psychosocial adjustment associated with traumatic brain injury: Statistics BNI neuro-rehabilitation must beat. *BNI Quarterly*, 3, 10–17.

Steambrook, M., Moore, A.D., Peter, L.C., Deviane, C., and Hawryluk, G.A. (1990). Effects of mild, moderate and severe closed head injury on long term vocational status. *Brain Injury*, 4(2), 1983–190.

Veach R., and Taylor M. (1989). Vocational placement of minor head injured survivors. *Cognitive Rehabilitation*, 4, 14–16.

Wood, F., Novack, T., and Long, C. (1984). Post-concussion symptoms: Cognitive, emotional and environmental aspects. *The International Journal of Psychiatry in Medicine*, 14, 277–283.

Young, M.E., Eisner-Leverenz, J., Ewing-Cobbs, L., and High, W. (1993). *Checklist for Writing Neuropsychological Reports in Functional Terms for Vocational Rehabilitation*. Southwest Regional Brain Injury Rehabilitation and Prevention.

Zasler, N.D. (1989). Employment outcomes of persons with traumatic brain injury. *Brain Injury*, 3(4), 331–333.

Zuger, R.R., and Boehm, M. (1993). Vocational rehabilitation counseling of traumatic brain injury: Factors contributing to stress. *Journal of Rehabilitation*, 59(2), 28–30.

APPENDIX A

A checklist designed to help neuropsychologists write reports of the most benefit to vocational rehabilitation counselors. Reprinted with permission.

Southwest Regional Brain Injury Rehabilitation and Prevention Center—Draft Checklist for Writing Neuropsychological Reports in Functional Terms for Vocational Rehabilitation

MARY ELLEN YOUNG, JOYCE EISNER-LEVERENZ, LINDA EWING-COBBS, AND WALTER HIGH

I. COGNITIVE OBSERVATIONS
  A. *Attention and concentration*
    1. How long can client focus on a task?
       _____ <5 min _____ 5–30 min _____ 30–60 min
       _____ # of hours
    2. Does client need breaks?
       _____ usually _____ sometimes _____ rarely
    3. Does client make impulsive errors?
       _____ usually _____ sometimes _____ rarely
    4. Is client distractable?
       _____ usually _____ sometimes _____ rarely
    5. Is client at increased risk in jobs involving specific hazardous conditions such as:

moving equipment	_____ yes	_____ no
electrical shock	_____ yes	_____ no
heights	_____ yes	_____ no
hazardous materials	_____ yes	_____ no
security/police duty	_____ yes	_____ no

  B. *Approach to Task and Problem-Solving Skills*
    1. Can client use organized approach to tasks?
       _____ usually _____ sometimes _____ rarely
    2. Can client recognize errors?
       _____ usually _____ sometimes _____ rarely
       _____ with prompts _____ without prompts
    3. Can client correct errors?
       _____ usually _____ sometimes _____ rarely
       _____ with prompts _____ without prompts
    4. Can client accept and use feedback?
       _____ usually _____ sometimes _____ rarely
    5. Can client generate problem-solving strategies?
       _____ usually _____ sometimes _____ rarely
       _____ with prompts _____ without prompts

6. Can client change approach if ineffective?

_____ usually _____ sometimes _____ rarely
_____ with prompts _____ without prompts

C. *Memory*

1. Does client have any problems remembering events that occurred or persons who were met prior to injury?

_____ yes _____ no

If yes, please indicate whether client has problems remembering:

minutes before injury?   _____ yes _____ no
hours before injury?   _____ yes _____ no
day before injury?   _____ yes _____ no
week before injury?   _____ yes _____ no
month before injury?   _____ yes _____ no

2. Does client have problems remembering current events or persons?

_____ yes _____ no

If yes, please indicate whether client has problems remembering things that have happened:

in the last minute?   _____ yes _____ no
in the last hour?   _____ yes _____ no
in the last day?   _____ yes _____ no
in the last week?   _____ yes _____ no
in the last month?   _____ yes _____ no

3. Does client have problems remembering one- or two-step directions? _____ yes _____ no

If yes, please indicate whether client has problems remembering:

for a minute?   _____ yes _____ no
for an hour?   _____ yes _____ no
for a day?   _____ yes _____ no
for a week?   _____ yes _____ no
for a month?   _____ yes _____ no

4. Does client have problems remembering more complicated directions? _____ yes _____ no

If yes, please indicate whether client has problems remembering:

for a minute?   _____ yes _____ no
for an hour?   _____ yes _____ no
for a day?   _____ yes _____ no
for a week?   _____ yes _____ no
for a month?   _____ yes _____ no

5. Are client's memory problems (check all that apply):

_____ global? _____ visual? _____ verbal?

6. Does client use memory aids?

_____ usually _____ sometimes _____ rarely
_____ with prompts _____ without prompts

7. Does client ask for clarification and repetition of directions?
   _____ usually _____ sometimes _____ rarely
8. Does client have more subtle problems remembering new information that impacts the ability to do more complex jobs or tasks?
   _____ Yes _____ No

D. *Insight*

1. Does client overestimate physical capacities?
   _____ usually _____ sometimes _____ rarely
2. Does client overestimate memory abilities?
   _____ usually _____ sometimes _____ rarely
3. Does client overestimate other cognitive abilities?
   _____ usually _____ sometimes _____ rarely
4. Does client underestimate behavioral changes?
   _____ usually _____ sometimes _____ rarely

II. WORKER TRAIT FACTORS

A. *Functional Reasoning Level* (Check one):

_____ 0 Does not use common sense, cannot follow simple instructions

_____ 1 Uses common sense, follows 1–2 step instructions in tasks with no variability

_____ 2 Uses common sense, follows simple written and oral instructions, minimal variability in tasks

_____ 3 Uses common sense, interprets instructions in written or diagram form, deals with several concrete variables

_____ 4 Solves practical problems within existing structure, deals with several concrete variables with limited standardization, interprets directions in all modalities

_____ 5 Defines problems, collects data, establishes facts, draws valid conclusions, interprets extensive instructions in any format, deals with both abstract and concrete variables

_____ 6 Applies logical or scientific thinking to solve wide range of abstract problems, may involve formulas and equations

B. *Physical Capacities/Sensory Modalities*

1. Status of motor system? (check all that apply)
   _____ hemiparesis   _____ right _____ left
   _____ hemiplegia   _____ right _____ left
   _____ paraplegia
   _____ quadriplegia
   _____ ataxia
   _____ apraxia

2. Problems noted in visual acuity?

_____ yes _____ no

3. Problems noted in perception?

visual scanning?   _____ yes _____ no
form perception?   _____ yes _____ no
clerical perception?   _____ yes _____ no

4. Visual fields intact?   _____ yes _____ no

If no, specify

_____

5. Does client have inattention to visual field (visual neglect?

_____ yes _____ no

If yes,   _____ right _____ left

_____ subtle _____ apparent

6. Problems with hearing?   _____ yes _____ no

7. Problems with sensation/touch?

_____ yes _____ no

C. *Language Skills*

1. Receptive—understands simple 1- to 2-step verbal instructions?

_____ usually _____ sometimes _____ rarely

2. Expressive:

Expresses basic needs (e.g. food, water, toileting)?

_____ usually _____ sometimes _____ rarely

Expresses more complex ideas (e.g. social relationships, abstract concepts)?

_____ usually _____ sometimes _____ rarely

For the next sections, circle the applicable rating based on the following scale, where appropriate:

1. Top 10% of general population
2. Top third of general population (exclusive of top 10%)
3. Middle third of general population
4. Bottom third of general population (exclusive of bottom 10%)
5. Bottom 10% of general population

3. Reading recognition	1	2	3	4	5
4. Reading comprehension	1	2	3	4	5
5. Written spelling	1	2	3	4	5

D. *Math Skills*

1. Calculation	1	2	3	4	5
2. Numerical reasoning	1	2	3	4	5

E. *Motor Execution*

1. Eye-hand coordination	1	2	3	4	5
2. Finger dexterity—left	1	2	3	4	5
right	1	2	3	4	5
both	1	2	3	4	5

   3. Manual dexterity—left   1 2 3 4 5
                            right   1 2 3 4 5
                            both   1 2 3 4 5
   4. If the above ratings are below average, is this due to:
      Slowness?   _____ yes _____ no
      Inaccuracy?   _____ yes _____ no
   5. Reaction time—upper extremities:
   _____ impaired _____ not impaired

III. BEHAVIORAL OBSERVATIONS
   A. Appropriate social interaction?
       _____ usually _____ sometimes _____ rarely
   B. Appropriate frustration tolerance?
       _____ usually _____ sometimes _____ rarely
   C. Appropriate dress?
       _____ usually _____ sometimes _____ rarely
   D. Appropriate hygiene?
       _____ usually _____ sometimes _____ rarely
   E. Punctual, e.g., for appointment and returning from breaks?
       _____ usually _____ sometimes _____ rarely
   F. Dependable, e.g., scheduled and kept appointments?
       _____ usually _____ sometimes _____ rarely
   G. Annoying habits?
       _____ usually _____ sometimes _____ rarely
   H. Disinhibition
       Verbal?   _____ usually _____ sometimes _____ rarely
       Physical?   _____ usually _____ sometimes _____ rarely
       Sexual?   _____ usually _____ sometimes _____ rarely

IV. RECOMMENDATIONS
   A. Recommend return to pre-injury job?
       _____ yes _____ no _____ unable to judge _____ N/A
       If yes, estimate time to return to work

   B. Is further recovery expected?   _____ yes _____ no
       Over what period of time?

   C. Is further rehabilitation recommended?
       _____ yes _____ no
       If yes, check what is recommended:
       _____ medical consultation
       _____ occupational therapy consultation
       _____ psychological/psychiatric services
       _____ physical therapy consultation
       _____ case management/social services
       _____ independent living evaluation
       _____ speech/language therapy

_____ educational services
_____ driving evaluation
_____ vocational assessment
_____ vocational counseling
_____ cognitive training
_____ behavioral training
_____ work adjustment services
_____ therapeutic recreation services
_____ supported employment/job coaching services
_____ substance abuse screening/treatment
Is counseling recommended? _____ yes _____ no
If yes, check type:
_____ individual
_____ marital
_____ family

D. Supervision needed in competitive job for:
Behavioral problems? _____ yes _____ no
Cognitive difficulties? _____ yes _____ no
Physical limitations? _____ yes _____ no
Other? _____ yes _____ no

V

SPECIAL POPULATIONS

12

Mild Traumatic Brain Injury
in Children

JENNIFER BLAIR THOMSON AND
KIMBERLY A. KERNS

Research regarding children with brain injuries, particularly mild traumatic brain injury (MTBI), has been comparatively slow to develop. Assessing the cognitive sequelae of pediatric brain injury has been difficult
due to a lack of sensitive measures, a limited understanding of the interaction of the injury with the neurodevelopment of the child, and the large
number of MTBI cases that go unreported. Indeed, the literature to date
is mixed regarding whether children who have sustained MTBI suffer
long-term neurocognitive sequelae.

The Need for a Developmental Approach

The impact of injury on developing neural systems precludes one from
assuming that the sequelae of TBI seen in child populations are the same
as that in adults. Although developmental factors are often acknowledged, their interactions with injury are not well understood.

Children's neural systems are immature and constantly changing.
Damage cannot be viewed solely in the present, but must also be considered in terms of possible compromise to future learning potential, skill
development, and behavior. Contrary to the "Kennard Principle" (Kennard, 1936, 1940), a long-held notion that a relatively plastic young brain
can effectively moderate the effects of a brain injury, deficits due to early
brain damage can have both immediate and long-term sequelae.

In fact, some research suggests that diffuse injury at earlier ages may
result in more deficits than that seen in older children (Anderson and
Moore, 1995; Levin et al., 1993). Some deficits may not be immediately
apparent, but are realized at the time at which the skills dependent upon
the damaged areas fail to emerge. This appears to be the case, for exam-

ple, with early frontal lobe damage. Because physiological maturation of the prefrontal cortex continues well into adolescence (Yakovlev and Lecours, 1967), deficits in functions subserved by the frontal lobes may become apparent only much later (Eslinger et al., 1992; Grattan and Eslinger, 1991; Goldman-Rakic, 1984; Mateer and Williams, 1991; Williams and Mateer, 1992). Thus, research regarding the functional outcome of children who have sustained MTBI must take into account not only sequelae from the present injury, but deficits that may not become apparent until months or even years post injury.

Differences across age groups also exist in the mechanisms of injury. Incidence statistics show that for infants, falls are the single greatest cause of injury (Di Scala et al., 1991), while sports-related injuries, pedestrian–motor vehicle, and bicycle accidents predominate in the 5 to 14-year-old age range (Klauber et al., 1981, 1986). Finally, motor vehicle accidents account for most injuries in adolescents and adults (Annegers et al., 1980). In fact, falls as cause of injury decrease almost linearly with age, while traffic-related accidents increase, until late adulthood when falls again increase (Di Scala et al., 1991). This change in the mechanism of injury undoubtedly plays a role in both the pathophysiology and the severity of injuries in child populations. Low velocity falls, in particular, may produce injuries that go unreported, since they are considered part of normal growing up (Segalowitz and Brown, 1991). Unfortunately, mechanism of injury is often not reported or controlled for in research studies.

Age at the time of injury also makes the effects of brain injury difficult to address. Research regarding executive functioning abilities, for example, must take into account the age at which these skills normally develop. By failing to consider normal development, one could falsely assume that deficits in function are attributable to early brain damage when, in fact, those functions have yet to develop normally.

A child's age also has implications for rehabilitation. Children have shorter learning histories, and thus smaller information stores, than adults. Younger children have less learned information to "fall back on" and have a greater need for new learning. Impaired learning and memory abilities will have a differential impact on children in comparison to adults, who have already done most of their "learning."

Accurate estimates of MTBI in children are difficult to obtain. There is confusion over what constitutes a brain injury, as opposed to an injury to the face or head that may spare the brain itself (Goldstein and Levin, 1987). Locating brain injury cases not reported to hospitals is also difficult, leading to underestimates of mild brain injuries. Since children who sustain injury are less likely to lose consciousness (Boll and Barth, 1981; Ewing-Cobbs et al., 1989), many cases of milder injury may go unreported to either medical or educational professionals. Most researchers, however, agree that from 1 million (Eiben et al., 1984) to 5 million (Di Scala et al., 1991) children sustain traumatic brain injury each year, with most cases being mild injuries. Among children ages 5 to 14 years, mild traumatic brain injuries are the most prevalent; severe and fatal head trauma make up only 10% of the injuries in this group (Annegers, 1986).

Review of Representative Literature

Despite the ubiquity of MTBI, a review of existing literature indicates considerable controversy regarding its long-term impact, if any, on children. Satz et al. (1997) reviewed research studies of mild head injury in children and adolescents from 1970 to 1995. A preliminary box tally revealed 13 adverse, 18 null, and 9 indeterminate findings related to neuropsychological, academic, or psychosocial outcome following MTBI in children. As noted earlier, differences in results may be accounted for by a failure to account for factors such as age at the time of injury, mechanism of injury, or failure to follow children for a sufficient length of time. Additionally, perhaps only a few children who sustain MTBI exhibit persistent cognitive difficulties. If this is the case, group comparison studies are not likely to demonstrate any significant effect of MTBI. Finally, failure to use measures, which are sufficiently sensitive to the types of cognitive sequelae seen following MTBI may result in incorrect conclusions.

Keeping in mind these limitations, some researchers have concluded that no effects of MTBI can be detected from available evidence. Rutter and his colleagues (Rutter et al., 1980; Brown et al., 1981; Chadwick et al., 1981a,b) were among the first to report that the mildly brain injured children in their prospective longitudinal study were at no increased risk for long-term cognitive sequelae, as evidenced through seven subtests of the Wechsler Intelligence Scale for Children (WISC), a reading task, and parental questionnaires. Although mild deficits were demonstrated by the MTBI group, no pattern of recovery was observed in this group (as with the more severely head injured cohort). Rutter posited that acute damage to the brain results in cognitive deficits that improve following the injury. The authors concluded that the deficits in the more severely injured children were a result of brain injury, as the deficits lessened with time. Cognitive deficits noted in the MTBI group did not change over time and thus were not seen as due to the injury, but rather as "premorbid characteristics." Unfortunately, several problems existed in this study. First, the MTBI group was not matched to the severe injury or control groups (for empirical comparison), nor were the same number of measures utilized for the MTBI group allowing for a full comparison. It also may be that above some threshold effect, it is harder to show recovery. Perhaps a moderately to severely injured child has "more room" for demonstrable improvement than a mildly injured child. Drawing conclusions regarding MTBI from this study is thus difficult.

In a subsequent study, Winogron et al. (1984) reported that neuropsychological profiles after severe injury are more distinctive, whereas profiles of either moderate or mild head injury in children are more similar. In their study using the Wechsler Intelligence Scale for Children-Revised (WISC-R), Peabody Picture Vocabulary Test, Wide Range Achievement Test, and portions of the Knights-Norwood Neuropsychological Test Battery, the highest number of deficits was seen in the severely injured children, with 50% of the children with normal deficit indices (DI's) having sustained mild injuries. Comparisons between these children and normal control children were not conducted.

Bijur et al. (1990) reported no differences between MTBI cases and controls on most measures of intelligence, mathematical and reading ability, and aggression. Fay et al. (1993) reported no clinically significant differences between MTBI and control children on a battery of tests including the WISC-R, motor/psychomotor skills, and adaptive/functional behaviors (as measured by the CBCL). Children were tested at 3 weeks and 1 year postinjury. Controls subjects were "matched" to the injured children by having teachers of the injured students select a child in the classroom of the same perceived ability level as the injured child before the injury.

Asarnow et al. (1995) reported on a large sample of 137 MTBI children who were compared with a sample of both noninjured controls, and a group of injured children admitted to the same hospital emergency room who had not experienced brain/head injuries. This study utilized a number of neuropsychological measures including tasks assessing executive functions, attention and memory, general intellectual functioning, and fine motor speed. Additionally, they compared measures of school achievement and parental report of behavior (CBCL's completed retrospectively) pre- and post injury. Cognitive testing was done at 1 month, 6 months, and 12 months following the injury. Preliminary results of this study suggest that children admitted to the emergency room with MTBI do not show clinically significant neuropsychological impairment at 1, 6, or 12 months post injury, nor do they exhibit any changes in academic functioning or behavior problems. Again, however, group average statistics may not capture individual children who might have suffered sequelae, as this group may be more likely to have greater variability.

Bijur et al. (1996) studied 1586 children with one mild head injury, 278 with two mild head injuries, 51 with three or more head injuries from birth to 10 years, and a group of controls without head injury matched by gender. At age 10 they found no evidence that multiple head injuries have a deleterious effect on a global measure of intelligence or academic achievement.

Although many studies have failed to detect deficits in the childhood MTBI population, to conclude that this group is deficit free is problematic. Many of these studies have used measures unlikely to reveal the cognitive deficits commonly seen from MTBI. Measures of intelligence, tasks from the Halstead-Reitan Neuropsychological Test Battery, and academic

achievement tests, although adequate (but not comprehensive) for revealing deficits in a severely injured population, may not be sensitive
enough to delineate subtle cognitive processing difficulties. In studies of
adults with MTBI, performance may break down when individuals are
required to perform tasks that tap higher level attention and concentration abilities, particularly when there are demands for speed and multiple simultaneous operations. An interaction between head injury and personality and psychosocial variables may also exist (Boll, 1983; Beers, 1992).

Another limitation exists in the assessment of problem-solving/exec-
utive functioning abilities. Mild TBI may result in disorders of executive
functioning often not revealed in a highly structured testing situation. In
addition, many tests currently used to assess executive functions for children are not well developed (Welsh and Pennington, 1988). Perhaps more
importantly, executive functioning deficits may only become apparent at
a much later age, when those functions become developmentally appropriate. As Johnson (1992) notes,

> "Tuber's dictum 'Absence of evidence is not evidence of absence' is most
> pertinent to the brain-injured child with outwardly good physical re-
> covery, but in whom the structural damage and metabolic dysfunction
> of the brain, and resulting aberrations, are hidden out of sight" (p. 408).

Perhaps, like adults, although most of the children who suffer MTBI do
not suffer long-term consequences, a minority of these children do have
residual deficits. Mittenberg et al. (1997) reported that when asked, children with MTBI report symptoms very similar to those seen in adults including, headache, memory loss, photosensitivity, trouble with attention,
and sensations of "spinning." Such symptoms were not reported by children with orthopedic injuries or noninjured controls.

Several researchers have demonstrated cognitive processing deficits
and behavior problems in children with MTBI. Gulbrandsen (1984) found
children with MTBI had significantly lower scores than a matched control sample on a number of cognitive measures, including selected subtests of the WISC and tasks from the Reitan-Indiana Neuropsychological
Test Battery for Children. Mild traumatic brain injury in this study was
defined as no loss of consciousness or a loss of consciousness for less than
5 minutes. Stringent exclusion criteria were utilized to eliminate children
with premorbid difficulties. The design of this study was similar to the
Fay et al. study (1993), in that children were matched by sex and age to
other children in their classroom felt to be at the same academic achievement level.

Hannay and Levin (1988) reported memory impairments in groups of
severely and mildly brain-injured children, and noted that about 9% of
children with milder injuries exhibited residual impairment on continuous recognition tasks large enough to be outside the range for normal

adolescents. Klonoff and his colleagues (Klonoff et al., 1977, 1993) also reported continuing complaints of learning and memory/attention deficits on a 5- and 23-year follow-up study of children with brain injuries, in a sample where most of the children appeared to have sustained mild injuries. Findings 1 year post injury revealed impairment on more than 50% of neuropsychological measures. More striking was that by the end of the 5-year period, 25% of the sample of younger children had failed an elementary grade or were in remedial services. About 70% of the older children who failed a grade or withdrew from school had no premorbid history of school problems. Unfortunately, injury severity was not clearly defined, limiting conclusions regarding MTBI.

Problems in academics are also frequently reported following brain injury. In a study examining the impact of MTBI on academic achievement, Adams (1990) found that deficits were persistent and remained long past the expected recovery period for MTBI. Deficits were noted on tasks with higher levels of complexity and tasks requiring less-entrenched skills. Segalowitz and Brown (1991) administered a self-report questionnaire to assess the prevalence of mild head injury (MHI) in a group of high school students. More than 31% of the sample reported they had sustained MHI, with half of those reporting some period of unconsciousness that would place their injuries in the mild range. Significant findings included a relationship between brain injury and grade repetition and the need for remedial services. The MHI group showed a higher degree of mixed-handedness. In addition, both hyperactivity and stuttering were related to having been unconscious, and a relationship between unconsciousness and difficulty in mathematics was noted.

Wrightson et al. (1995) compared 78 preschool children with 86 controls with similar socioeconomic status (SES), developmental status and family status. No differences were seen in cognitive tests soon after insult, although subjects scored less than controls on a visual closure task when retested at 6 months and 1 year, and were more likely to have had another mild head injury. When tested again at age 6.5 years, subjects still scored more poorly than controls, their reading ability was related to their visual closure score at 1 year, and they were more likely to have needed help with reading. The authors suggest that MTBI in the preschool years does not affect already established skills, so that no group differences are seen in the first few weeks after injury, but that the children with MTBI do not develop some skills as effectively later on.

Segalowitz and colleagues (1995) compared a sample of 10 well-functioning university students with a history of MTBI (onset averaged 6.4 years before testing) with matched controls on a series of standard neuropsychological measures of attention, memory, thinking, and on a series of auditory vigilance tasks, during which event-related potentials (ERPs) were also recorded. Results indicated that MTBI students performed as well as the control students on all the standard neuropsychological measures, but performed more slowly and less accurately on the most difficult of the auditory vigilance tasks (a complex oddball paradigm). Despite the overall solid performance of the MTBI group, ERPs revealed substantially and significantly reduced P300 amplitudes and subsequent attenuation on all the oddball tasks, both easy and difficult. These data suggest that despite excellent behavioral recovery, students with a history of MTBI displayed subtle information processing deficits involving attention, that were not apparent on standard neuropsychological measures, but were evident long after the original injury.

Several studies have also been conducted documenting adjustment difficulties post-MTBI in children. Asarnow et al. (1991) reported a higher incidence of behavior problems in mildly injured children (compared with published norms of the CBCL), but no impairment in adaptive functioning. Bijur et al. (1990) also reported a small but significantly increased rating of hyperactivity in mildly brain injured children. Polissar and colleagues (1994) found that when statistical corrections for multiple comparisons were made, statistically significant (but weak) associations were found with MTBI and a number of neurobehavioral variables both initially and 1 year following the injury. Their results suggest that MTBI has a weak effect on a spectrum of neurobehavioral skills, rather than having substantial effects in any single area.

Roberts et al. (1995) presented longitudinal data on a child who sustained a whiplash type injury at 7 years of age without any loss of consciousness or apparent neurological effects. However, neurobehavioral symptoms developed and increased in severity and frequency during the 2 years following the accident, and persisted for 4 years post trauma. Interestingly, upon further investigation, this child's PET scan was judged to be abnormal and the child responded very well to a course of anticonvulsant medication. Fuld and Fischer (1977) described a child who suffered an MTBI and evidenced continuing and serious intellectual impairments and personality changes, including aggressive behavior, in spite of normal EEG patterns and neurological examinations.

The identification of emotional and behavioral problems among children with MTBI has led to the suggestion that children who incur mild head injuries have a higher prevalence of premorbid characteristics such as maladjustment or risk taking than do children in the community. Pelco et al. (1992) have directly tested this hypothesis. They found that children with mild injuries did not have significantly more premorbid emotional or behavioral problems than other children in the community, and had significantly fewer problems than children referred to a psychiatric outpatient clinic.

In summary, although most children may recover uneventfully from MTBI, it is clear that some children who suffer an MTBI will experience adverse cognitive, academic, and behavioral sequelae. Further research is called for before reaching conclusions about the effects of age, mechanism of injury, and long-term outcome of this population. In addition, the evaluation of any differences between those children who do suffer lasting sequelae and those who do not, to identify risk or protective factors will be important. Long-term prospective studies should be designed within a developmental framework to clarify these issues.

Most children who do suffer from the lasting effects of an MTBI are likely to be under-served in the educational and rehabilitation settings, as they often go unrecognized or misidentified due to difficulties with behavior management. Even if a child's deficits are appropriately reported to school personnel, services may be unavailable due to a lack of education regarding the effects of brain injury or to scarce or inaccessible resources.

The rehabilitation professional must thus be able to provide: (1) pertinent information regarding a child's cognitive status through a comprehensive assessment, and (2) a plan for appropriate remediation.

Assessment

A variety of problems may be noted after a child sustains brain injury. Parents and/or teachers may express concern regarding a child's declining schoolwork, difficulties with attention and concentration skills, or changes in mood and personality (including increased frustration and anger). Children with MTBI who are having more difficulty with schoolwork than before injury often become increasingly frustrated and depressed.

The most important domains of assessment in a child with known or suspected MTBI are attention/concentration, speed of processing, memory, and new learning, and executive functions. Neuropsychologists should familiarize themselves with a variety of new measures of attention, memory, and executive function appropriate for use with children. Tasks must be sensitive and place sufficient demands on cognitive processing to capture deficits (Gordon et al., 1986; Johnson et al., 1988). Executive functions are particularly difficult to evaluate within a structured testing situation. Consequently, using behavioral observations is particularly important, and interviews with parents and teachers to identify difficulties with behavior, self-regulation, alterations in mood, or social interaction are warranted.

Rehabilitation

The primary goal for a child in the school setting is to be become an "effective learner." Thus, for a child with MTBI, delineating impaired cognitive processes and aiming interventions at improving those basic processes is paramount. Mateer and colleagues (1996) provided a comprehensive review of rehabilitative strategies used with children and adolescents with all ranges of TBI severity.

The majority of services or interventions a child with MTBI receives are likely to be delivered within a school system. For example, if a child is trained in the use of a memory compensation system, the actual monitoring and prompting for use of that system is likely to be done in the classroom. Thus, much of cognitive rehabilitation involves devising accommodations that can be provided within the school setting.

Education of family, school personnel, and other individuals involved with the child regarding the effects of MTBI is an integral step in the cognitive rehabilitation process. For example, a child's limitations in attentional abilities must be explained to family and teachers so that inattentive behavior is not assumed to be intentional or functional in nature (i.e., problems with motivation, not trying hard enough, or underachievement).

Cognitive remediation strategies may encompass a combination of direct interventions aimed at improving functional ability, compensations for abilities that cannot be remediated, and changes in the environment when appropriate and possible.

Direct Retraining

One promising area for the rehabilitation of children with attention deficits is direct training of attentional skills. Studies of the efficacy of Attention Process Training (Sohlberg and Mateer, 1986) in children with attention problems (Semrud-Clikeman et al., in press; Williams, 1989) have demonstrated improved attention skills and increased performance on measures of academic efficiency. Attention process training was used with a small sample of adolescents who had sustained TBI who also showed some improvement following treatment (Thomson and Kerns, submitted).

The development of pediatric attention training materials and the evaluation of their effectiveness is currently in progress. These materials have been successfully utilized to increase speed of processing, selective attention, and performance on a measure of academic efficiency in children with ADHD (Kerns et al., submitted; Eso and Kerns, 1998). In case studies of brain injured children, downward extensions of APT materials have been shown to be effective for the direct retraining of attention and concentration skills, suggesting that further investigation of this approach is warranted.

Direct retraining of memory, visual processing, and executive functioning impairments, as outlined in accompanying chapters, have yet to be empirically validated in children. Although many computer software programs are available for such pursuits (particularly regarding memory building), information regarding the validity of such approaches to rehabilitation is currently unavailable.

Compensation Training

Training of compensatory strategies to improve functioning, despite impaired abilities, is another frequently used technique. Compensation for attentional difficulties can be affected through behavioral approaches using commercial devices such as the Attention Training System (Gordon et al., 1991), wherein a teacher or aide can discreetly signal the child via a remote-controlled device when lapses in attention take place. Simpler behavioral systems include a teacher and student mutually devising acceptable "signals" (e.g., a touch on the shoulder, calling the child's name twice) for lapses in the child's attention. For younger children, a "star sheet" system is often helpful. In this case, a teacher draws a "star" on a sheet (attached to the student's desk) when the youngster is noted to be attending. "Stars" can later be traded for various rewards agreed upon in advance by teacher, child, and parent. Systems that provide rewards for on-task behavior are more likely to generalize and to become internalized behaviors.

Giving a child notes from a teacher or from a peer "note-taker" can be very helpful for children with difficulties in attention, memory, or processing speed. A peer note-taker or "study-buddy" system is often useful; older children can learn to tape classes or lectures. Memory deficits may be particularly amenable to compensation training through the utilization of a memory or assignment notebook. It is insufficient to simply give a child an assignment sheet and assume that it will remediate difficulties with memory for class assignments. Training in the use of memory notebooks must be carried out systematically. The authors have found the use of a "daily checklist" in the beginning of a memory system or notebook to be helpful (Kerns and Thomson, in press). On this checklist, daily behaviors should be listed (e.g., "write down math assignment," "get notes from my friend," "bring home math book") in chronological order. The page can be covered with a plastic protector so that each activity can be "checked-off" with a grease pencil as it is carried out. In this fashion, the child can visually monitor which activities have been, and need to be, carried out. Eventually, daily activities should become routine, and this page of the memory notebook may be eliminated on a trial basis. The sheet with school assignments is also imperative for a child with MTBI.

Changing the Environment

Many treatment strategies for children with MTBI will involve changing the environment to address cognitive deficits. A variety of practical treatment options within the school and home environments are outlined in Appendix A.

Education

Often classroom teachers are unaware that a child has been injured, or may have little information regarding the impact of such an injury on the child's ability to learn. Several available books and pamphlets are aimed at giving educators information regarding TBI and its impact on childrens' learning. The following are examples of such references the authors have found helpful:

"A Teacher's Guide: Managing Children With Brain Injury in the Classroom" (Pollock et al., 1993),
"An Educator's Manual: What Educators Need to Know About Students with Brain Injury" (Savage & Wolcott, 1995),
"Traumatic Brain Injury in Children and Adolescents: A Source Book for Teachers and Other School Personnel" (Mira et al., 1992),
"An Educational Challenge: Meeting the Needs of Students with Brain Injury" (Deboskey, 1996).

Behavioral Interventions

Changes in personality and emotional functioning are frequent sequelae of MTBI, with parents often reporting significant changes in this area as the most striking outcome of the injury. A thorough discussion of techniques for the management of problematic behaviors is beyond the scope of this text. Readers are referred to several texts aimed specifically at addressing these issues (Barin et al., 1985; Horton, 1994; Lehr, 1990; Ylvisaker et al., 1998).

Generalization

Generalization of direct retraining approaches can be ensured through good communication with the child's parents and teachers, along with occasional assessments. Informal (via interview) or more formal (via rating scales or psychometric testing) monitoring of attentional behaviors at school and in the home can provide a good indication of treatment efficacy in the child's everyday environment. Keeping adequate records of a child's performance on training tasks is imperative, along with data from outside sources designed to tap generalization of skills into the natural environment. Data keeping of this sort is integral in the determination of generalization of skills. If a child improves on treatment tasks (e.g., attention training), but not on functional skills thought to reflect improvement in the natural environment (e.g., parental report of improved attention, more actual time spent on tasks in the school environment), the utility of retraining needs to be evaluated.

When utilizing compensation strategies such as memory notebooks, generalization must be planned. The clinician needs to ensure that these strategies are used throughout the child's day. Training of compensation strategies can initially take place in the outpatient environment, but the clinician must then monitor the school and home environment to determine whether strategies are being effectively incorporated. Appropriate training techniques for the use of compensation strategies will increase the probability that compensation strategies will be used appropriately. Training of family members and school personnel in the use of such a system to ensure generalization and consistency of performance in different environments is important.

Case Studies

Case 1

Due to problematic behaviors and difficulty in school, EC, a 9-year-old girl, was referred for neuropsychological evaluation and subsequent treatment approximately 16 months after she was involved in a pedestrian–bicycle accident. Review of her medical and educational history did not reveal any apparent difficulties before injury. In fact, strong skills were noted on entering kindergarten and placement in a gifted program was recommended.

EC was struck by a bicycle as she stepped out of a minivan when she was 7 years old, and at the end of her 2nd grade year. There was no loss of consciousness. EC's mother reported that after discharge from the hospital, EC was very emotional and cried often. She was also very demanding and "mean" in her manner. EC's mother became most concerned when EC appeared to show memory impairments and difficulties with concentration, math, and reading.

EC's overall intellectual abilities were in the superior range (WISC-III Full Scale Intelligence Quotient (IQ) (FSIQ) = 121), with above average range verbal abilities [Verbal IQ (VIQ) = 113] and superior range nonverbal abilities performance IQ (PIQ) = 126]. Deficits, relative to predicted ability, were seen on measures sensitive to working memory, vigilance, distractibility, and executive function (e.g., self-regulation, planning).

Treatment included a combination of education with parents regarding the effects of MTBI and direct attention training for EC over a period of eight 1-hour weekly sessions. EC performed a variety of attention tasks including taped exercises, alphabetizing sentences, card sorting, and serial counting. During the initial training course, EC was noted to make little gain on the training materials. Though she appeared to be putting forth adequate effort, the tasks appeared frustrating and the expected improvement was not occurring. After the third session, it was decided that the materials selected were too difficult for EC. The tasks were simplified and EC's performance on these new tasks (as measured through speed and number of errors) began to show the expected trend of improvement. At treatment's end, EC had surpassed those tasks at the level of the materials she originally was started with and was showing expected gains.

This case illustrates the importance of tracking performance and matching materials to the level of the child. Unlike adult populations, assumptions about overlearned behaviors cannot be made with children. They may lack prerequisite skills necessary to easily perform the basic requirements of some training materials. It is imperative that the therapist carefully match treatment materials to both the child's area of difficulty and his/her cognitive developmental level. For example, a task frequently utilized for improving attention and working memory is one in which the client is required to alphabetize the individual words in progressively longer sentences. If a child has not yet learned to alphabetize, then working with this type of task would not be influencing attention, but rather training a new skill.

Retesting was completed with EC approximately 3 months after treatment. It revealed considerable improvement on the Gordon Diagnostic System—Distractibility Task (45/45 correct), and normal performance on the Attentional Capacity Test. EC's parents also noted some improvement in attention and concentration behavior in the home. EC's initial evaluation took place over 12 months post-injury, at a time when neurocognitive sequelae would likely have stabilized, increasing the likelihood that gains were related to training. Treatment tasks were all very dissimilar to assessment tasks.

Case 2

RE was a 17-year-old girl referred for a neuropsychological evaluation and subsequent treatment approximately 5 months after she was kicked by a horse and fell to the ground. Whether she struck her head was uncertain, and observers at the scene reported she did not lose consciousness. She went on to ride the horse, and later when asked about the injury she had no recall of the episode. RE continued to display posttraumatic amnesia and was taken to the emergency room by her parents. She was diagnosed as suffering a concussion and discharged to her home with head injury precautions.

Immediately following the incident, her mother noted a number of changes in her functioning, including considerable fatigue, difficulty retaining new information, repetitive speech patterns, and difficulty focusing her attention. She also suffered from dizziness and frequent headaches. At the time of the neuropsychological assessment, both RE and her mother reported that RE continued to forget things, such as conversations with friends, that she had difficulty remembering to complete tasks, and that she was retaining less information and thus having more problems in school. Both she and her mother also said that RE was more emotionally labile and frequently became angry for no reason at family and friends. Her mother was quite distressed over the changes in her daughter's functioning.

Review of RE's medical history was unremarkable. Her mother reported that she had always done well in school and had been at the top of her class. She was currently attending a private school and had already been accepted to a college in an engineering program for the following year. Testing indicated average range verbal abilities, and above average nonverbal abilities. She had difficulty on tasks requiring shifting mental set and dealing with distractions. Her performance on measures sensitive to executive function (self-regulation and planning) were in the borderline range. On measures of memory she scored in the average range on recall of visual information, but in the impaired range on multiple measures requiring recall of verbal information.

RE was seen weekly on eight occasions for 1-hour sessions. Treatment consisted of direct intervention with attention training materials and compensation training with a memory system. Information regarding her injury and the consequences was shared with appropriate school personnel and educational materials were provided to her parents. After two sessions, it was recommended that RE and her mother attend counseling to deal with changes in RE's emotional functioning and her mother's reaction to the injury. Psychosocial treatment continued throughout and beyond cognitive therapy. Goals included better adjustment to the injury related changes, improved communication, and anger management.

During cognitive therapy, RE made considerable progress on all treatment tasks. She performed a variety of attention tasks including taped exercises, alphabetizing sentences, card sorting, and computer tasks aimed at improving speed of response as well as sustained attention. She instituted the use of a compensatory memory system for class and project planning, and for her own social calendar.

RE was seen for follow-up testing approximately two months following treatment. Upon reevaluation, she exhibited improvement on measures of attention/concentration and executive functioning, so that her performance now fell in the average range on all measures administered. On measures of new learning and memory, she also made significant improvement. She now scored in the average range on immediate recall of verbal information. Her initial recall improved and was in the low end of the average range. Delayed recall remained below average, though it improved over pretreatment testing (on an alternate form of the test).

It was felt that RE's lowered performance on measures of memory and new learning was probably due, at least in part, to impaired concentration ability. After treatment, immediate recall of information did improve, though there was still some evidence of lowered retention of information over time. RE benefited from not only direct intervention strategies, but also from education with her family and school, introduction of a compensatory memory system, and involvement in appropriate psychosocial counseling with her family.

In conclusion, it is felt that cognitive rehabilitation therapies with children suffering from MTBI is warranted. The authors are also involved in the modification of materials for attention training with children and the assessment of the efficacy of those materials. Certainly, the two cases outlined above suggest that such treatment may be efficacious, but more research in this area is necessary.

References

Adams, W. (1990). Effects of mild head injury on children's academic performance. Paper presented at the North Coast Society of Pediatric Psychology, Detroit, MI.

Anderson, V., and Moore, C. (1995). Age at injury as a predictor of outcome following pediatric head injury: A longitudinal perspective. *Child Neuropsychology, 1*(3), 187–202.

Annegers, J.F. (1986). The epidemiology of head trauma in children. In K. Shapiro (Ed.), *Pediatric Head Trauma*. Mt. Kisco, NY: Futura.

Annegers, J.F., Grabow, J.D., Kurland, L.T., and Laws, E.R. (1980). The incidence, causes, and secular trends of head trauma in Olmstead County, Minnesota, 1935–1974. *Neurology, 30*, 912–919.

Asarnow, R.F., Satz, P., Light, R., Lewis, R., and Neumann, E. (1991). Behavior problems and adaptive functioning in children with mild and severe closed head injury. *Journal of Pediatric Psychology, 15*, 543–555.

Asarnow, R.F., Satz, P., Light, R., Zaucha, K., Lewis, R., and McCleary, C. (1995). The UCLA study of mild closed head injury in children and adolescents. In S. H. Broman and M.E. Michel (Eds.), *Traumatic Head Injury in Children*, New York, NY: Oxford Press.

Barin, J.J., Hanchett, J.M., Jacob, W.L., and Scott, M.B. (1985). Counseling the head injured patient. In M. Ylvisaker (Ed.), *Head Injury Rehabilitation: Children and Adolescents*. Austin, TX: ProEd, Inc.

Beers, S. (1992). Cognitive effects of mild head injury in children and adolescents. *Neuropsychology Review, 3*, 281–320.

Bijur, P.E., Haslum, M., and Golding, J. (1990). Cognitive and behavioral sequelae of mild head injury in children. *Pediatrics, 86*, 337–344.

Bijur, P.E., Haslum, M., and Golding, J. (1996). Cognitive outcomes of multiple head injuries in children. *Journal of Developmental and Behavioral Pediatrics, 17*(3), 143–148.

Boll, T.J. (1983). Minor head injury in children: Out of sight but not out of mind, *Journal of Clinical Child Psychology, 12*(1), 74–80.

Boll, T.J., and Barth, J.T. (1981). Neuropsychology of brain damage in children. In S.B. Filskov, and T.J. Boll (Eds.), *Handbook of Clinical Neuropsychology* New York, NY: John Wiley & Sons, Inc.

Brown, G., Chadwick, O., Shaffer, D., Rutter, M., and Traub, M. (1981). A prospective study of children with head injuries: III. Psychiatric sequelae. *Psychological Medicine, 11*, 63–78.

Chadwick, O., Rutter, M., Brown, G., Shaffer, D., and Traub, M. (1981b). A prospective study of children with head injuries: II. Cognitive sequelae. *Psychological Medicine, 11*, 46–61.

Chadwick, O., Rutter, M., Shaffer, D., and Shrout, P.E. (1981a). A prospective study of children with head injuries: IV. Specific cognitive deficits. *Journal of Clinical Neuropsychology, 3*, 101–120.

De Boskey, D.S. (1996). An educational challenge: meeting the needs of students with brain injury. Alexandria, VA: The Brain Injury Association, Inc.

Di Scala, C., Osberg, S., Gans, B.M., Chin, L.J., and Grant, C.C. (1991). Children with traumatic head injury: Morbidity and postacute treatment. *Archives of Physical Medicine Rehabilitation, 72*, 662–666.

Eiben, C.F., Anderson, T.P., Lockman, L., Matthews, D.J., Dryja, R., Martin, J., Burrill, C., Gottesman, N., O'Brian, P., and Witte, L. (1984). Functional outcome of closed head injury in children and young adults. *Archives of Physical Medicine Rehabilitation, 65*, 168–170.

Eslinger, P.J., Grattan, L.M., Damasio, H., and Damasio, A.R. (1992). Developmental consequences of childhood frontal lobe damage. *Archives of Neurology, 49*, 746–769.

Eso, K., and Kerns, K.A. (1998). Efficacy of a new attention training program in children diagnosed with ADHD. *Journal of the International Neuropsychological Society, 4*(1), 43.

Ewings-Cobb, L., Miner, M.E., Fletcher, J.M., and Levin, H.S. (1989). Intellectual, motor, and language sequelae following closed-head injury in children and adolescents. *Journal of Pediatric Psychology, 14*, 531–547.

Fay, G., Jaffe, K.M., Polissar, N.L., Liao, S., Martin, K.M., Shurtleff, H.A., Rivara, J.B., and Winn, H.R. (1993). Mild pediatric traumatic brain injury: A cohort study. *Archives of Physical Medicine Rehabilitation, 74*, 895–901.

Fuld, P.A., and Fisher, P. (1977). Recovery of intellectual ability after closed head-injury. *Developmental Medicine and Child Neurology, 19*, 495–502.

Goldman-Rakic, P. (1984). The frontal lobes: Uncharted provinces of the brain. *Trends in Neurosciences*, 412–429.

Goldstein, F.C., and Levin, H.S. (1987). Epidemiology of pediatric closed head injury: Incidence, clinical characteristics, and risk factors. *Journal of Learning Disabilities, 202*, 518–525.

Gordon, M., McClure, F. D., and Post, E. M. (1986). *Interpretive Guide to the Gordon Diagnostic System.* Syracuse, NY: Gordon Systems, Inc.

Gordon, M., Thomason, D., Cooper, S., and Ivers, C. (1991). Non-medical treatment of ADHD/Hyperactivity: The attention training system. *Journal of School Psychology, 29*, 151–159.

Grattan, L.M., and Eslinger, P.J. (1991). Frontal lobe damage in children and adults: A comparative review. *Developmental Neuropsychology, 7*(3), 283–326.

Gulbrandsen, G.B. (1984). Neuropsychological sequelae of light head injuries in older children 6 months after trauma. *Journal of Clinical Neuropsychology, 6*, 257–268.

Hannay, H.J., and Levin, H.S. (1988). Visual continuous recognition memory in normal and closed-head-injured adolescents. *Journal of Clinical and Experimental Neuropsychology, 11,* 444–460.

Horton, Jr. A.M. (1994). *Behavioral Interventions with Brain-Injured Children.* New York, NY: Plenum Press.

Johnson, D.A. (1992). Head injured children and education: A need for greater delineation and understanding. *British Journal of Educational Psychology, 62,* 404–409.

Johnson, D.A., Roethig-Johnston, K., and Middleton, J. (1988). Development and evaluation of an attentional test for head injured children—1. Information processing capacity in a normal sample. *Journal of Child Psychology and Psychiatry, 29*(2), 199–208.

Kennard, M.A. (1936). Age and other factors in motor recovery from precentral lesions in monkeys. *American Journal of Physiology, 115,* 138–146.

Kennard, M.A. (1940). Relation of age to motor impairments in man and in subhuman primates. *Archives of Neurology and Psychiatry, 44,* 377–397.

Kerns, K.A., Eso, K., and Thomson, J. (1998). *Investigation of a direct intervention for improving attention in young children with ADHD.* Manuscript submitted for publication.

Kerns, K.A., and Thomson, J. (In Press). Implementation of a compensatory memory system in a school-aged child with severe memory impairment. *Pediatric Rehabilitation.*

Klauber, M.R., Barrett-Connor, E., Hofstetter, C.R., and Micik, S.H. (1986). A population-based study of nonfatal childhood injuries. *Preventive Medicine, 15*(2), 139–149.

Klauber, M.R., Barrett-Connor, E., Marshall, L.F., and Bowers, S.A. (1981). The epidemiology of head injury: A prospective study of an entire community—San Diego County, California, 1978. *American Journal of Epidemiology, 113,* 500–509.

Klonoff, H., Clark, C., and Klonoff, P.S. (1993). Long-term outcome of head injuries: A 23-year follow-up study of children with head injuries. *Journal of Neurology, Neurosurgery, and Psychiatry, 56,* 410–415.

Klonoff, H., Low, M.D., and Clark, C. (1977). Head injuries in children: A prospective five year follow-up. *Journal of Neurology, Neurosurgery, and Psychiatry, 40,* 1211–1219.

Lehr, E. (1990). *Psychological Management of Traumatic Brain Injuries in Children and Adolescents,* Rockville, MD: Aspen.

Levin, H.S., Culhane, K.A., Mendelsohn, D., Lilly, M.A., Bruce, D., Fletcher, J.M., Chapman, S.B., Harward, H., and Eisenberg, H.M. (1993). Cognition in relation to magnetic resonance imaging in head-injured children and adolescents. *Archives of Neurology, 50,* 897–905.

Mateer, C.A., Kerns, K.A., and Eso, K.L. (1996). Management of attention and memory disorders following traumatic brain injury. *Journal of Learning Disabilities, 29,* 618–632.

Mateer, C.A., and Williams, D. (1991). Effects of frontal lobe injury in childhood. *Developmental Neuropsychology, 7*(2), 359–376.

Mira, M.P, Tucker, B.F., and Tyler, J.S. (1992). *Traumatic Brain Injury in Chil-*

dren and Adolescents: A Source book for Teachers and Other School Personnel. Austin, TX: Pro-Ed, Inc.

Mittenberg, W., Wittner, M.S., and Miller, L.J. (1997). Postconcussion syndrome occurs in children, *Neuropsychology, 11*(3), 447–452.

Pelco, L., Sawyer, M., Duffield, G., Prior, M., and Kinsella, G. (1992). Premorbid emotional and behavioral adjustment in children with mild head injuries. *Brain Injury, 6,* 29–37.

Polissar, N.L., Fay, G.C., Jaffe, K.M., Liao, S., Martin, K.M., Shurtleff, H.A., Rivara, J.B., and Winn, H.R. (1994). Mild pediatric traumatic brain injury: adjusting significance levels for multiple comparisons, *Brain Injury, 8*(3), 249–264.

Pollock, E., Fue, L.D., and Goldstein, S. (1993). *A Teacher's Guide: Managing Children with Brain Injury in the Classroom.* Salt Lake City, UT: The Neurology, Learning and Behavior Center.

Roberts, M.A., Mandshadi, F.F., Bushnell, D.L., and Hines, M.E. (1995). Neurobehavioral dysfunction following mild traumatic brain injury in childhood: A case report with positive findings from positron emission tomography (PET). *Brain Injury, 9*(5), 427–436.

Rutter, M., Chadwick, O., Shaffer, D., and Brown, G. (1980). A prospective study of children with head injuries. I. Design and methods. *Psychological Medicine, 10,* 633–645.

Satz, P., Zaucha, K., McCleary, C., and Light, R. (1997). Mild head injury in children and adolescents: A review of studies. *Psychological Bulletin, 122* (2), 107–131.

Savage, R.C. and Wolcott, G.F. (1995). An educator's manual: what educators need to know about students with brain injury. Alexandria, VA: The Brain Injury Association, Inc.

Segalowitz, S.J., Bernstein, D.M., and Lawson, S. (1995). Lower amplitude P300 in mild head injury in the absence of objective behavioral sequelae. *Psychophysiology, 32,* S67.

Segalowitz, S.J., and Brown, D. (1991). Mild head injury as a source of developmental disabilities. *Journal of Learning Disabilities, 24,* 551–559.

Semrud-Clikeman, M. Nielsen, K.H., Clinton, A., Sylvester, L., Parle, N., and Connor, R. (In press). An intervention approach for children with teacher and parent identified attentional difficulties. *Journal of Learning Disabilities.*

Sohlberg, M.M., and Mateer, C.A. (1986). *Attention Process Training (APT).* Puyallup, WA: Association for Neuropsychological Research and Development.

Thomson, J., and Kerns, K.A. (1998). *Rehabilitation of high school-aged individuals with traumatic brain injury through utilization of an Attention Training Program.* Manuscript submitted for publication.

Welsh, M.C., and Pennington, B.F. (1988). Assessing frontal lobe functioning in children: Views from developmental psychology. *Developmental Neuropsychology, 4,* 199–230.

Williams, D., and Mateer, C.A. (1992). Developmental impact of frontal injury in middle childhood. *Brain and Cognition, 20,* 196–204.

Williams, D.J. (1989). *A process-specific training program in the treatment of attention deficits in children.* Ph.D. Dissertation, University of Washington, Seattle, WA.

Winogron, H.W., Knights, R.M., and Bawden, H.N. (1984). Neuropsychological deficits following head injury in children. *Journal of Clinical Neuropsychology, 6,* 268–279.

Wrightson, P., McGinn, V., and Gronwall, D. (1995). Mild head injury in preschool children: Evidence that it can be associated with a persisting cognitive defect, *Journal of Neurology, Neurosurgery and Psychiatry, 59*(4), 375–380.

Yakovlev, P.I, and Lecours, A.-R. (1967). The myelogentic cycles of regional maturation of the brain. In A. Minkowski (Ed.), *Regional Development of the Brain in Early Life.* Oxford: Blackwell Scientific, pp. 126–139.

Ylvisaker, M., Feeney, T.J., and Szekeres, S.F. (1998). Social-environmental approach to communication and behavior. In M. Ylvisaker (Ed.) Traumatic Brain Injury Rehabilitation: Children and Adolescents. Second Edition. Boston, MA: Butterworth-Heinenann, pp. 271–302.

APPENDIX A

A list of suggested interventions for dealing with a child with mild brain injury in the school and home environments.

A. Inattentiveness
1. Cue the child to pay attention to important information.
2. Allow the child to take frequent breaks.
3. Present information in a short and concise format.
4. Provide several repetitions of information in order to allow for fluctuations in attention.
5. Speak slowly and distinctly, and face the child when speaking.
6. Stop periodically to summarize important points.
7. Seat the child in an area free of distractions, such as near the front of the classroom, or away from noises such as heating vents, clocks, or fans and away from window and doors.
8. Allow the child to use earplugs or a headset during independent work time.
9. Keep the child's desk or other work area free from clutter.
10. Work with the child in small groups whenever possible in order to minimize distractions from other students.
11. Prepare the child for new situations in advance.
12. Allow sufficient time between tasks.
13. Require the child to attend to only one activity at a time.

B. Motor Restlessness
1. Allow the child to stand while working.
2. Assign the child active jobs, such as erasing the blackboard or handing out papers.

C. Language Processing
In addition to environmental modifications recommended by the child's speech and language therapist, the following may be helpful:
1. Utilize paraphrasing, repetition, and summarizing.
2. Provide concrete and concise verbal information.
3. Allow nonverbal communication such as gesturing or signing.
4. Ask nonthreatening questions that require only a short or one-word response.
5. Allow the student time to formulate a response.
6. Provide opportunities for verbal expression in a small group.
7. Provide alternative options for responding.
8. Supplement oral instructions with written instructions and/or visual information such as pictures or maps.

D. Memory and Learning:.
1. Utilize the "three R's": Repetition, Review, and Rehearsal.
2. Ensure that previously learned information can be recalled over time before presenting new information.

3. Use mental imagery techniques when appropriate.
4. Teach memory mnemonics.
5. "Anchor" new learning to previous experience.
6. Use overlearning.
7. Avoid the use of multistep instructions or provide written instructions.
8. Have the child repeat information immediately to check accuracy.
9. "Reteach" material, such as including a few old spelling words on new spelling lists or reintroducing facts in another context.
10. Post information to be remembered like schedules of assignments.

E. Executive Functioning and Problem-Solving Skills
   1. Provide a highly structured and consistent environment.
   2. Use well-defined goals and objectives.
   3. Provide assistance with identification of appropriate solutions.
   4. Provide assistance with shifting solutions.
   5. Shorten or simplify tasks when necessary.
   6. Help the child break down assignments, and estimate how much time he/she will need to complete each part.
   7. Assign a classroom "buddy" who can assist the student when confused or experiencing problems.

13

Cognitive Remediation of Mild Traumatic Brain Injury in an Older Age Group

SARAH A. RASKIN

The occurrence of MTBI in older individuals can be complicated by many factors. There are differences in the cause of injury, increased risk of premorbid medical conditions, age-related differences in brain functioning, and social and emotional factors.

Some evidence suggests that age differentially affects the rate and extent of recovery after any brain injury (Miller, 1984; Rutherford et al., 1979) and there is speculation that the neuroanatomical changes associated with cognitive remediation may be different in the older brain (Goodman and Englander, 1992). Symptoms following MTBI have been found to be greater in older individuals (Wilson et al., 1987; Russell and Smith, 1961). As for outcome, one study reported that at admission, 53% of older individuals with MTBI were living at home alone and 32% were at home with family; in the follow-up study, 72% had experienced a change in functional status such that increased family involvement and use of community support services was necessary (Wilson et al., 1987).

Neuroanatomical changes that occur with aging may predispose the individual to greater impairment when MTBI is superimposed. Three kinds of age-related changes have been identified in the brain (Squire, 1987). First, as the individual ages, the number of neurons decreases, most markedly in the substantia nigra, locus coeruleus, parts of the limbic system (including the hippocampus), and prefrontal cortex (Selkoe, 1992). Axonal atrophy can occur even in cells that survive. Apparently, axons and cell bodies that secrete acetylcholine are most susceptible. Second, total brain weight decreases and there is atrophy particularly in cerebral cortex, thalamus, basal forebrain, and hippocampus (Vroman et al., 1989). Due to this decrease in cortical size, shearing in the bridging veins from the cerebral cortex to the dura occurs more frequently, leading to subdural and subarachnoid hemorrhage. Third, pathologic changes such as neurofibrillary tangles begin to develop with advancing age, which may lead to less efficient neurotransmission. Plaques develop in the extracellular spaces of the hippocampus, the cerebral cortex, and the meninges (Squire, 1987). The myelin sheath itself may also become altered.

Demographic Variables

Individuals who incur MTBI after age 65 are different in many ways from younger survivors (Roy et al., 1986). Although the percentage of all TBI that are MTBI (84%) is the same in those over 65 years of age as in those under 65 (Miller and Jones, 1990), MTBIs in older individuals are likely to lead to greater disability (Goodman and Englander, 1992; Katz et al., 1990).

In a study of MTBI in the elderly by Roy et al. (1986), falls were reported to be responsible for two-thirds of the injuries in older persons, as compared to motor vehicle accidents for MTBI in general. Because the elderly are more prone to falls, they are more likely to experience focal injuries after MTBI (Hernesniemi, 1979; Katz et al., 1990). Of note, medical conditions other than the MTBI were present in 96 cases (66%) (Roy et al., 1986). These conditions included extracranial injury (24%), cardiac disease (12%), dementia (5%), respiratory disease (5%), other neurological disease (4%), and gastrointestinal disease (3%). Fifteen patients had previous brain injuries, 10 had preexisting dementia, and 18 had other preexisting neurological disorders.

Other preexisting conditions can also affect the pathophysiology of MTBI in older individuals. Long-term use of alcohol or of antiinflammatory medications can increase risk for hemorrhage as can diabetic, atherosclerotic, amyloid, or hypertensive vasculopathy. Lowered cardiac output or poor intracerebral collateral circulation can lead to cerebral infarction. Respiratory difficulties can lead to hypoxic encephalopathy. Alcohol use, exposure to neurotoxins earlier in life, and previous neurologic disorders (TBI, stroke, dementia) can all reduce the "cerebral reserve" and lead to a much greater degree of dysfunction than might otherwise be expected (Galbraith, 1987). Thus, even mild TBI, when added to preexisting impairment, can cause severe cognitive deficits. Moreover, the physician may be more likely to focus on medical disorders, which can obscure the diagnosis of brain injury (Galbraith, 1987). Thus, an older individual brought in confused after a fall may be treated for the cause of the fall (e.g., cardiac dysfunction) and the brain injury may be missed. In addition, older individuals may be more prone to delayed symptoms such as hematoma and Alzheimer's disease-like pathology (Goldstein et al., 1994).

In addition to relatively severe cognitive changes in the elderly with MTBI, compared with younger survivors, they may also exhibit acute behavioral changes typically seen with dementia. These include agitation, delusions, hallucinations, illusions, restlessness and wandering, rage and anger, sleep disturbances, sun downing, disinhibition, personality changes, and compulsive behaviors (Rapp et al., 1992). Moreover, these difficulties are often treated with pharmacological agents, such as chlorpromazine, which have sedative and anticholinergic effects.

Assessment

When doing an assessment of cognitive function in the elderly, being aware of complicating sensory or perceptual factors is important. These include poor hearing, poor visual acuity, visual field cuts or glaucoma, and difficulty speaking due to reduced motor control or missing teeth. Physical illness, pain (including minor pain or chronic pain from arthritis), or lack of sleep can greatly impair concentration, attention, and judgment. There may be periods of disorientation on awakening, the "postlunch dip" or sun downing (Broughton, 1975), so, if possible, testing at different times of the day can be instructive. There are reversible causes of cognitive dysfunction that may be missed in cases with MTBI, including electrolyte disturbance, drug side effects, hypoxia, and paroxysmal nocturnal dyspnea, which should be carefully evaluated (Goodman and Englander, 1992). The examiner should take into account cardiac and pulmonary reserve.

Older individuals are likely to have prescribed medications, such as hypnotics, sedatives, or narcotic analgesics (Goodman and Englander, 1992). Anticonvulsants, which may be prescribed prophylactically, may produce lethargy. Tranquilizers and antidepressants can cause both cognitive changes and lethargy (Boop, 1990).

In one study, 148 individuals who met the criteria for MTBI were administered a neuropsychological battery (Raskin et al., 1998). The complete battery is presented in Chapter 4. Correlational analyses revealed significant ($p < 0.01$) relationships between age and a number of neuropsychological variables, most being measures of general intelligence and of attention tasks within a test of long-term memory retention. Therefore, the sample was broken into two groups (more than 40 years of age and 40 years of age or less). Students' t-tests revealed significant differences in general intelligence and attention.

Overall, the older subjects were superior on tests of general intelligence, possibly due to age corrections. In contrast, their performance was relatively impaired on tests of attention. These results are presented in Table 13.1. These data suggest a greater relative likelihood of decline in attention after MTBI with advancing age.

This finding is supported by a study involving a dual task paradigm to measure attention (Stablum et al., 1996). These authors also reported greater impairment in older individuals with MTBI as compared with

Table 13-1 Test Results Demonstrating Significant Differences Between Two Age Groups

	Mean (Standard deviation)		
	≤40	>40	t
WAIS-R Information	15.80 (5.86)	20.14 (5.23)	4.45**
WAIS-R Vocabulary	40.01 (12.25)	49.90 (10.64)	4.57**
WAIS-R Digit Symbol	57.65 (12.38)	50.72 (10.77)	3.48**
CVLT Trial I	7.35 (2.36)	6.40 (1.91)	2.69*
CVLT Trial V	13.94 (2.06)	12.96 (2.32)	2.61*
CVLT List B	7.19 (1.95)	6.10 (1.95)	3.30**
CVLT Cued Recall I	12.93 (2.41)	11.57 (2.96)	2.93*
WAIS-R Arithmetic	10.98 (3.54)	12.60 (3.33)	2.71*

WAIS-R, Wechsler Adult Intelligence Scale-Revised; CVLT, California Verbal Learning Trial.
**$p \le .001$.
*$p \le .01$.

younger individuals with MTBI. In addition, the effect was demonstrated over a 2-year period following the injury.

In assessing an older individual with MTBI, many standard tests of cognitive functions for the elderly are available. These include self-report measures and objective tests. Gilewski and Zelinski (1986) describe the value of self-report questionnaires in this population. As mentioned in Chapter 5, self-reports can help determine treatment goals and measure improvement in treatment. These authors then review 10 memory questionnaires, including Sunderland et al.'s Everyday Memory Questionnaire (Sunderland et al., 1983), which has been used with both brain injury survivors and the elderly, and metamemory questionnaires (e.g., Dixon & Hultsch, 1983).

Several brief scales were designed to measure cognitive and emotional changes over time in the elderly. These can be helpful to track deterioration in patients suspected of having a superimposed dementing illness, and for tracking improvement in individuals undergoing treatment. The Brief Cognitive Rating Scale (Reisberg et al., 1983) is one. The Brief Psychiatric Rating Scale (Overall and Gorham, 1962) measures psychiatric symptoms and has been used extensively to measure the effectiveness of medications in the elderly. Raskin (1988) designed the Inventory of Psychic and Somatic Complaints in the Elderly with both measures of cognitive functions and psychiatric symptoms. Cognitive items from this scale were demonstrated to correlate with standard psychometric tests (Reisberg et al., 1981).

To assess cognitive functions in older persons with MTBI, it is sometimes helpful to begin with a gross screening test, such as the Dementia Rating Scale (Mattis, 1988). This test provides only gross information but samples most functional domains, and if the individual is severely impaired this may be as much as he/she can do.

To assess memory functioning, the Fuld Object-Memory Test (Fuld, 1977) was designed to be used with the elderly. It has high face validity as it deals with common objects. For verbal learning and recall, Brandt (1991) developed the Hopkins Verbal Learning Test that has six parallel forms, allows for identification of semantic categorization, and has been used with older individuals.

As in all subjects with MTBI, measures of complex attention and of memory should be administered. Studies of the Consonant Trigrams Test (Peterson and Peterson, 1959), for example, are available to demonstrate performance by subjects with MTBI and subjects with varying degrees of dementia (Corkin, 1982) and norms are available for older subjects on other tests sensitive to MTBI, such as the Paced Auditory Serial Addition Task (Brittain et al., 1991) and the Rey-Osterreith Complex Figure (Berry et al., 1991). Care should be given to avoid tests that require a speeded response and to use appropriate norms. To rule out dementia, tests for anomia (Boston Naming Test [Goodglass and Kaplan, 1983]) and apraxia (Test of Oral and Limb Apraxia [Helm-Estabrooks, 1992]) can also be administered.

Beyond the initial diagnosis, considering changes in functioning in older individuals over time is also important. Thus, many diagnoses can be confirmed only by examining whether the individual's pattern of deficits follow in the predicted sequence.

Mental Health

Depression poses a particular difficulty in the assessment and treatment of the elderly individual with MTBI. Elderly persons who are depressed, but have no evidence of neurologic impairment or dementia have been demonstrated to be impaired on tasks of attention, memory recall, and abstraction (King et al., 1991; Raskin, 1986). Typically, however, the pattern of deficits may be very different. There is some evidence that older individuals with depression do poorly at recall tasks, but are unimpaired when given a recognition format, for example (Raskin, 1986). The pattern of impairment on recall tasks may also be different, with depressed patients showing a slower rate of forgetting and more primacy effect (Gainotti and Marra, 1994). In addition, those with depression rarely demonstrate confusion, recent memory impairment, reduced alertness, or confabulation (Salzman and Gutfreund, 1986).

While depression is generally a frequent sequelae of MTBI, as an individual ages, one is likely to experience considerable losses, changes, and unexpected challenges. One must take a multidimensional approach that considers the biological, cultural, historical, sociological, environmental, and personality variables involved in mood (Hazlewood and Fielstein, 1990). Many commonly used scales of emotional functioning do not necessarily have age-appropriate test items or norms. Therefore, examining each individual's life and level of functioning is important.

Alexopoulos et al. (1988) developed the Cornell Scale to measure depression in elderly patients, with or without dementia. The Geriatric Depression Scale has been used specifically to differentiate the depressed demented from the nondepressed demented (Sheikh and Yesavage, 1986). The three-area severity of depression scales is a brief clinical measure designed to screen for depression and has also been used to follow change in symptoms of depression with treatment (Raskin, 1988).

Normal Aging

Considerable controversy exists about the effects of normal aging on memory functioning, which illustrates the need to use age-appropriate norms in documenting change following MTBI. Age-associated memory impairment in otherwise healthy individuals over age 50 may be related to changes in the cholinergic system (Bartus et al., 1982) or to a loss of noradrenergic function (McEntee and Crook, 1990).

Dementia

An individual who is in the early stages of dementia may not be aware of cognitive changes. The trauma of a fall or motor vehicle accident may serve to focus attention on the person's cognitive functions. Thus, decline in functioning, which has in fact been progressive, may be incorrectly attributed to an MTBI. To make a diagnosis, looking for the primary cognitive changes seen in Alzheimer's disease may be necessary, which include decline in overall level of intellectual functioning, significantly higher Verbal IQ as compared to Performance IQ, memory impairment, constructional apraxia, decreased verbal fluency, and anomia (McKhann et al., 1984; Rosen, 1989) and to follow any cognitive changes over time to determine whether there is progressive decline.

Rehabilitation

Often social issues are of great importance and older individuals with MTBI may need greater social and physical support. Social status appears to effect more directly the outcome in older survivors than in younger ones. In a group of patients over 60, those living with family and friends before the injury were more likely to survive and have a more complete recovery than those living alone or in institutions (Hernesniemi, 1979). As approximately one-half of the elderly TBI survivors live alone (Roy et al., 1986); they may end up hospitalized for MTBI due to safety concerns. This is, of course, a further stressor. Generally, people prefer to be at home, and the elderly person, in particular, may have difficulty with strange environments (Galbraith, 1987).

There are also age cohort issues. This includes asking older male individuals to comply with young female therapists or using cooking as a goal in a person who has never cooked before. The survivor may choose to limit mobility due to realistic fear and anxiety of reinjury, and aiding him or her in gradual return to pleasurable activities may be necessary.

In elderly cases, rehabilitation staff members may frequently deem the individual poorly motivated and end treatment, rather than recognize the influence of neuropsychological variables on motivation (Hesse and Campion, 1983). In part, ensuring that the treatment goals and materials are meaningful to the person, and providing more time to complete tasks and the opportunity to self-pace take on greater importance in rehabilitation efforts (Hesse and Campion, 1984).

The goals for rehabilitation of older persons are also likely to differ from those for younger people. Return to work is less likely to be a goal as age increases (McMordie et al., 1990). In contrast, returning to drive is often a complicated issue. On the one hand, the ability to drive may be the only route to independence for older individuals who live outside of urban areas. On the other hand, on testing, they may demonstrate cognitive impairments that raise concern about ability to drive safely. We combine a careful neuropsychological assessment of attention, speed of processing, abstract thinking, and visual perception with several test-drives in a dual control car to determine appropriateness of driving. We also counsel on issues of fatigue, time of day, and driving on fast highways vs. using other roads where people can drive more slowly and there is less traffic. Some states allow for "modified" licenses (i.e., limit driving after 9 P.M.).

Few studies have focused on remediation of older survivors of MTBI. Lessons may be learned, however, from studies of treatment for dementia and the healthy elderly. Results of formal traumatic brain injury inpatient rehabilitation with severely brain-injured patients over 50 years of age were reported by Davis and Acton (1988). Fifty-eight percent were discharged to home after an average rehabilitation stay of 70 days (range of 15–77 days). No information was provided about the type of treatment administered. No analyses were performed, but there did not appear to be an appreciable change in Ranchos Los Amigos scale following treatment. However, it was reported that the elderly group had significantly worse Ranchos score both at admission and at discharge than a younger comparison group. Follow-up was performed from two to 5 years after discharge. At follow-up 85% were living at home. None were employed.

All patients reported continued cognitive deficits. Fourteen of 23 patients were independent in activities of daily living at follow-up, 9 required supervision. This demonstrates the need for careful tracking of community integration after inpatient discharge.

Dementia

Many studies have been published documenting attempts to remediate memory deficits in individuals with dementia. Some techniques are aimed merely at specific tasks such as list-learning, with limited practical applications (Bird and Luszcz, 1993). In one study, prompting and reinforcement were used with the method of vanishing cues, and the authors concluded that training was more effective when multiple modalities, especially physical practice, were employed (McEvoy and Patterson, 1986).

Behavior management techniques have also been used. Rapp et al. (1992) present behavior management techniques, used previously with young traumatic brain injury survivors, and adopted for use with demented elderly individuals. These techniques were successful in reducing dementia-related behavioral difficulties, such as paranoia and agitation, but were not focused on aiding cognitive difficulties.

Normal Aging

A large number of studies have been published on memory intervention strategies for healthy older adults (Yesavage et al., 1989; Zarit et al., 1981). The use of mnemonics, encoding strategies, and repetition have all been tried in memory-impaired elderly subjects but with limited generalization (Beck, 1990).

Vroman et al. (1989) describe a program of cognitive rehabilitation for the elderly that relied on computer programs. The patients were all 65 years of age or older, complained of memory problems, and participated for several months to a year. The initial study involved weekly sessions for 15 weeks. A wide variety of computer programs were used. Specific cases were presented in which improvements on tasks were observed, with maintenance of these gains after interruption in treatment. The authors argued that computers particularly lend themselves to facilitating the observation of strengths and weaknesses in oneself. This improves metacognitive awareness and allows for the recognition and use of metacognitive strategies, such as organization of material and specific mnemonics. In addition, by giving immediate feedback, and providing tasks within their level of mastery, sense of control can be developed by the individuals. Thus, rather than being frightened and confused by losing objects and getting lost, they can begin to predict troublesome situations and avoid them or use strategies to help them get through them. Self-instructional training has also been used with older adults to help with problem-solving (Meichenbaum, 1974), which may be a particularly good procedure for ensuring generalization.

Medications

A variety of medications have also been used to attempt to improve cognitive performance in the elderly. Motivation in elderly patients was improved with amphetamine treatment, most likely due to the stimulant properties (Clark and Mankikar, 1979). Cholinergic agents have also been tried, but most have had unremarkable results. These are reviewed by Feeney and Sutton (1979). Agents are currently being investigated to inhibit enzymes that liberate beta-amyloid protein from its precursor, thereby preventing inflammatory or neurotoxic responses (Selkoe, 1992).

Generalization

As mentioned previously, it is perhaps more important with older survivors of MTBI than with younger ones to insure that treatment tasks and goals are meaningful in the person's daily life. Research on rehabilitation suggests that older adults are less interested in participating in long-term rehabilitation focused on improving individual skills. In addition, return to work is less likely to be a long-term goal. Instead, generalization can better be measured in terms of return to previously enjoyed activities and integration into the community. Being able to continue to live independently is an important goal, as is maintaining the ability to drive. Because of the interaction of MTBI with other neurological and medical complications, it is extremely important to continue to monitor the individual well after discharge.

We have found home-based services to be of particular use in this population, due to the higher likelihood of relying on functional skills training and due to the ability to increase awareness of deficits if they are demonstrated within activities that the individual performs in his/her daily life. Environmental restructuring, providing cues within the environment, can also be very helpful. For example, keys can be color coded with matching colors on the locks; doors can be labeled with pictures of what is in the room; increased contrast between light and dark can be used to highlight salient features, such as dark place settings on a white tablecloth (Beck, 1990). External memory aids, such as lists of things to do each day, diaries, and alarm watches have also been used in the elderly (Beck, 1990) and are described in detail in Chapter 6.

Case Studies

Case 1

HH is a 72-year-old widowed woman who is living independently. She graduated from high school and worked in the home and in raising her son. Her prior medical history was significant for a mastectomy, but the oncologist verified that no cognitive changes were observed following the surgery for 1 year until the accident. HH was driving when she was struck by another vehicle from behind. She called her son, who drove her home. He reported that she seemed "stunned and somewhat confused" immediately after the accident, but she did not report any loss of consciousness. Two days later she contacted her primary care physician, complaining of neck pain.

Neuropsychological evaluation was administered 3 months after the accident, at the request of her son. Her son drafted a letter saying that his mother had changed drastically after the accident. He stated that she had been completely independent before and extremely organized with good memory abilities. Since the accident, she was extremely disorganized, her living conditions were messy and she was forgetful of appointments, bills, and telephone conversations. He found her easily distracted and confused. On evaluation she demonstrated a superior range performance in verbal, and a high-average range performance in nonverbal reasoning and problem-solving. However, her attention and memory processes were in the impaired range. She also exhibited significant anxiety. Six months later (9 months after the accident) a reevaluation was done. Computerized tomography scan performed in the interim, to rule out other neurologic disorders, was normal. At this time, her intellectual functioning remained high, with no evidence of decline. However, she continued to exhibit severe deficits in attention and memory. Her mood appeared to have stabilized. Cognitive remediation was recommended to focus on organizational strategies and memory aids.

When HH was first interviewed for treatment, however, she expressed virtually no awareness of her deficits and little need for treatment. Even when recent examples were presented (she had forgotten one scheduled appointment and come at the wrong time for another), she stated that she never had difficulty with functioning in her daily life. Therefore, it was not judged to be appropriate to coerce her into a long-term full-time treatment program.

Instead, a home-based evaluation was done. It was hoped that by demonstrating real-life problems and strategies in her daily life, her awareness and interest in treatment strategies would increase. It was pointed out to her in the evaluation that she frequently repeated herself without awareness of having done so. She had also forgotten the appointment for the home visit, despite having written it down. She was given practical strategies, such as keeping a large calendar in a place that she would see it every day (such as the refrigerator or inside the front door). In addition, her son was consulted and given strategies to use that might be helpful for her. Three months later, a follow-up home visit was performed. At this time both HH and her son were reporting that her symptoms were slowly improving. She had begun to implement some strategies that had been discussed and was less defensive about needing to use them.

Case 2

JH is a 76-year-old right-handed woman. She graduated from high school and worked in a clerical position until she retired at age 67. She was in good health until she was involved in a head-on motor vehicle collision. She struck her head and had bruising above both eyes. She does not believe that she lost consciousness but has no recall of the impact. She was taken to the emergency room and discharged after a few hours. Computerized tomography scan of the head was negative. Over the next few days she contacted the hospital several times complaining of head pain and back pain. One week following the accident she called complaining of dizziness.

She was referred for neuropsychological evaluation $1^1/_2$ months after the accident. She complained of word-finding difficulties, difficulty following directions, and difficulty following conversations. She felt her mind was slower than before and that her memory was impaired. Her son reported that she had been "pretty sharp" mentally before the accident. For example, she could follow her stocks and dividends and do all aspects of daily living. Following the accident, he reported that she was easily confused, forgetful, and tended to be overwhelmed by day to day events.

During the evaluation, many paraphasias were noted in her spontaneous speech, she was a poor historian of the events since the accident, and she frequently repeated the same stories. Toward the end of the day she became noticeably more confused and required repetition of directions. On testing, she displayed severely impaired memory processes. She had been started on a course of antidepressants with no change in her cognitive functioning. It was judged likely that she was, in fact, suffering from a slowly progressive dementing illness, possibly exacerbated by the accident.

However, to determine the effects of any brain injury, a reevaluation was performed. This reevaluation was completed 6 months following the accident. On this evaluation she demonstrated continued impairments in visual attention, visual perception, naming, executive functions, and memory. However, she showed minor improvement in auditory attention and memory. Since there had been no further decline, but rather minor improvement, it appears that her cognitive deficits were the result of the MTBI.

References

Alexopoulos, G., Abrams, R., Young, R., and Shamoian, C. (1988). Use of the Cornell Scale in nondemented patients. *Journal of the American Geriatric Society*, 36, 230–236.

Bartus, R., Dean, R., Beer, B., and Lippa, A. (1982). The cholinergic hypothesis of geriatric memory dysfunction. *Science, 217,* 408–417.

Berry, D., Allen, R., and Schmitt, F. (1991). Rey-Osterreith Complex Figure: Psychometric characteristics in a geriatric sample. *The Clinical Neuropsychologist, 5,* 143–153.

Bird, M., and Luszcz, M. (1993). Enhancing memory performance in Alzheimer's disease: Acquisition assistance and cue effectiveness. *Journal of Clinical and Experimental Neuropsychology, 15,* 921–932.

Boop, W. (1990). Pain management in the geriatric patients. In F. Maloney and K. Means (Eds.), *Rehabilitation and the Aging Adult.* Physical Medicine and Rehabilitation: State of the Art Reviews. Philadelphia, PA: Hanley & Belfus, Inc., pp. 93–124.

Brandt, J. (1991). The Hopkins Verbal Learning Test: Development of a new memory test with six equivalent forms. *The Clinical Neuropsychologist, 5,* 125–142.

Brittain, J., La Marche, J., Reeder, K., Roth, D., and Boll, T. (1991). Effects of age and IQ on Paced Auditory Serial Addition Task Performance. *The Clinical Neuropsychologist, 5,* 163–175.

Broughton, R. (1975). Biorhythmic variations in consciousness and psychological functions. *Canadian Psychological Review, 16,* 217–239.

Clark, A., and Mankikar, G. (1979). d-Amphetamine in elderly patients refractory to rehabilitation procedures. *Journal of the American Geriatric Society, 27,* 174–177.

Corkin, S. (1982). Some relationships between global amnesiacs and the memory impairment in Alzheimer's disease: A report of progress. In S. Corkin et al. (Eds.), Alzheimer's disease: A report of progress. Aging (Vol. 19). New York, NY: Raven Press, pp. 21–47.

Davis, C., and Acton, P. (1988). Treatment of the elderly brain-injured patient: Experience in a traumatic brain injury unit. *Journal of the American Geriatric Society, 36,* 225–229.

Dixon, R., and Hultsch, D. (1983). Structure and development of metamemory in adulthood. *Journal of Gerontology, 38,* 682–688.

Feeney, D., and Sutton, R. (1979). *CRC Critical Reviews in Neurobiology, 3,* 135–197.

Fuld, P. (1977). *Fuld Object-Memory Evaluation.* Stoelting Co.

Gainotti, G., and Marra, C. (1994). Some aspects of memory disorders clearly distinguish dementia of the Alzheimer's type from Depressive Pseudo-Dementia. *Journal of Clinical and Experimental Neuropsychology, 16,* 65–78.

Galbraith, S. (1987). Head injuries in the elderly. *British Medical Journal, 294,* 325.

Gilewski, M., and Zelinski, E. (1986). Questionnaire assessment of memory complaints. In L. Poon (Ed.), *Handbook for Clinical Memory Assessment of Older Adults.* Washington, DC: American Psychological Association.

Goldstein, G., Levin, H., Presley, R., Searcy, J., Colohan, A., Eisenberg, H., Jann, B., and Bertolino-Kusnerik, L. (1994). Neurobehavioral consequences of closed head injury in older adults. *Neurology, 57,* 961.

Goodglass, H., and Kaplan, E. (1983). *Boston Naming Test.* Malvern, PA: Lea & Febiger.

Goodman, H., and Englander, J. (1992). Traumatic brain injury in elderly individuals. In S. Berrol (Ed.), *Physical Medicine and Rehabilitation Clinics of North America: Traumatic Brain Injury, 3*(2), 441–459. Philadelphia, PA: W.B. Saunders Company.

Hazlewood, M., and Fielstein, E. (1990). Psychological aspects of aging. In F. Maloney and K. Means (Eds.), *Rehabilitation and the Aging Adult.* Physical Medicine and Rehabilitation: State of the Art Reviews. Philadelphia, PA: Hanley & Belfus, Inc.

Helm-Estabrooks, N. (1992). *Test of Oral and Limb Apraxia.* Boston, MA: Riverside Publishing Company.

Hernesniemi, J. (1979). Outcome following head injuries in the aged. *Acta Neurochir, 49*, 67–79.

Hesse, K.A., and Campion, E.W. (1983). Motivating the geriatric patient for rehabilitation. *Journal of the American Geriatrics Society, 31*(10) 586–589.

Katz, D., Kehs, G., and Alexander, M. (1990). Prognosis and recovery from traumatic brain injury: The influence of advancing age. *Neurology, 40*, 276.

King, D., Caine, E., Conwell, Y., and Cox, C. (1991). The neuropsychology of depression in the elderly: A comparative study of normal aging and Alzheimer's disease. *Journal of Neuropsychiatry, 3*, 163–168.

Mattis, S. (1988). *Dementia Rating Scale.* Odessa, FL: Psychological Assessment Resources, Inc.

McEntee, W., and Crook, T. (1990). Age-associated memory impairment: A role for catecholamines. *Neurology, 40*, 526–530.

McEvoy, C., and Patterson, R. (1986). Behavioral treatment of deficit skills in dementia patients. *The Gerontologist, 26*, 475–478.

McKhann, G., Drachman, D., Folstein, M., Katzman, R., Price, D., and Stadlan, E. (1984). Clinical diagnosis of Alzheimer's disease, *Neurology, 34*, 939–944.

McMordie, W., Barker, S., and Paolo, T. (1990). Return to work after head injury. *Brain Injury, 4*, 57–69.

Meichenbaum, D. (1974). Self-instructional strategy training: A cognitive prothesis for the aged. *Human Development, 17*, 273–280.

Miller, E. (1984). *Recovery and Management of Neuropsychological Impairments.* Chichester: John Wiley & Sons, Inc.

Miller, J.D., and Jones, P.A. (1990). Minor head injury. In M. Rosenthal, M.R. Bond, E.R. Griffith, and J.D. Miller (Eds.), *Rehabilitation of the Adult and Child with Traumatic Brain Injury*, 2nd Ed. Philadelphia, PA: F.A. Davis, pp. 236–247.

Overall, J., and Gorham, D. (1962). The Brief Psychiatric Rating Scale. *Psychological Reports, 10*, 799–812.

Peterson, L., and Peterson, M. (1959). Short-term retention of individual verbal items. *Journal of Experimental Psychology, 58*, 193–198.

Rapp, M., Flint, A., Herrmann, N., and Proulx, G. (1992). Behavioral disturbances in the demented elderly: Phenomenology, pharmacotherapy, and behavioral management. *Canadian Journal of Psychiatry, 37,* 651–657.

Raskin, A. (1986). Validation of a battery of tests designed to assess psychopathology in the elderly. In G. Burrows, T. Norman, and L. Dennerstein (Eds.), *Clinical and Pharmacological Studies in Psychiatric Disorders.* London: John Libbey and Co., Ltd., pp. 57–71.

Raskin, S., Mateer, C., and Tweeten, R. (1998). Neuropsychological assessment of individuals with mild traumatic brain injury. *The Clinical Neuropsychologist, 12,* 21–30.

Reisberg, B., Ferris, S., de Leon, M., and Crook, T., and Gershon (1981). The relationship between psychiatric assessments and cognitive test measures in mild to moderately cognitively impaired elderly. *Psyopharmacology Bulletin, 17,* 99–101.

Reisberg, B., Schneck, M., Ferris, S., Schwartz, G., and de Leon, M. (1983). The Brief Cognitive Rating Scale: Findings in primary degenerative dementia. *Psychopharmacology Bulletin, 19,* 47–50.

Rosen, W. (1989). Assessment of cognitive disorders in the elderly. In E. Perecman (Ed.), *Integrating Theory and Practice in Clinical Neuropsychology.* Hillsdale, NJ: Lawrence Erlbaum Associates, pp. 381–394.

Roy, C., Pentland, B., and Miller, J. (1986). The causes and consequences of minor head injury in the elderly. *Injury, 17,* 220–223.

Russel, W., and Smith, A. (1961). Post-traumatic amnesia in closed head injury. *Archives of Neurology, 5,* 16.

Rutherford, W., Merrett, J., and McDonald, J. (1979). Symptoms at one year following concussion from minor head injuries, *Injury, 10,* 225–230.

Salzman, C., and Gutfreund, M. (1986). Clinical techniques and research strategies for studying depression and memory. In L. Poon (Ed.), *Clinical Memory Assessment of Older Adults.* Washington, DC: American Psychological Association, pp. 257–268.

Selkoe, D. (1992). Aging brain, aging mind. *Scientific American,* (September) 135–142.

Sheikh, J., and Yesavage, J. (1986). Geriatric Depression Scale (GDS): Recent evidence and development of a shorter version. In T. Brink (Ed.), *Clinical Gerontology: A Guide to Assessment and Intervention.* New York, NY: Haworth Press.

Squire, L.R. (1987). *Memory and Brain.* New York, NY: Oxford University Press.

Stablum, F., Mogentale, C., and Umilta, C. (1996). Executive functioning following mild closed head injury. *Cortex, 32,* 261–278.

Sunderland, A., Harris, J., and Baddeley, A. (1983). Do laboratory tests predict everyday memory? A neuropsychological study. *Journal of Verbal Learning and Verbal Behavior, 22,* 341–357.

Vroman, G., Kellar, L., and Cohen, I. (1989). Cognitive rehabilitation in the elderly: A computer-based memory training program. In E. Perecman (Ed.), *Integrating Theory and Practice in Clinical Neuropsychology.* Hillsdale, NJ: Lawrence Erlbaum Associates, pp. 395–416.

Wilson, J., Pentland, B., Currie, C., and Miller, J. (1987). The functional effects of head injury in the elderly. *Brain Injury, 1,* 183–188.

Yesavage, J., Lapp, D., and Sheikh, J. (1989). Mnemonics as modified for use by the elderly. In L. Poon, D. Rubin, and B. Wilson (Eds.), *Everyday Cognition in Adulthood and Late Life.* Cambridge: Cambridge University Press.

Zarit, S., Cole, K., and Guider, R. (1981). Memory training strategies and subjective complaints of memory in the aged. *The Gerontologist, 21,* 158–162.

14

Issues of Gender, Socioeconomic Status, and Culture

SARAH A. RASKIN

In managing the cognitive and emotional symptoms of mild traumatic brain injury (MTBI), it is important to be aware not only of the premorbid personality and medical history of each client, but also of personal variables that can affect symptom presentation, assessment, and treatment. Individuals with MTBI may differ in their symptom presentation, and appropriate treatment needs to be based on their own background, and the needs and expectations inherent in their own life roles. These variables include gender differences, socioeconomic differences, lifestyle differences, and cultural differences. Some assessment issues are lack of standardized tests for specific populations, absence of appropriate norms, and difficulty in using translators.

Gender Differences in Assessment and Treatment

Social Differences

Providers of treatment to individuals with MTBI need to be aware of gender variations regarding rehabilitation needs, expectations, and goals. Many such differences are imposed by societal constraints. For example, the ability of women and men to return to work after injury may be disparate. One study reported that 44% of white disabled men participate in the workforce, while only 24% of white disabled women do, and that the gap between disabled women and nondisabled women is greater then that between disabled men and nondisabled men (Fine and Asch, 1988). Not surprisingly, disabled women earn less than either disabled men or nondisabled women, regardless of age or educational attainment. Clearly a complicated interaction exists, and may reflect both the premorbid likelihood of lower employment status for women and difficulties due to the disability. However, women receiving rehabilitation services are substantially more likely to be closed in a nonwage-earning capacity, less likely to be referred for vocational training, and more likely to be channeled into homemaking than men, regardless of premorbid occupational status (Fine and Asch, 1988).

Men and women who have a MTBI may be treated differently by medical professionals. Fidell (1980) showed that medical professionals hold beliefs about the personalities and behaviors of women that may result in women receiving less aggressive treatment than men. In particular, physicians are more likely to attribute symptoms to psychogenic causes or malingering in women than in men (Lennane and Lennane, 1973) and they are more likely to prescribe mood-modifying drugs to women than to men. Mental health professionals have a tendency to attribute problems and behaviors of men to external sources, and problems of women to internal biological or psychological sources (Tavris, 1992). Such attributions are particularly likely to occur in conditions that do not have clear objectively measurable medical signs or symptoms, such as MTBI.

Self perception can also be affected by physical changes. Even mild TBI can lead to feelings of awkwardness, balance problems, and reduced coordination, and such injuries are frequently associated with prolonged pain, immobility, or stiffness. These feelings and conditions have different effects in the two genders. Women who are awkward may appear less attractive and graceful, which can affect opportunities for both work and intimate relationships (Fine and Asch, 1988). Men who lose some motor coordination and/or experience neck and back pain may no longer be able to participate in physical activities. Many men, in particular, have commented that, before injury they used physical exertion as a coping mechanism for release of anger and anxiety, and as a source of self-esteem.

As MTBI tends to occur in middle age, it disrupts ongoing behavior and well-established roles (Meyerowitz et al., 1988). Socially, women in middle age are likely to be sensitive to the fact that, as they are aging, they may be viewed by others as less attractive. If there is an expected social role of women as nurturers and caregivers, women who are themselves in need of assistance or who appear unable to care for others may be rejected. Men, conversely may have established roles that involve financial and physical independence. Men are more likely to have interpersonal relationships in which problems, especially physical or mental weaknesses, are not discussed. As a result, friendships may suffer from a lack of understanding and an inability to participate fully in group activities.

Social differences also exist between heterosexual and homosexual brain injury survivors. Mapou (1990) provides a guide to issues about the rehabilitation of gay and lesbian individuals with traumatic brain injury. Confronting the staff's own ignorance about the prevalence and unique needs and challenges of gay and lesbian TBI survivors is essential. Particular problems often involve client or staff's awkwardness around discussions of sexuality, or difficulty involving intimate partners in the rehabilitation process. The latter may be particularly troublesome if the partner and other family members have conflicts.

Neuroanatomical/Chemical Differences

Increasing evidence suggests differences in brain organization between men and women (Kimura, 1992). There is also evidence of gender differences in neurochemistry (Heninger, 1997) and growing support for the role of hormonal influences on brain function (Kimura, 1992), though the implications of these differences for cognitive, behavioral, emotional, and social functioning are not well understood.

Early indications of gender differences in cognitive functioning came from observations that more boys than girls have dyslexia and women recover more quickly and to a greater degree from strokes than do men. In general, men perform better than women on spatial tasks, tasks that require mental rotation, mathematical reasoning, and route navigation. Women, however, perform better than men on tasks that require the rapid matching of items, verbal fluency, arithmetic calculation, recalling landmarks on a route, and fast precision manual tasks (Kimura, 1992). Notably, however, variability of performance within each sex is greater than that between the sexes.

In our sample of 148 individuals with MTBI (80 women and 68 men) a complicated relationship was found when gender analyses were performed (see Chapter 3 for a complete description of the sample) (Raskin et al., 1998). Overall, men and women performed differently on neuropsychological measures (F = 4.62, $p < 0.001$), but not on emotional (MMPI) ones. The most consistent cognitive difference was a better performance by women than men on measures of verbal learning. This reinforces the need to compare subjects to gender-specific norms.

Differences in Coping

Gender differences were also reported in a study of persistent problems and coping strategies 18 months to 33 years after brain injury (Willer et al., 1991). The men reported their greatest continued difficulties to be loss of independence, loss of roles as husband, father, and provider, and difficulty recognizing and accepting post-TBI changes and limitations. Women with TBI reported their greatest difficulties to be loss of autonomy (including employment, mobility, and self-esteem), loneliness and depression, including a general discomfort in social settings, and decreased interest in sex, including feelings of inadequacy as sexual partners. Their partners also differed in terms of problems identified. Men with wives who had brain injury reported the greatest difficulties to be the wife's loss of autonomy, mood swings, insecurities, and social isolation. Women with husbands who had brain injury reported the greatest difficulties to be changes in personality and cognitive abilities, lack of insight, and reduced emotional and financial support.

Gender differences in coping strategies were present, as well. Women with TBI used coping strategies of relying on the support of spouses and others, support groups, memory aids, and reassuming family responsibilities. Men with TBI reported relying on increasing their participation in family decisions, learning to understand the needs of others, becoming involved with activities outside the home, and learning to develop a realistic appraisal of abilities. These strategies may be more or less successful, of course, depending upon the social support available. Unfortunately, divorce, decreased sexual relations, and withdrawal of support are frequent results of MTBI.

Socioeconomic Status

Several studies have suggested that individuals with higher socioeconomic status (SES) experience less impairment in functional status after MTBI (Binder, 1986; Rimel et al., 1981). Employers of those with low SES are apparently more likely to fire an individual outright. However, as Kay (1992) points out, socioeconomic status can work either way. Individuals with higher socioeconomic status are more likely to have an understanding employer and a work schedule and demands that are flexible. However, some higher socioeconomic occupations require high levels of attention, memory, planning, and problem-solving abilities as well as self-initiation, which may be especially impaired after MTBI. This is not to assume, however, that lower SES jobs do not require these skills. Many lower SES jobs are in fact physically dangerous and require a fast response for safety. We have been surprised, for example, at the number of survivors who have received the suggestion to work at a fast-food restaurant. Such work typically requires fast response times, efficient working memory, and considerable sustained and divided attention.

Additionally, access to comprehensive TBI rehabilitation is often easier for those with higher socioeconomic status. Unfortunately, most brain injury rehabilitation programs are by necessity quite expensive or at least require adequate insurance coverage. Thus, the ability to obtain treatment is often based solely on ability to pay (Zahara and Cuvo, 1984). There is currently a two-tiered level of care for people with brain injuries in this country. The wealthy and well-insured have access to a comprehensive system of care that is denied to those on public assistance and many individuals who are patrons of the larger health care insurers (Brody, 1988). Many survivors we encounter initiate litigation against their own insurance companies only to pay for rehabilitation services. Those without insurance are left with what little care is available on a pro bono basis from a limited number of practitioners and public hospitals. Those on public assistance generally can find some therapists within public hospitals, but this is frequently not an integrated rehabilitation program.

We have found disparities in rehabilitation goals possibly depending on socioeconomic status. Those with lower status and fewer financial reserves are more likely to request short-term treatment focused on immediate return to work at any level, while survivors with greater resources may be more interested in a long-term, process-specific plan with concurrent greater likelihood of generalization, and are more focused on return to work at the same occupation.

Cultural Differences

Differences in cultural background include not just language differences, but also differences in group identity, individual identity, beliefs, and values (Dana, 1993), which influence the use of services, the presentation of symptoms, the assessment techniques used, and all aspects of treatment. For example, multicultural clients are more likely to end treatment prematurely due to frustration, misunderstanding, role ambiguities, and differences in priorities of treatment (Sue and Zane, 1987).

Dana (1993) provides brief descriptions of these differences. Group identity refers to the culture consciousness, which includes the behaviors sanctioned by the group. Some members of the culture may identify with their culture, some reject their original cultural group and identify with the dominant culture, some identify with both cultures, and some reject both. Individual identity or self-concept includes culturally mediated norms about assertiveness, aggression, expression of emotion, and individual goal-attainment vs. sacrificing for the greater good. Beliefs include ideas about illness and how much responsibility and control the individual has over health (as opposed to spiritual figures). Values include varieties of problem-solving. As the process of reidentifying the self-concept is primary in rehabilitation after MTBI, it is extremely important that it is not only the norms of the dominant culture that are reinforced.

A review of difference among individual cultures is beyond the scope of this chapter. However, a brief description of key differences between the largest cultural groups in the United States is provided and is taken largely from Dana (1993).

Anglo-American culture values independence and autonomy with the idea that each person potentially controls their environment and their own well-being. There is a strong ethic of competition with an emphasis on winning, and decision-making occurs in a hierarchical and linear manner. Communication is dependent on eye contact, limited physical contact, and controlled emotion. There are accepted ideas of hard work, rigid time schedules, planning, delayed gratification, and the value of progress.

African Americans may have difficulty identifying with either the traditional culture or the dominant culture. There may be a unique subculture with distinct values designed to fight against the prevalent poverty, racism, discrimination, limited opportunities and education, poor health, and violence. Differences exist in linguistic code and physical style. Widespread shame may still be associated with mental illness (Zea et al., 1996), although there is also evidence that African Americans avoid mental health services primarily due to bad experiences with professionals who were not culturally competent (Pugh and Mudd, 1971).

As in other cultures, there are a variety of traditional remedies, and information passed orally may be given more credibility than in European culture (Bowser, 1992). There may be an official name, a name within the family, a name among friends, and a name for the street. The use of a particular name by a health professional can lead to distance or mistrust. The individual is also likely to be involved in a collective network with a wide range of social relations. Property is readily shared and help is readily given. If rehabilitation efforts serve to isolate the individual from the collective they will be much less effective than if they work within the cultural context.

Asian Americans constitute many different nationalities with different cultural backgrounds. Manifestations may include focusing on somatic concerns rather than mood in depression because the expression of emotion was considered dangerous (Tseng, 1979). In Chinese culture, the cause of mental distress is likely to be sought in relations to others and disharmony there rather than within an individual and traditional medicines might be employed. Japanese Americans may identify depression with nervousness and may manifest as exaggerated anxiety concerning minor changes in physical and mental functioning (Rin et al., 1973).

Latino Americans also constitute a variety of cultural, racial, and ethnic backgrounds. In general, those with Latin American cultural backgrounds may be accustomed to attributing mental changes to external causes or physical symptoms (Zea et al., 1996) and may be more comfortable with directive therapy than other cultural groups (Dana, 1993). They may also continue to have strong beliefs in traditional healing methods and may have a strong belief in Christian religion.

Assessment

Assessment and treatment, when possible, are best done in the favored language. In addition, it is important that the tests used not be simply translated versions of English tests, but be linguistically and culturally appropriate and use appropriate norms (Ostrosky-Solis et al., 1989). Several batteries specific to Spanish-speaking subjects are in the early phases of development (Ostrosky-Solis et al., 1989; Pontón et al., 1996; Sano et al., 1994) and many individual tests exist (Beck, 1993a,b; Garcia and Azan, 1984; Roselli et al., 1990; Wechsler, 1968). Ardila et al. (1994) provide an excellent battery of tests and include cultural, educational, and language considerations for each cognitive domain to be assessed.

Chinese translations have been developed for some tests and shown to be valid indicators of brain injury (Chiu et al., 1993). There are some Japanese assessment materials designed especially to measure neurotoxin exposure (e.g., Yokoyama et al., 1990).

In addition, there may be a complicated interaction of culture, socio-economic status, gender (Ostrosky-Solis et al., 1989), education, and age (Lowenstein et al., 1993; Rosselli et al., 1990). These are reflected in dif-ferences on individual tests, such as motor speed (Ardila et al., 1994) and Digit Span due possibly to different syllabic length of digits in different languages, and different encoding styles for numbers (Lowenstein et al., 1993; Olazaran et al., 1996).

For all individuals, assessment and treatment is best conducted in the preferred language, although this is often impossible. If foreign language interpreters are used, it is desirable that these are trained interpreters, rather than friends or family members. This is because interpreting is, in fact, a much more complex skill than merely being bilingual. Moreover, using family members as interpreters may be problematic because of a patient's modesty (Haffner, 1992).

Additionally, if a child is used to relay difficult or emotionally charged information, especially about a parent's deficits, this can place a large bur-den on that person and can be directly counter to accepted family roles. Furthermore, other issues may surface for the survivor that she or he may not want to discuss in front of significant others. Finally, family and friends may try to "cover" for errors the survivor makes, especially if they believe the survivor "really" knows the correct answer. A trained inter-preter should also be able to provide some valuable information on cul-tural differences to the therapist. Finding an interpreter who is knowl-edgeable in issues of neuropsychological functioning is rare. Therefore, meeting with the interpreter separately is crucial to explain the types of tests to be given and the importance of reporting responses verbatim.

Problems may arise, however, even with a trained interpreter. Dikengil et al. (1993) provide examples of interpreters both protecting a patient and discounting a patient because she or he was from lower social classes or due to other prejudices. A useful set of guidelines for the use of inter-preters in brain injury rehabilitation is provided.

If rehabilitation materials are to be developed, like assessment materi-als, it is important that they are not merely translated from English lan-guage materials. The practice of translation and back-translation can help ensure that the linguistic content is accurate, but again, cultural and ed-ucational considerations should be taken into account (Brislin, 1970).

Differences in rehabilitation with individuals from another culture might involve using therapists in the community of the same culture, es-pecially for psychosocial counseling, differential involvement of family members, willingness to work with traditional healers, with culture-specific healers or healing techniques, and use of in-home and community sessions and services. Therapists must be accepting of different communication styles and nonverbal patterns.

Of course, if most members of a clientele are of a particular cultural background, it is essential that the therapists also be from the same background and that members of the community be integrated in decision-making processes to ensure adequate treatment and community integration at discharge.

Conclusions

With the many demands and breadth of knowledge necessary for practicing rehabilitation, individual differences can be overlooked. Therefore, imposing one's own value system in terms of conceptualizing deficits, adopting a style of presentation, selecting treatment techniques, and framing treatment goals is easy. However, sensitivity to differences due to gender, socioeconomic status, or culture can improve access to rehabilitation and the ability to profit from rehabilitation for a wide variety of people with MTBI.

References

Ardila, A., Rosselli, M., and Puente, A. (1994). *Neuropsychological Evaluation of the Spanish Speaker*. New York, NY: Plenum Press.

Beck, A. (1993a). *Beck Anxiety Inventory: Spanish Translation*. San Antonio, TX: The Psychological Corporation.

Beck, A. (1993b). *Beck Depression Inventory: Spanish Translation*. San Antonio, TX: The Psychological Corporation.

Binder, L. (1986). Persisting symptoms after mild head injury: A review of the postconcussive syndrome. *Journal of Clinical and Experimental Neuropsychology, 8,* 323–346.

Bowser, B. (1992). African-American culture and AIDS prevention. In Cross-Cultural Medicine—A Decade Later [Special Issue]. *Western Journal of Medicine, 157,* 286–289.

Brislin, R. (1970). Back-translation for cross-cultural research. *Journal of Cross-Cultural Psychology, 1,* 185–216.

Brody, B.A. (1988). Justice in the allocation of public resources to disabled citizens. *Archives of Physical Medicine and Rehabilitation, 69,* 333–336.

Chiu, W., Lin, W., Lin, L., Hung, C., and Sh'h, C. (1993). Neurobehavioral manifestations following closed head injury. *Journal of the Formos Medical Association, 92,* 255–262.

Dana, R. (1993). *Multicultural Assessment Perspectives for Professional Psychology*. Boston, MA: Allyn and Bacon.

Dikengil, A., Jones, G., and Byrne, M. (1993). Orientation of foreign language interpreters working with brain-injured patients. *The Journal of Cognitive Rehabilitation, July/August,* 10–11.

Fidell, L. (1980). Sex role stereotypes and the American physician. *Psychology of Women Quarterly, 4,* 313–330.

Fine, M., and Asch, A. (1988). *Women with Disabilities.* Temple University Press: Philadelphia, PA.

Garcia, R., and Azan, A. (1984). *Inventario Multifasico de la Personalidad-Minnesota.* Minneapolis, MN: The University of Minnesota.

Haffner, L. (1992). Translating is not enough: Interpreting in a medical setting. In Cross-Cultural Medicine—A Decade Later [Special Issue]. *Western Journal of Medicine, 157,* 255–259.

Heninger, G. (1997). Serotonin, sex, and psychiatric illness. *Proceedings of the National Academy of Sciences, 94,* 4823–4824.

Kay, T. (1992). Neuropsychological diagnosis: Disentangling the multiple determinants of functional disability after mild traumatic brain injury. In L. Horn and N. Zasler (Eds.), *Rehabilitation of Post-Concussive Disorders, Physical Medicine and Rehabilitation: State of the Art Reviews.* Philadelphia, PA: Hanley and Belfus, pp. 109–128.

Kimura, D. (1992). Sex differences in the brain. *Scientific American,* **267**(3), 119–125.

Lennane, K., and Lennane, R. (1973). Alleged psychogenic disorders in women—a possible manifestation of sexual prejudice. *New England Journal of Medicine, 288*(6), 288–292.

Lowenstein, D., Arguelles, T., Barker, W., and Duara, R. (1993). A comparative analysis of neuropsychological test performance of Spanish-speaking and English-speaking patients with Alzheimer's Disease. *Journal of Gerontology: Psychological Sciences, 48,* P142–P149.

Mapou, R. (1990). Traumatic brain injury rehabilitation with gay and lesbian individuals. *Journal of Head Trauma Rehabilitation, 5,* 67–72.

Meyerowitz, B., Chaiken, S., and Clark, L. (1988). Sex roles and culture: Social and personal reactions to breast cancer. In M. Fine and A. Asch (Eds.), *Women with Disabilities.* Philadelphia, PA: Temple University Press, pp. 72–89.

Olazaran, J., Jacobs, D., and Stern, Y. (1996). Comparative study of visual and verbal short-term memory in English and Spanish speakers: Testing a linguistic hypothesis. *Journal of the International Neuropsychological Society, 2,* 105–110.

Ostrosky-Solis, F., Quintanar, L., and Ardila, A. (1989). Detection of Brain Damage: Neuropsychological Assessment in a Spanish Speaking Population. *International Journal of Neuroscience, 49,* 141–149.

Pontón, M., Satz, P., Herrera, L., Young, R., Ortiz, F., Elia, L., Furst, C., and Namorow, N. (1996). Development of a Neuropsychological Screening Battery for Hispanics. Presented at the International Neuropsychological Society, Chicago, IL.

Pugh, T., and Mudd, E. (1971). Attitudes of Black women and men toward using community services. *Journal of Religion and Health, 10,* 256–277.

Raskin, S., Mateer, C., and Tweeten, R. (1998). Neuropsychological Assessment of Individuals with Mild Traumatic Brain Injury. *The Clinical Neuropsychologist, 12,* 21–30.

Rimel, R., Giordani, B., and Barth, J. (1981). Disability caused by minor head injury. *Neurosurgery, 9*, 221–228.

Rin, H., Schooler, C., and Caudill, W. (1973). Symptomatology and hospitalization: Culture, social structure, and psychopathology in Taiwan and Japan. *Journal of Nervous and Mental Disease, 157*, 296–312.

Roselli, M. Ardila, A., Florenz, A., and Castro, C. (1990). Normative data on the Boston Diagnostic Aphasia Examination in a Spanish-speaking population. *Journal of Clinical and Experimental Neuropsychology, 12*, 313–322.

Sano, M., Wilson, J., Stern, Y., and Rosen, W. (1994). A Spanish Version of the Alzheimer's Disease Assessment Scale: Development of Preliminary Validation. Paper presented at the International Neuropsychological Society.

Sue, S., and Zane, N. (1987). The role of culture and cultural techniques in psychotherapy. *American Psychologist, 42*, 37–45.

Tavris, C. (1992). *The Mismeasure of Woman*. New York, NY: Simon & Schuster.

Tseng, W. (1979). The nature of somatic complaints among psychiatric patients, the Chinese case. *Comparative Psychiatry, 16*, 313–336.

Wechsler, D. (1968). *Escala de Inteligencia Wechsler para Adultos*. New York, NY: The Psychological Corporation.

Willer, B., Allen, K., Liss, M., and Zicht, M. (1991). Problems and coping strategies of individuals with traumatic brain injury and their spouses. *Archives of Physical Medicine and Rehabilitation, 72*, 460–464.

Yokoyama, K., Araki, S., Osuga, J., Karita, T., Kurokawa, M., and Koda, K. (1990). Development of Japanese edition of NES and WHO NCTB. *Sangyo-Igaku, 32*, 354–355.

Zahara, D.J., and Cuvo, A.J. (1984). Behavioral applications to the rehabilitation of traumatically head-injured persons. *Clinical Psychology Review, 4*(4), 477–491.

Zea, M., Belgrave, F., Townsend, T., Jarama, S., and Banks, S. (1996). The influence of social support and active coping on depression among African Americans and Latinos with disabilities. *Rehabilitation Psychology, 41*, 225–242.

Index